Polymers:
The Pathway to Versatile Technology

Edited by Anthony J. O'Lenick Jr.

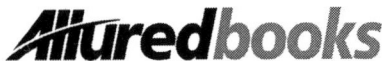

Polymers: The Pathway to Versatile Technology

ISBN: 978-1-932633-76-4

Copyright 2011, by Allured Business Media. All Rights Reserved.

Editorial

Book Editor: Angela C. Kozlowski
Indexer: Joy Dean Lee
Cover Design: Bryan Crowe
Page Layout: Bryan Crowe, Beth Hagenberg

Administration

Publisher: Marian Raney
Book Sales Executive: Marie Kuta
Book Coordinator and Web Support: Anita Singh

Neither this book nor any part may be reproduced or transmitted in any form by any means, electronic or mechanical, including photocopying, microfilming and recording, or by any information storage retrieval system, without permission in writing from the publisher.

NOTICE

To the best of our knowledge the information in this book is accurate. However, in a time of rapid change, it is difficult to ensure that all information provided is entirely accurate and up-to-date. Therefore, the author and the publisher accept no responsibility for any inaccuracies or omissions and specifically disclaim any liability, loss, or risk, personal or otherwise, which is incurred as a consequence, directly or indirectly, of the use and/or application of any of the contents of this book. Mention of trade names or commercial products does not constitute endorsement or recommendation for use by the Publisher.

Alluredbooks

A division of Allured Business Media
336 Gundersen Drive, Suite A, Carol Stream, IL 60188 USA
Tel: 630-653-2155 • Fax: 630-653-2192
www.AlluredBooks.com
E-mail: books@allured.com

Table of Contents

Introduction

SECTION 1 – Polymer Types

1. Radical Polymers
   O'Lenick 1

SECTION 2 – Natural Polymers

2. Recent Advances in Biopolymers and Biomedical Materials
   Lochhead, et al 15
3. Fluid Gels Based On Natural Polymers For Cosmetic Applications
   Willams, et al 35
4. A Surfactant/Biopolymer Stabilizer for Emulsions
   Tadros, et al 49
5. Castor Polyesters for Personal Care
   O'Lenick and LaVay 63
6. Rhizobium Gum: A Novel Cosmetic Ingredient from Soil to the Skin
   Bresin, et al 75

SECTION 3 – Polymers in Hair Care

7. Recent Polymer Technologies for Hair Care
   Ridley, et al 87
8. Deposition from Conditioning Shampoo: Optimizing Coacervate Formation
   Lochhead, et al 113
9. Advances in Polymers for Hair Styling
   Lochhead and Huizinga 121
10. Advances in Polymers for Hair Coloring
    Lochhead 135

11. Innovations in Hair Styling Technology
   Schueller and Romanowski 149

12. Protecting the Hair with Natural Keratin Biopolymers
   Roddick-Lanzilotta, et al... 161

13. Advances in Polymers for Hair Conditioning Shampoos
   Lochhead and Huisinga 175

14. Polyquaternium-74: An Advanced Hair Conditioning Polymer
   Leroy 189

15. Evaluating Polyimide-1, a Styling Resin for Gel and Mousse Formulations
   Clements 205

16. Polyurethane-14 AMP-Acrylates Copolymer: A Hair Fixative Technology with "Memory"
   Martino, et al 219

17. Using Polyquaternium-64 to Condition Damaged Hair
   Shimada, et al 233

18. New Dimension in Hairstyling—VP/Methacrylamide/Vinyl Imidazole Copolymer
   Wood, et al 247

19. Testing Polysilicone-19 for Claims of Hair Conditioning and UV Protection
   Herrwerth, et al 261

20. New Hybrid Polymer for Hair Spray Formulations
   Schwarzwälder, et al 275

SECTION 4 – Polymers in Skin Care

21. Peptides, Amino Acids and Proteins in Skin Care?
   Lintner.. 289

22. Hyperbranched Polyalphaolefins Enhance Anhydrous Stick Formulations
   Nicholas and Brooks... 301

23. Enhancing the Feel of Vegetable Oils with Silicone
   Girboux and Courbon 315

24. Formulating with Surfactant Silicones
   O'Lenick 327

SECTION 5 – Polymers in Sun Care

25. Film-forming Polymers as a Strategy for Sunscreen Efficacy
   Davis, et al 339

26. Silicones Bring Multifunctional Performance to Sun Care
   Van Reeth, et al 351

SECTION 6 – Polymers in Nail Care

27. Thermoplastic Silicone Elastomers Improve Nail Polish Performance
   Schlosser and Hassenzahl 369

28. Silicone Compounds - New Formulation Possibilities
   O'Lenick 377

29. Equilibration Reaction of Silicone Fluids
   O'Lenick, et al 387

30. Stimuli-responsive Polymer Systems: A Review of Thermo-associative Thickening
   Lochhead 397

SECTION 7 – Polymer Technology

31. Citrate Polyesters
   O'Lenick 415

Index 433

Introduction

Polymers are a broad class of compositions that are becoming increasingly important in the area of personal care formulation. They are compositions rather than compounds, meaning polymers are made up of a distribution of compounds of differing molecular weight, depending upon the type of polymerization used.

Polymer function is manifold, including conditioning, film formation, waterproofing, thickening, delivery, glossing, fixatives, and much more. It is quite common to find several polymers in a formulation providing different functionality.

Polymers can be anionic, cationic, nonionic or amphoteric. The ionic nature is important in formulation both in terms of function and interaction with other formulation ingredients. The interaction in formulation is an interesting and ever-developing area in personal care. Specifically, coacervate technology and complexation offer methods of improved efficiency of polymers from formulations.

Polymers can be green, sustainable and renewable, or they can be synthetic, or contain elements of both. In fact, biopolymers are becoming more and more important in our industry. Living systems make use of biopolymers quite commonly. Proteins, DNA, starches, sugars, and cellulose are very common biopolymers. Biopolymers can find application in formulations as ingredients in and of themselves, or may be deriviaized into bio-organic polymers.

The processes used to make polymers are both numerous and diverse. The processes can include radical polymerization of vinyl monomers, ring opening reactions, equilibration reactions, condensation polymers or combinations of these. Each process has its own inherent advantages and disadvantages. Each has its own oligomer distributions, residual catalysts, residual monomers, content and functionality.

The analysis of the exact composition in a polymer can be problematic, in turn making alternate supply of an identical material problematic.

The INCI names for polymers are generic to the monomers uses and lack definition of the number of each monomer relative to each other and the total number present in the polymer.

All these factors make polymers a topic that should be of keen interest to formulators, marketers, raw material suppliers, regulators and researchers in the personal care market.

This compilation is intended to provide the reader with articles from *Cosmetic and Toiletries* magazine that describe polymers of interest to the personal care market. The reader is encouraged to look more deeply into the topic with a questioning mind.

There are many opportunities to use existing polymers in combination with other ingredients to provide cosmetically elegant products heretofore unknown.

Happy reading.

Tony O'Lenick

CHAPTER 1

Radical Polymers

Thomas O'Lenick
University of Tennessee
Anthony J. O'Lenick Jr.
Siltech LLC

Background

There are many types of reactions that result in polymers. There are advantages and disadvantages to each type. Some use vinyl monomers and react using radical mechanisms. Others are addition polymers that use more traditional organic chemistry, like esterification, ring opening and amidification.

We have divided the type of reactions into radical polymers and non-radical mechanisms. There are a variety of new cleaner types of radical polymerizations that are seen primarily in academic environments, but we believe they will become more main stream as time progresses. The main reason why we believe this is that the polymers are more pure and have less unreacted monomers.

Theory

Conventional Radical Polymerization

Conventional radical polymerization, which is most commonly used commercially, uses a chain-growth mechanism. There are two advantages for conventional radical polymerization:

- High molecular weight is obtained at low monomer conversion (because every monomer adds directly to the chain end).
- Unlike condensation polymerizations, radical polymerizations have no by-products.

There are two major problems with conventional radical polymerization:
- The polymerization needs an oxygen-free environment.
- Termination is a major problem, effecting polydispersity and chain branching.

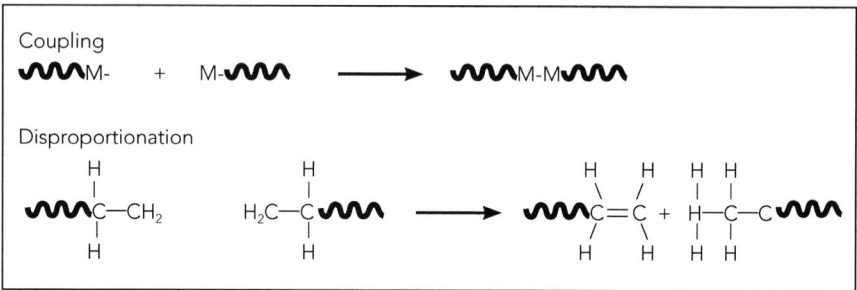

Figure 1. Two types of termination in radical polymerization.

There are two major types of termination: disproportionation and coupling (See **Figure 1**).

Coupling involves two active chain ends coming together to form a sigma bond. This simply combines two active chains and destroys the active radical, therefore stopping the polymerization. Disproportionation occurs when two active chain ends come together and exchange a hydride. One polymer chain becomes unsaturated while the other end becomes saturated. The saturated polymer chain can no longer participate in the polymerization, but the unsaturated polymer canpolymerize further and will add a tail to the head. This means that this polymer will have a branch point in the polymer backbone. The last key feature is an initiator needed to start the polymerization. There are many types of initiators for free radical polymerization. Careful consideration must be taken to find the best initiator for a specific environment.

Kinetics

A series of assumptions must be made to examine the kinetics of the polymerization. First, the reactivity of each radical is independent of chain length; this means that an activated radical on the end of the polymer chain will have the same reactivity as a single monomer radical. This is referred to as equal reactivity.

Initiation: $R_i = 2fk_d[I]$
Propagation: $R_p = k_p[M][M·]$
Termination: $R_t = k_t[M]^2$

Second, we assume that initiation and termination are equal. This is the steady state assumption.

Where f is the initiator efficiency, [M] is the monomer concentration and [M] is the active radical. Controlled-living polymerizations are effective by limiting the amount of active radical ([M]). The radical concentration shows up in two formulas: propagation and termination. By decreasing the amount of radical in the reaction mixture, we decrease both the propagation and termination steps; however, the termination step is greatly decreased because the radical concentration is raised to the power of two. Example: if we decrease the radical concentration from 1M to 0.50M, the propagation step is 0.50kp, while the termination is now 0.25kt. This is the major principal behind controlled-living polymerizations. The degree of polymerization and average kinetic chain length is not affected by the decrease in radical concentration.

Controlled "Pseudo-living" Radical Polymerization

Radical polymerizations have some major advantages over condensation polymers. Radical polymerization is a type of chain polymerization, meaning the polymer chain grows only at the active chain end. Molecular weight grows very rapidly at low monomer concentration, and vinyl monomers can be polymerized easily. Polymer morphology can also be controlled with ease. Though this makes radical polymerization very appealing to the industry, there are a few problems with conventional radical polymerizations.

The major problem is termination. These reactions must be carried out in the absence of oxygen and solvents that can act as a chain transfer agent. There are two major types of termination: disproportionate and coupling. Several methods have been developed to limit the amount of termination in radical polymerization. These methods are called controlled-living radical polymerizations or pseudo-living radical polymerizations. There are three major types of controlled-living radical polymerizations: Atom Transfer Radical Polymerization (ATRP), Nitroxi-Mediated Radical Polymerization (NMRP) and Reversible-Addition Fragmentation Transfer Radical Polymerization (RAFT).

These techniques can provide great control of polydispersity (as low as 1.05) and molecular weight (Mn). Each of these styles of polymerization uses a different technique to decrease the radical concentration. A brief look at the kinetics of radical polymerizations will show why these techniques work. The ability to have extremely low PDI and controlled molecular weights make these polymerizations very appealing in the drug delivery industry.

Atom Transfer Radical Polymerization (ATRP)

ATRP or Atom Transfer Radical Polymerization is a living polymerization reaction involving free radicals. It was introduced as an extension to Atom Transfer Radical Addition (ATRA) by Jin-Shan Wang and Matyjaszewski (1995) and Sawamoto et al (1994/5). It allows the reaction to be carried out in a controlled way, and can be used to obtain polymers with high molecular weight and low polydispersity index.

This control result is from the use of a transition metal-based catalyst. This catalyst provides equilibrium between active and propagating polymers, as well as an inactive form of the polymer, known as the dormant form. Since the dormant state of the polymer is vastly preferred in this equilibrium, side reactions are suppressed. By lowering the concentration of radicals, termination is suppressed and control is achieved.

This technique uses an oxidation/reduction mechanism to control the amount of radicals in the reaction (See **Figure 2**).

ATRP uses the exchange of a halogen from one oxidation state to another. This process involves a metal halide, ligand (to coordinate the metal and monomer), monomer and initiator. One of the most commonly used metals is copper (I) bromide (CuBr). The monomer then exchanges a Br radical to oxidize the copper to copper (II) bromide (CuBr2). This prevents the concentration of radicals in the solution, because CuBr2 cannot initiate the polymerization. This allows a very low concentration of active radical and propagation with very low termination. There are some problems with ATRP, the first being the reaction conditions. To achieve a successful polymerization, the correct solvent, initiator and ligand have to be selected. The second problem is the removal of CuBr and CuBr2 from the reaction mixture. This means taking several steps to remove the copper from the polymer. This post reaction clean up is most commonly accomplished using aluminum oxide chromatography. These additional steps along with small amounts of polymer lost in the processing will increase the cost of the final polymer.

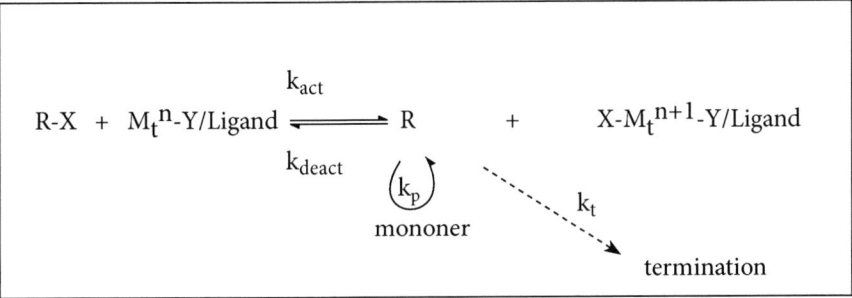

Figure 2. Transition-Metal-Catalyzed ATRP.[1]

Reversible Addition-Fragmentation Transfer (RAFT)

RAFT is a form of reversible addition–fragmentation chain transfer polymerization that was discovered by the CSIRO in 1998. This is a new method for the synthesis of living radical polymers. RAFT polymerization uses thiocarbonylthio compounds, such as dithioesters, dithiocarbamates, trithiocarbonates and xanthates, in order to mediate the polymerization via a reversible chain-transfer process.

This allows access to polymers with low polydispersity and high functionality. RAFT also allows for the production of complex architectures such as block, star, graft, comb and brush (co)polymers.

---

1. Atom Transfer Radical Polymerization, Krzystof Matyjaszewski and Jianhui Xia; Chem. Rev, 2001, 101, 2921-2990. Department of Chemistry, Carnegie Mellon University, Pittsburgh, Pennsylvania 15213.

RAFT is also known for its compatibility with a great variety of monomers. See **Figure 3** for the RAFT process.

RAFT utilizes the chain-transfer mechanism to control the radical concentration. The chain transfer agent, most commonly a thioester, is easily attacked by an activated radial. The thioester radical then kicks off another radical that is used in the propagation step. Normal free radical initiators can be used in the polymerization technique. AIBN is the most commonly used initiator for this technique. AIBN is a commonly used shorthand for Azobisisobutyronitrile, a very efficient radical catalyst. The properties of AIBN are shown in **Table 1**.

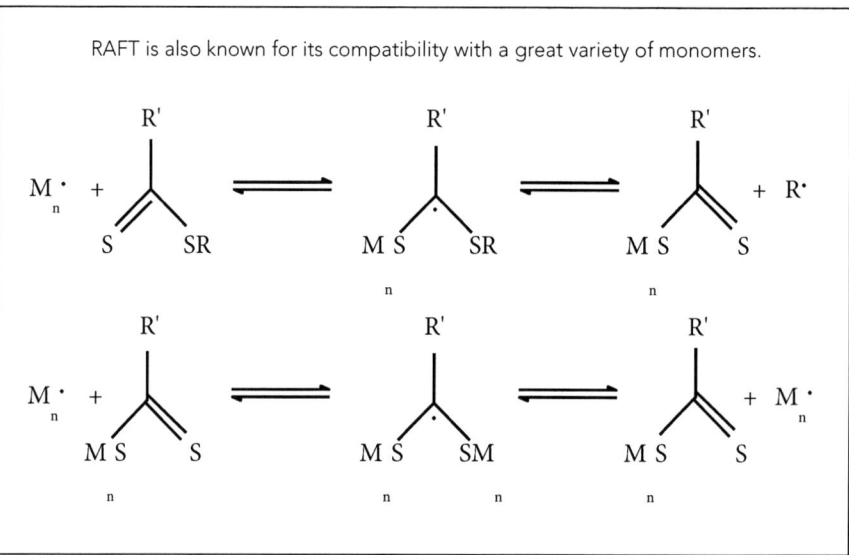

Figure 3.

Table 1
AIBN Properties Azobisisobutyronitrile

Systematic name	2,2-Azobis (2-methylpropionitrile)
Other names	Azobisisobutyronitrile
	AIBN
Molecular formula	$C_8H_{12}N_4$
Molar mass	164.2 g/mol
Appearance	white crystalline
CAS number	78-67-1

Nitroxi-Mediated Radical Polymerization (NMRP)

NMRP uses a unique initiator system to control the radical concentration. This is called the persistent radical effect. By introducing a radical that does not initiate a polymer chain, it will force the equilibrium back to the products. This means that the only radical in the system is the active polymer chain (See **Figure 4**).

The phenol radical will start the polymerization, while the nitroxide radical will not.

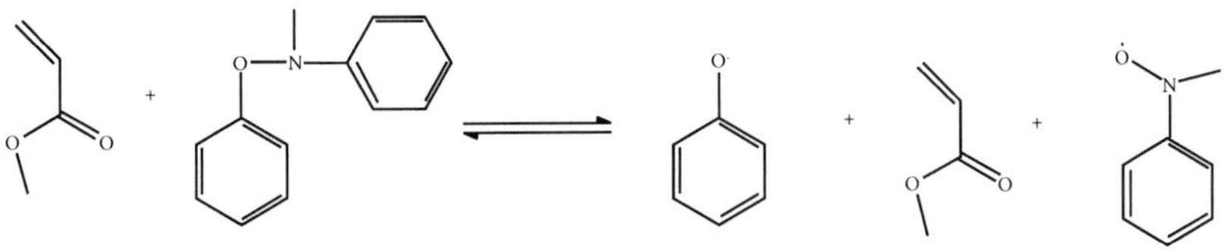

Figure 4. NMRP mechanism

While controlled radical polymerization gives improvement in polydispersity and unreacted vinyl monomer content, the ability to prepare polymers usingthis technology is more complicated in terms of solvents, reagents and control. Although primarily the venue of university laboratories at present, we believe this technology or related, but not yet developed, technologies will become more and more common in the cosmetic arena. This is because this type of polymerization has a higher cost, but fewer by-products. Presently, the premium for this type of polymerization limits its use to pharmaceutical applications, where the cost is more easily absorbed. As the cost decreases more cosmetic applications will develop, first in the premium brands, and later in the mass market. The requirement for ever lower levels of unreacted monomer will drive the industry to new technologies.

Practice

Non-Living Polymerization General Considerations
US Patent 5,162,472 issued November 10, 1992, to O'Lenick, titled Free radical silicone polymers, teaches a general polymerization procedure as follows:

The polymerization of the vinyl-containing compounds is achieved by utilizing free radical catalyst in a low oxygen-containing solvent, most commonly water. The choice of solvent will depend upon the solubility of the reactants. Generally, a solvent is chosen in which all reactants are soluble. This improves contact and leads to a more uniform polymer. Sparging with nitrogen is common to remove dissolved oxygen contained therein immediately prior to use. Then the specified amount of the treated solvent is added to a suitable glass vessel. Most commonly, 50–80% of the total weight of the batch is water. The specified amount of the specified monomers is then added under agitation. Nitrogen is continuously sparged, and the temperature is raised to about 50°C.

Other Polymers

Theory
Condensation polymers are any class of polymers formed through a condensation reaction, releasing (or condensing) a small molecule by-product such as water or methanol, as opposed to addition polymers, which involve the reaction of unsaturated monomers. Types of condensation polymers include polyamides and polyesters.

Condensation polymerization, a form of step-growth polymerization, is a process by which two molecules join together with the loss of a small molecule—often water. The type of end product resulting from a condensation polymerization is dependent on the number of functional end groups of the monomer that can react.

Monomers with only one reactive group terminate a growing chain, giving end products with a lower molecular weight. Linear polymers are created using monomers with two reactive end groups and monomers with more than two end groups give three-dimensional polymers, which are crosslinked.

Polyesters

Polyesters are molecules that possess multiple ester bonds. The ester bond is:

$$-O-\overset{\overset{\displaystyle O}{\|}}{C}-R-$$

The molecule can be thought of as a progressive condensation of carboxylic groups with hydroxyl groups to produce a larger molecule and a molecule of water.

$$HO\overset{\overset{\displaystyle O}{\|}}{C}-CH_2CH_2\overset{\overset{\displaystyle O}{\|}}{C}OH + HO-CH_2CH_2OH \xrightarrow{180\text{-}200°C}$$

$$\underset{\text{Carboxy}}{HO\overset{\overset{\displaystyle O}{\|}}{C}-CH_2CH_2}\underset{\text{Ester}}{\overset{\overset{\displaystyle O}{\|}}{C}O-CH_2CH_2}\underset{\text{Hydroxy}}{OH} + H_2O$$

The molecule has a hydroxyl group and a carboxylic group that will subsequently react to make larger polymers.

$$HO\overset{\overset{\displaystyle O}{\|}}{C}-CH_2CH_2\overset{\overset{\displaystyle O}{\|}}{C}O-CH_2CH_2(O\overset{\overset{\displaystyle O}{\|}}{C}-CH_2CH_2\overset{\overset{\displaystyle O}{\|}}{C}-OCH_2CH_2)xOH$$

The inclusion of mono-functional acids or alcohols can be used to cap the molecule at one end.

Polyamides

Polyamides are analogues of polyesters. They are molecules that possess multiple amide bonds. The amide bond is:

$$-R'-N-\overset{\overset{O}{\|}}{C}-R-$$

Amides differ fundamentally from esters in two respects. First, amide groups can differ in the degree of substitution around nitrogen (the 'R' group above); hydroxyl groups cannot. Second, since amines are bases, they form salts when combined with amines. Hydroxyl groups do not form salts with carboxylic acids.

$$R-NH_2 \quad CH_3\overset{\overset{O}{\|}}{C}OH \rightarrow R^1\overset{\overset{H}{|}}{N^+}-H\ ^-O\overset{\overset{O}{\|}}{C}-CH_3 \xrightarrow{Heat} R^1NH-\overset{\overset{O}{\|}}{C}-CH_3 + H_2O$$

Amine   Carboxylic   Salt   Amide   Water
        Acid

All amines form salts, regardless of substitution, but only primary and secondary amines form amides. Tertiary amines do not form amides (See **Table 2**).

Mechanistically, however, the reaction to make polyamides can be thought of like the polyester reaction: a progressive condensation of carboxylic groups with amino groups to produce a larger molecule and a molecule of water.

$$HO\overset{\overset{O}{\|}}{C}-CH_2CH_2\overset{\overset{O}{\|}}{C}OH \ + \ H_2N-CH_2CH_2NH_2 \xrightarrow{180°C}$$

$$HO\overset{\overset{O}{\|}}{C}-CH_2CH_2\overset{\overset{O}{\|}}{C}NH-CH_2CH_2NH_2 + H_2O$$
Carboxy   Amide   Amine

The molecule has a hydroxyl group and a carboxylic group that will subsequently react to make larger polymers.

Table 2
Amine Reactions

Amine	Type	Product
RNH_2	Primary amine	$R_1NHC(=O)-CH_3$ Amide
R_1NH-R_2	Secondary amine	$R_1N(R_2)C(=O)-CH_3$ Amide
$R_1N(R_2)-R_3$	Tertiary amine	$R_1N^+H(R_2)-R^3$ $^-OC(=O)-CH_3$ Salt

$$HOC(=O)-CH_2CH_2C(=O)NH-CH_2CH_2(NHC(=O)-CH_2CH_2C(=O)-NHCH_2CH_2)xNH_2$$

Polyamide

Polyamides made by living organisms are called polypeptides or proteins. They are synthesized using enzymes. Proteins and polypeptides are very important classes of molecules, which include enzymes—structural components of cells. The cosmetic chemist is interested in these materials because they are used in the makeup and treatment of hair and skin.

Proteins consist of amino acids, which have a carboxy group and an amino group. When the amino group reacts with the carboxyl group in living systems, a peptide bond is formed. The peptide bond is an amide. Amino acids are linked to each other by a complex DNA-controlled process. Amino acids are the basic building blocks of enzymes, hormones, proteins and body tissues. A peptide is a compound consisting of two or more amino acids. Oligopeptides have ten or fewer amino acids. Polypeptides and proteins are chains of ten or more amino acids. Peptides consisting of more than 50 amino acids are classified as proteins.

Polyurethanes

Urethanes are a class of compounds prepared by the following reaction:

$$ROH + CH_3N{=}C{=}O \rightarrow CH_3N\underset{H}{-}\overset{\overset{O}{\|}}{C}-OR$$

Alcohol   Methyl Isocyanate   Urethane

When the alcohol is a poly-hydroxy compound and the isocyanate is a polyisocyanate, polyurethanes are formed. Isocyanates are classified in two ways. First, by the number of reactive groups present, and second, by the presence or absence of aromatic groups (See **Table 3**).

Table 3
Isocyanate Selection

Classification	Aromatic	Aliphatic
Monoisocyanate	Toluene Monoisocyanate	Methyl Isocyanate
Diisocyanate	Methylene Diphenyl Diisocyanate Toluene-2,4-diisocyanate	1.6-hexane Diisocyanate Isophorone Diisocyanate

Conclusion

The chemistry of polymers is critically important to the future of the personal care market. The products are a direct result of the processes and raw materials used to make them.

As the personal care market is driven more to sustainable, green, consumer friendly products the pressure will be not only for polymers that are REACH compliant, but polymers that use sustainable, green, consumer friendly monomers. The formulator needs to be very cognisant of the chemistry and consider the impact on product performance and the environment.

CHAPTER 2

Recent Advances in Biopolymers and Biomedical Materials

Robert Y. Lochhead, Stephen F. Foster, Ashley L. Cox, Margaret B. Lochhead, Vipul Padman and Emily A. Hoff
University of Southern Mississippi, Hattiesburg, MS USA

KEY WORDS: *Filmstrips, aloe vera pectin, hydrogels for tissue engineering, mucoadhesive gels, controlled delivery, nanofibers*

ABSTRACT: *This overview of literature provides a snapshot of research trends in biopolymers and biomedical polymers. To improve product efficacy, the personal care industry often looks to other sectors for innovative materials and ideas. Here, the authors encourage readers to innovate by technology transfer and by gaining a better understanding of biopolymers.*

In this overview of recently published scientific literature, the authors provide a snapshot of current research trends in biopolymers and biomedical polymers. During the trial-and-error process to improve product benefits, the personal care industry eagerly formulates with new and different materials and ideas. Sometimes these new materials are generated within the industry while other time, they are borrowed from other sectors. By reviewing the current scientific literature, the authors hope to encourage readers to innovate by technology transfer and by gaining a better understanding of biopolymers at a time when they are escalating in importance.

Renewable Resources

Rising oil prices and environmental concerns have focused public interest and scientific research on renewable material sources, produced from agriculture and biological stock. The drive within the scientific community is to meet the current thermal and mechanical properties of standard petroleum materials with that of materials produced from agricultural sources such as corn or soybeans. With this in mind, a recent scientific publication in biomacromolecules[1] focused on analyzing the material properties as well as phase separation in copolymer blends of poly(3-hydroxybutyrate) with poly(L-lactic acid) and poly(ε-caprolactone).

Poly(3-hydroxybutyrate) (PHB) is a polymer that is synthesized from bacteria and poly(L-lactic acid) can be obtained from agricultural resources such as corn. The polymers PLA and poly(ε-caprolactone) (PCL) were blended with PHB in varying weight ratios of 15 to 85 percent. This publication compared the copolymer blends of PHB/PLA to PHB/PCL in both mechanical properties as well as phase behavior. The mechanical properties were determined by using a miniaturized stretching machine at a 10% strain/min setting. FT-IR imaging was used to detect phase separation in the cast films by using calibration curves.

Both of these copolymer blends have similar mechanical properties with PHB content less than approximately 40%, resulting in elongation to break percentages >100%. It is interesting that for PHB/PCL copolymers, the elongation to break did not result in values of 100% until the PHB content was below 35%. PHB/PLA copolymer possesses higher mechanical deformation properties than PHB/PCL copolymers. Analyzing the copolymers for phase separation behavior reveals that both copolymer systems become phase separated at weight concentrations of approximately 50/50.

For the PHB/PLA composition range, phase separation occurred from 45% to 65% PHB weight values. The miscibility gap in the PHB/PCL copolymers occurred over a smaller range of approximately 45% to 55% PHB weight values. The mechanical property values measured from the copolymers demonstrated that substitution of a petroleum based polymer, PCL, with a polymer produced from an agricultural source can yield similar or better mechanical properties.

Micropackaging of Aroma, Flavor in Filmstrips

Packages for cosmetic products are ideally designed to contain the product and prevent losses due to evaporation; they should also protect the product from degradation by the intrusion of external contaminants such as oxygen or microorganisms. There currently is an emerging trend toward the delivery of fragrance and flavors from filmstrips, which is expected to be boosted by restrictions on liquids and gels by airport security. Edible packaging is used to provide thin, protective layers that keep ingredients like flavors and fragrances localized and prevent them from intermingling prior to the point of use. These barrier films can be made from hydrocolloids, i.e., proteins and polysaccharides.

The requirements of a film for this purpose are good film cohesion, good mechanical properties, impermeability to target fragrances and flavors, and good water-barrier properties. The films can also be in the form of a "solid" emulsion in which lipid-encapsulated flavor and fragrance are dispersed in a hydrocolloid film. Crystallization of the lipid waxes in such films decreases water transfer and, if the lipid globules are small, the water permeability deceases when the lipid concentration in the film is close to 30%.[2]

Edible films made of iota(*i*)-carageenan offer the advantages of good mechanical properties, emulsion stabilization and decreased oxygen permeability; this biopolymer also has recently been evaluated as a hydrocolloid film former for edible aroma emulsion films[a].[3]

Carrageenans are sulfated polysaccharides obtained by extraction from seaweed (see **Figure 1**).

There are three major classes, namely kappa, iota and lambda carrageenan. This classification is based on the number and position of sulfate groups on the disaccharide repeat unit of the polysaccharide with kappa, iota and lambda carageenans being 20%, 33% and 41%, respectively. The ready availability and reasonable cost of the carrageenans has resulted in their wide use the food industry as thickeners and texturizers. *i*-Carrageenan is soluble in hot water and gels below 50ºC . The gel structure is a network in which the junction zones are aggregated double-helix coils. When cast, carrageenan produces a dense film of helices 1.39 nm apart.

---

[a] The Gelsite polymer is a product and registered trademark of Delsite Biotechnologies, Irving, Tex., USA.

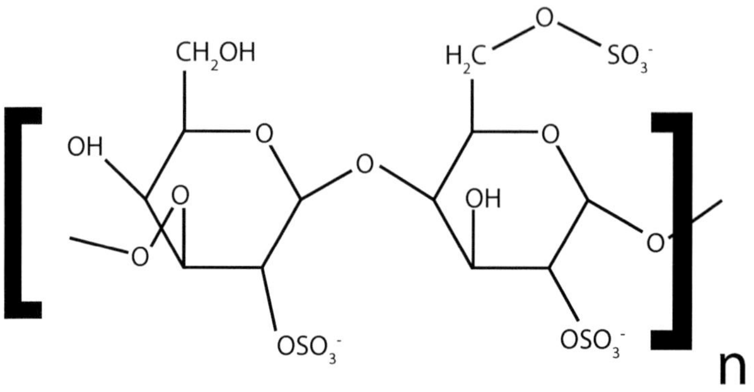

Figure 1. Carrageenan is a sulfated polysaccharide

Emulsion films were prepared by the inventor by solubilizing the fragrance, *n*-hexanal, in a mixture of glyceryl mono- and di-acetates and beeswax. This aroma fat-blend was homogenized into an *i*- carrageenan solution and the mixture was cast as a film. The aroma compound, *n*-hexanal, changed the structure of the carrageenan gel, raising the sol-gel transition temperature from 50ºC to 85 ºC, and the water-vapor permeability increased while oxygen permeability was unchanged. These changes were attributed to plasticization of the film by *n*-hexanal, and wavelength shifts in FTIR of the films indicated that the aldehyde group of the *n*-hexanal interacted with the –OH or sulfate groups of the *i*-carrageenan molecules.

This plasticization by *n*-hexanal apparently increased the mesh-size of the film sufficiently to allow the intrusion of water molecules but not enough to allow permeation of the larger oxygen molecules. Thus, oxidation of the fragrance would be slowed or prevented by the film's gel network but the ready intrusion of water would favor the release of aroma on demand.

Polysaccharide Gels: Pectin from a New Source

Like carrageenan, pectin is another polysaccharide that is commonly used as a gellant and texturizer in the food industry. The properties of pectin extracted from aloe vera have recently been disclosed.[4]

Pectins are anionic polysaccharides consisting primarily of 1,4 α-D galacturonic acid repeat units with 1,2 rhamnose branch points (see **Figure 2**).

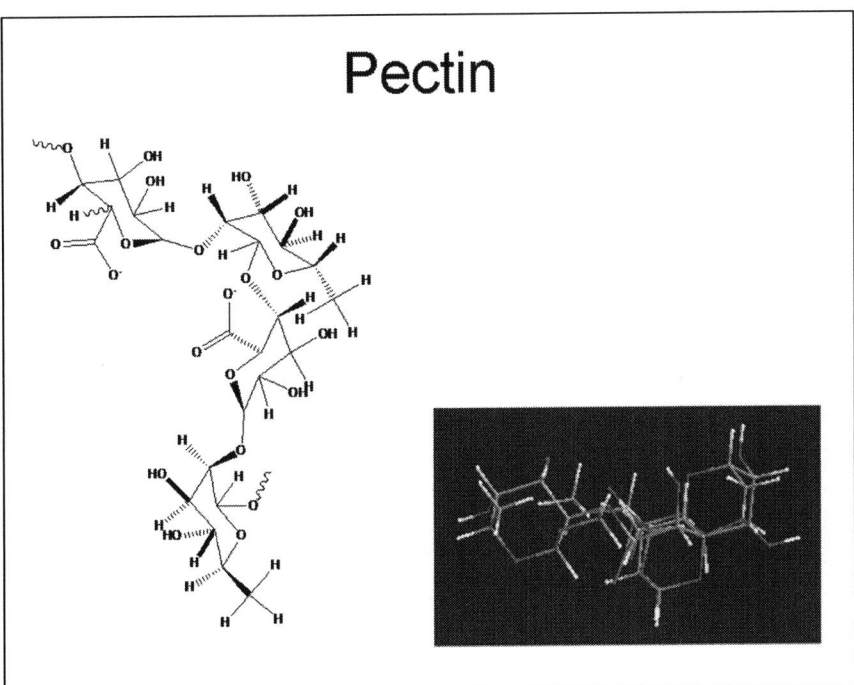

Figure 2. Depiction of pectin structure

Similarly to alginates, pectins gel in the presence of calcium ions. In these gelled structures the calcium ions are located specifically between the polyelectrolyte chains like eggs in an egg carton.[5-7] By measuring the intrinsic viscosity as a function of ionic strength, it was shown that aloe vera pectin has an inherently stiff polymer backbone; the intrinsic viscosity is an indication of a polymer's molecular hydrodynamic volume in solution.

Zeta potential measurements showed that, in aqueous solution, the potential on the pectin molecule is high and the polymer molecules interact strongly with to the water and generally avoid each other. However, above a sodium chloride concentration of only 0.1M, the potential drops to a level that allows the polymer molecules to interact with each other, and if the concentration is above the polymer's critical overlap concentration, a gel network can be established. This is shown by the "scaling" of the electrolyte solution's intrinsic viscosity with pectin concentration.

The exponent of 10.9 is much larger than the theoretical value of 4. In this concentration regime hydrophobic junction zones between the pectin molecules have been detected by the fluorescent probe 8-anilino naphthalenesulfonic acid, confirming that the gel structure is a hydrophilic polymer network linked by hydrophobic junction zones.

It is interesting though, that, even in the absence of salt and above the critical overlap concentration, the intrinsic viscosity rises faster with concentration than would be predicted (8.6) for a random coil polymer, indicating that even when the polymer molecules effectively repel one another, the flow of the system is constrained. In the presence of calcium the gel had a higher shear storage modulus than loss modulus, indicating that it was more solid-like than liquid-like. Moreover, aloe vera pectin at only 0.20% w/w exhibits almost the same values of elastic modulus as other pectins tested at higher concentrations (2.0% w/w) and higher calcium concentrations (10mM).

Polymers for Tissue Engineering

In medical sciences, tissue engineering has become a highly researched area focusing on the repair of damaged cells and restoration of function to damaged areas of the human body.[8] One key area that has inherent difficulties is that of nerve repair, since nerve damage is notorious for being difficult if not impossible to heal.

Scientists have begun researching new "smart" materials, or materials that perform a specific function upon external stimulus such as light, electric currents, pH, ionic strength and temperature, and have used these stimuli triggers to develop materials that could be useful in tissue engineering. In a recent article submission,[9] researchers synthesized an electroactive copolymer (PLAAP) using poly(L-lactide) (PLA) and aniline pentamer (AP) with the goal of creating a copolymer that could be used as a nerve repair scaffold material. The conjugated ring backbone of the aniline pentamer allows the polymer to be electroactive—a property that has been demonstrated as useful in proliferation or differentiation of various cell types.

This copolymer is soluble in relatively inexpensive solvents such as THF and $CHCl_3$ and is capable of forming films in either. The contact angles of various films formed in these solvents are relatively independent based on film formation in solvents THF and $CHCl_3$. The contact angle of the films are approximately 90 degrees but after the introduction of camphor sulfonic acid to emeraldine PLAAP, the contact angle lowers to almost 50 degrees. This contributes to the copolymer the right surface properties for biocompatibility of rat neuronal pheochromocytoma PC-12 cells, and results in the cells being able to spread across the surface of the PLAAP copolymer.

According to the study, two substrates were seeded with PC-12 cells, a PLAAP substrate and a tissue-culture-treated polystyrene (TCPS), and an electrical stimulus of 0.1V was applied across them using platinum microwire electrodes for 1 hr every day. Two more substrates were seeded, but not electrically stimulated so as to provide a contrasting sample group. It was shown that after 4 days, neurite extension occurred only in the PLAAP substrate stimulated by electrical stimulus and demonstrated that the electroactive PLAAP copolymer can accelerate the differentiation of nerve cells through electrical stimulus. This study proved that PLAAP copolymers can be modified so that they are biocompatible with PC-12 cells and then electrically stimulated to differentiate the nerve cells. The copolymer solubility in inexpensive solvents allows relative ease of processing for practical application, and the electroactivity of the copolymer provides the capability for cellular adhesion, growth and proliferation.

Scaffolds are artificial extracellular matrices used in tissue engineering to integrate tissues and organs and to provide a structure for cells to propagate, migrate and differentiate and become integrated with intrinsic body tissues. Collagen is the most abundant protein in vertebrates and Type I collagen is the most widely used scaffold material because it is abundant, biocompatible, bioabsorbable and it is not antigenic.[10] Monomeric collagen self-assembles to form fibrils in vitro under physiological conditions, the fibrils confer enhanced mechanical properties and biological stability, and the properties are further improved by crosslinking.

Collagen biomaterials are usually produced by sequential processing in which fibrils are allowed to form. They subsequently are crosslinked;[11] however, the mechanical properties of scaffolds formed by this process are inadequate for tissue engineering of hard tissues. Simultaneous processing in which the fibrils are grown and simultaneously crosslinked produces collagen gels with improved mechanical properties.[12]

The structure of these collagen gels, crosslinked with 1-ethyl-3-(3-dimethylaminopropyl)-carbodiimide, was recently studied by scanning electron microscopy and atomic force microscopy and it was discovered that, despite their improved mechanical properties, simultaneously processed collagen gels had fewer fibrils than those that had been sequentially processed. AFM showed that nonfibrous collagen filled the spaces between the fibrils in the simultaneously processed gels. It was postulated that the improved properties resulted from crosslinking of the fibrils with nonfibrous collagen.[13]

Hydrogels are promising scaffolds for cell adhesion, spreading and proliferation, and also for the repair and regeneration of tissues and organs.[14,15] In order to be used as cell-growth scaffolds for tissue engineering, hydrogels must be biocompatible, must have the correct mechanical properties and pore-size, and must be compatible with surrounding living cells.[16] pH sensitive hydrogel copolymers of cross-linked acrylic acid, ε-caprolactone and 2-hydroxyethylmethacrylate showed good biocompatibility, good biodegradation by the enzyme lipase, and good cell adhesion.[17]

However, natural physiological tissue regeneration during wound healing involves the simultaneous appearance of multiple growth factors in controlled amounts.[18] Conventional inert hydrogels are severely limited in their capability to deliver multiple proteins because these gels cannot distinguish between proteins of similar size nor can they govern the release rate of a smaller protein and simultaneously maintain a constant rate of release of a larger protein.

In order to mimic the natural process, layer-by-layer polymeric composites capable of the simultaneous but individually controlled release of two or more proteins have been developed.[19]

Despite many studies, the effect of charge density on multilayer growth is still unclear. For example, very thick films can be prepared form weak polyelectrolytes at high salt concentrations. The exponential growth of these films has been attributed to diffusion of the polyelectrolytes in and out of the multilayer during the B process of layer deposition.[20] This knowledge gap prompted a recent study of the formation of multilayer adsorption of alternating layers of chitosan and pectin as a function of degree of acetylates of pectin. During the process of deposition of chitosan, it was discovered that the chitosan diffused in and out of the film, and as the fresh become more charged and more water-soluble, this effect was magnified. Due to the excess of positive charge, the interaction between pectin and chitosan did not lead to 1:1 stoichiometric complexes.[21]

In addition to these fundamental difficulties, the layer-by-layer composites are fabricated by a series of complex steps; thus, a simpler approach is desirable. Ideally this simpler approach would be monolithic inert hydrogels—however, the tuned-free, diffusive delivery of different actives from an inert hydrogel is almost impossible.

As a consequence of these shortcomings of inert hydrogels, polymer networks with specific protein affinity sites have been developed to release target molecules at a rate determined by the association constant of the site-target molecule couple rather than the passive diffusion of the target molecule through a matrix.[22] Recently, a proof of concept study of monolithic affinity hydrogels for controlled protein release was reported.[23]

These hydrogels are prepared by copolymerizing poly(ethylene glycol) diacrylate [PEGDA] with glycidylmethacrylate-iminodiacetic acid [GMIDA]. The metal binding capabilities of iminodiacetic acid [IDA] have been used extensively for protein purification and this nondegradable hydrogel uses the ligand of IDA capability to tune the simultaneous delivery of two proteins histidine-tagged green fluorescent protein and lysozyme. For example, the affinity binding of histidine-tagged proteins and GMIDA ligands is mediated by metal ions such as nickel but nickel at low concentrations does not significantly affect lysozyme release from the hydrogel. Use of this dual-release mechanism allows the release to be tuned for each protein separately. As a corollary, complete and immediate release of the bound protein can be achieved by merely adding a metal chelating agent such as EDTA. Perhaps well-designed hydrogels such as these will someday trickle beneficial agents from topically-applied compositions.

It is interesting that Chen et al. reported that bovine fetal aorta endothelial cells could spread and proliferate on poly(acrylic acid) without any cell adhesive protein modification.[24] Another shortcoming of in vitro cell growth scaffolds is that they are irreversible physical gels of materials extracted from cells or tissue, chemically cross-linked gels or nanofiber networks, and it is difficult to remove cells from the matrices of these existing gels without damaging the cells in the process. In order to address this issue, thermoresponsive hydrogels have been developed as matrices that would allow facile harvesting of intact cells for implantation.[25]

The advent of living free-radical polymerization has made possible the synthesis of precise molecularly-designed block copolymers for this purpose. Amphipathic BAB block copolymers in which the A block is hydrophilic and the B block is thermoresponsively hydrophobic are preferred for this application. A recent study reported that the synthesis and characterization of such amphipathic molecules having a poly(N-isopropylacrylamide) and a hydrophilic inner a block of poly(N,N-dimethylacryamide).[25] Poly(N-isopropylacrylamide) was chosen because its lower critical solution temperature (LCST) of 32°C is close to the human physiological temperature (37°C); this polymer is soluble in water below 32°C and it phase-separates when the solution temperature is raised above this threshold.

For this block copolymer, the B-blocks become relatively hydrophobic and this causes them to aggregate above the LCST to form the core of polymer micelles. When the concentration is low, the micelles are isolated in solution and the composition is liquid-like; however, above a critical concentration, a network structure forms with the micelle cores becoming junction zones in the gel and the rheology becomes more solid-like; the elastic modulus becomes larger than the loss modulus.

The formation of the gel was shown on a molecular level in this case by measuring the diffusion coefficient of water by pulsed field gradient NMR and by contour microscopy using the fluorescent probe 8-anilino-1-naphthalenesulfonic acid. The apparent diffusion coefficient was high at short times, but it dropped with time of observation and plateaued at 400 milliseconds indicating that the water was being bounded, probably by a gel network. The hypothesis of a gel network was further supported by measurement of the fluorescence observed by confocal microscopy. The fluorescence intensified at elevated temperatures and the image showed large hydrophobic domains separated by tens of micrometers. These are assigned as the micelle core junction zones in the gel. This type of thermoreversible gel could form the basis of a topical treatment that could be removed by merely rinsing with cold water (see **Figure 3**).

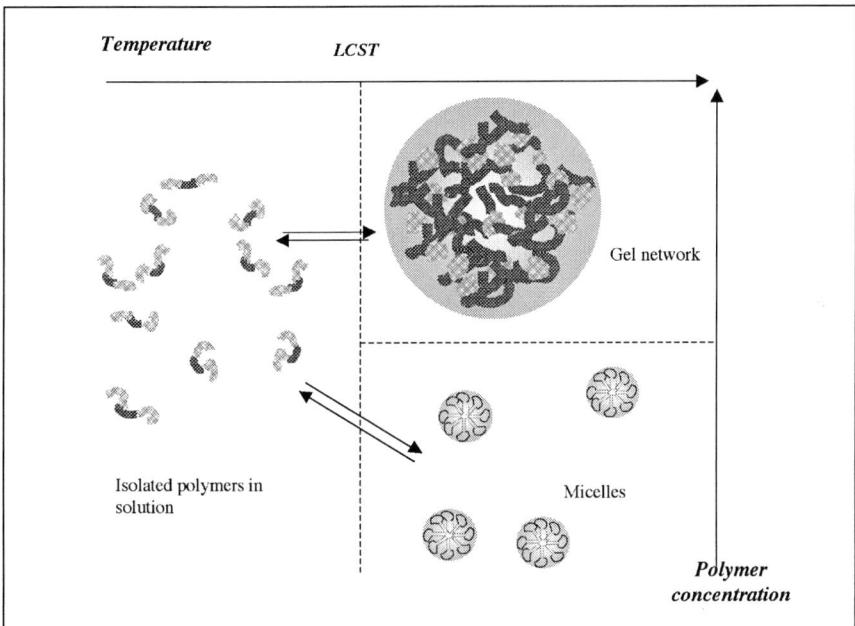

Figure 3. Thermoresponsive block copolymers are a) isolated at low temperatures and b) above the "trigger" temperature, they form micelles at low concentrations and gels at high concentrations. The transitions are reversible.

Mucoadhesive Gels

The emergence of antibiotic-resistant pathogens has the potential of driving civilization back to the pre-penicillin era, when relatively minor infections were life-threatening. In such an environment, even the administration of injections could compromise the body's natural barrier and allow the ingress of undesirable bacteria. In order to meet this challenge, the pharmaceutical industry is directing research attention to more efficient and advanced drug excipients, controlled release systems and bioadhesives. This is because of lower adminstration and dosage frequencies, longer retention times and the possibility of site specific drug delivery. One attractive route is via the mucus membranes of, for example, the nasal or buccal cavity. Mucus membranes are relatively thin and well served with blood vessels; this makes them attractive targets for penetration of drugs into the vascular system.

The polymer poly(acrylic) acid has been heavily researched for bioadhesion and mucoadhesion application. Poly(acrylic) acid contains a high number of carboxylic groups, providing a criticial characteristic of bioadhesion through hydrogen bonding (see **Figure 4**).

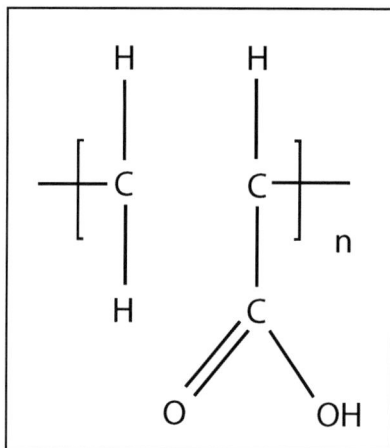

Figure 4. Poly(acrylic) acid

Organogels of a dispersion of poly(acrylic acid), nonaqueous solvent and a model antimicrobial agent have been formed with the application of an antimicrobial implant in the buccal cavity in mind. The proposed mechanism of mucoadhesion for these organogels is initial secondary interactions between the poly(acrylic) acid and the nonaqueous solvent, and once introduced into the oral cavity, interactions between poly(acrylic) acid and mucin.

The rheological properties, specifically pseudoplastic flow, of a mucoadhesive gel are critical to the success of drug delivery because of application ease and manufacturing ease. The quick structural recovery of pseudoplastic materials also aids in retention of the gel in the oral cavity. Because of swallowing and a constant flow of saliva, retention time of a mucoadhesive gel in the buccal cavity poses a major challenge. Correlations between viscoelastic properties and mucoadhesion were found in the poly(acrylic) acid organogels, where highly structured gels exhibited high mucoadhesion, because of molecular polymer chain entanglements. As the concentration of poly(acrylic) acid increased in the bioactive organogels, loss modulus, storage modulus, dynamic viscosity, compressibility, mucoadhesion and drug release rate also increased. Choice of nonaqueous solvent also affected the physiochemical parameters. The organogel with 5-10% w/w poly(acrylic) acid and the nonaqueous solvent PEG 400 maintained the most potential as an antimicrobial implant.[26]

Controlled Delivery from Micellar Aggregates and Vesicles

While micelle-aggregated gels are being developed for tissue engineering, the need for better chemotherapeutic agents is driving the reach for precise tailoring of the interactions between hydrophilic polymers and vesicles. In this context, it has recently been shown that polyaspartylhydrazide copolymers containing butyl moieties and/or (carboxypropyl)trimethylammonium moieties bind to the surface of phosphatidylcholine/cholesterol vesicles and this causes the vesicles to bind more strongly to cancer cells to increase the effectiveness of chemotherapy.[27]

Since the 1960s it has been known that cholesterol fills the voids in the palisade layer of lecithin monolayers and the scientific community understands that one of the roles of cholesterol in cells is to strengthen the phospholipid structure of the cell membranes.

Recently, it has been shown that hydrophobic matching between the cholesterol and fatty acid is required for the formation of lamellar liquid ordered phases.[28]

It has also been demonstrated by nearest neighbor recognition methods that cholesterol-rich fluid bilayers have an ordered bilayer structure a which free cholesterol and longer chain phospholipid homodimer co-exist in equilibrium with a stoichiometric complex composed of one molecule of cholesterol for every two molecules of longer chain phospholipid homodimer.[29] It is not surprising, therefore, that attempts have been made to decorate hydrophilic polymers with cholesterol mesogens to enhance their interaction with lipid membranes and vesicles. Langmuir trough studies showed that, for a homopolymer formed from cholesterol acrylamidobutyrate (CAB), the preferred configuration of the cholesterol rings is to lie flat at the air-water interface (see **Figure 5**).[30]

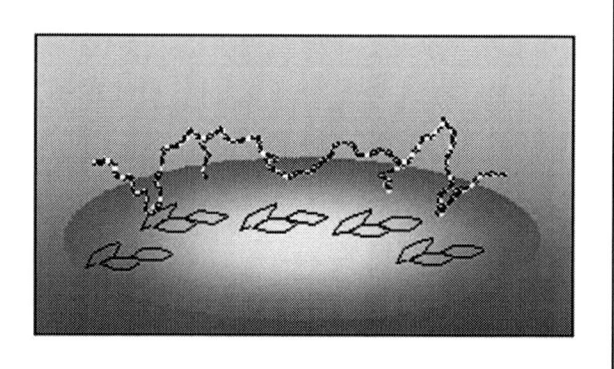

Figure 5. When present in the polymer in excess of 15 mole%, cholesterol side chains lie flat at the air/water interface. This may indicate that they would adopt this conformation at the surface of vesicles.

The inference to be drawn from this finding is that presumably the cholesterol rings of such a homopolymer would also lie flat at the surface a lipid bilayer. If this happened, the cholesterol rings would be sterically restricted from insertion between the lipid molecules of the bilayer and the resulting polymer-lipid interaction would be weak. A copolymer of CAB and 2-acrylamido-2-methylpropanesulfonic acid AMPS gave a similar surface configuration of the cholesterol when the mole ratio of CAB:AMPS was 15:85. However, a copolymer containing 10 mole percent CAB gave a close-packed surface structure with the cholesterol rings being organized side-by-side with a vertical orientation to the surface. The inference in this case is that this copolymer would be ideal for interacting with, and perhaps stabilizing, phospholipid bilayers (see **Figure 6**).

The precision with which these molecules have to be designed to fit their function is demonstrated by the finding that when the cholesterol mesogens content of the copolymer was reduced to 5 mole percent, the polymer tended to form bilayers and micelle assemblies. Similarly, the introduction of cholesterol mesogens to carboxymethylchitosan caused this polymer to form nanomicelles that could function as injectable drug carriers.[31]

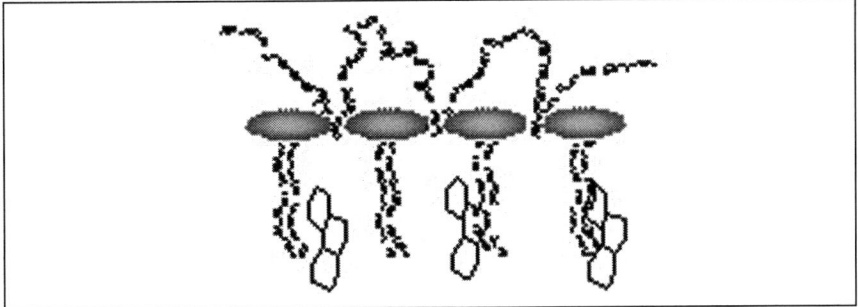

Figure 6. At 10 mole% cholesterol, the cholesterol side groups aligh in close-packed vertical conformation at the air/water interface. Presumably, these polymers would be structured appropriately to interpenetrate the palisade layers of vesicles.

Nanofiber Materials

Scaffolds for tissue engineering can be formed by the self-assembly of peptides into β-pleated sheets[32-34] and it has been shown that configurational and conformational organization of peptides can lead to self assembly into complex hierarchical structures such as nanotubes,[35] nanofibers[36] and helical fibrils.[37] An interesting development has been the demonstration that β-sheet-forming wheel-like synthetic peptides self assemble into nanofibers in phosphate buffer and rodlike structures in acid and alkaline media.[38] The nanofiber structures were clearly visible in transmission electron micrographs of specimens stained with phosphotungstic acid or uranyl acetate. An emphatic increase of fluorescence on binding with thioflavin T showed that the nanofibers self-assemble as β-pleated sheets and increase in fluorescence upon binding 8-anilino-1-naph-thalenesulfonic acid indicated that the outside of the nanofibers were hydrophilic (see **Figure 7** and 8).

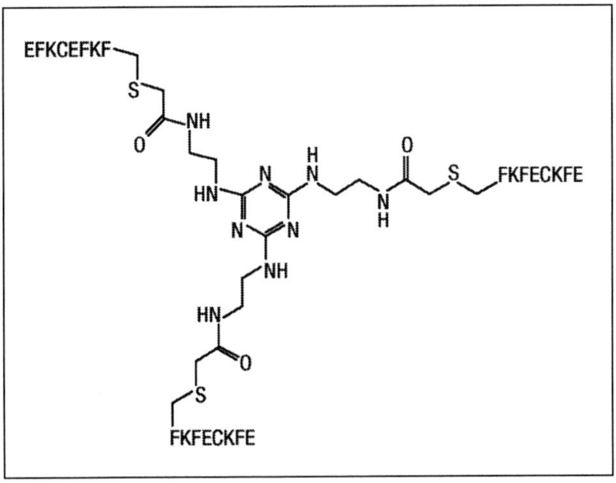

Figure 7. A ß-sheet-forming wheel peptide

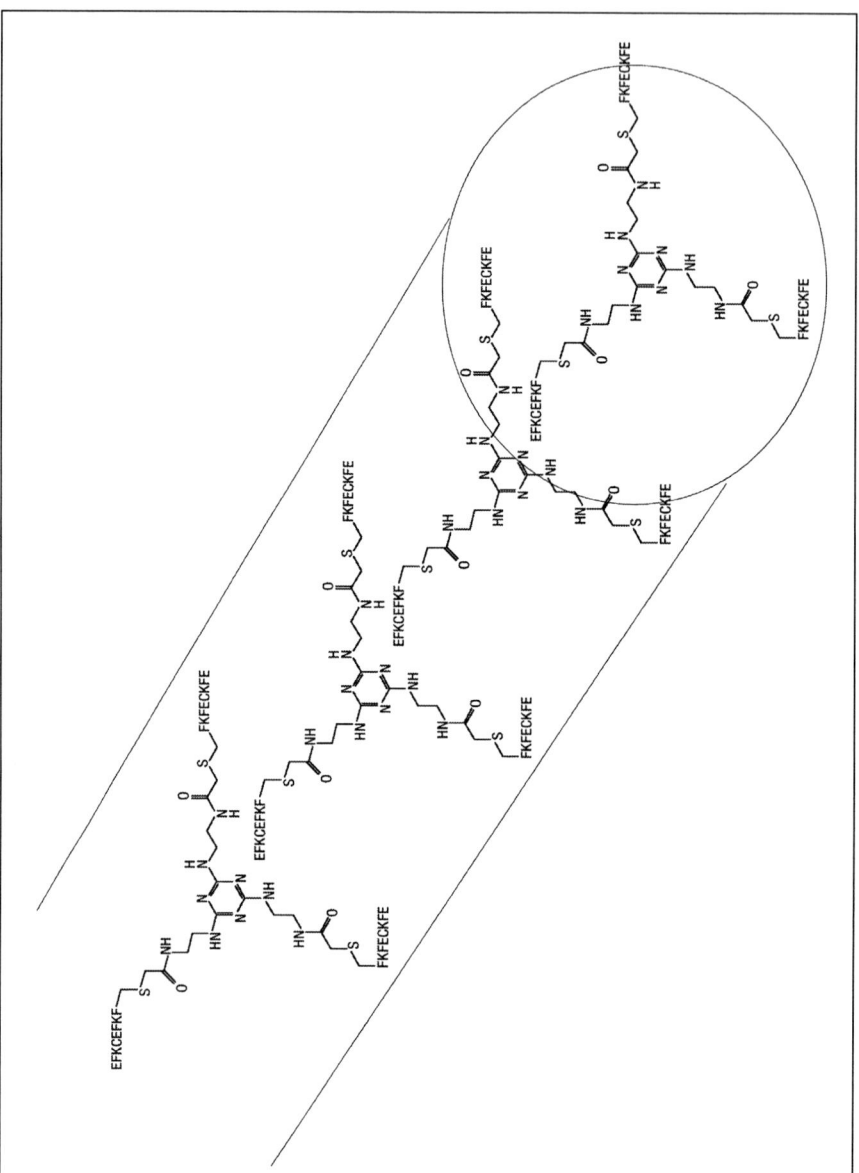

Figure 8. Wheel-like peptides can self-assemble to form nanofibers

Modified microcrystalline celluloses are used extensively as rheology modifiers in personal care and also in foods. The rheology conferred by these materials is attributed to the formation of composite network structures between cellulose microcrystalline fibrils and soluble polymers.

A recent study on the interaction between cellulose nanofibers may shed some light on exactly what is happening between the crystalline microfibrils when they form higher order structures.[39] The nature of the surface of cellulose nanocrytals differs depending upon the method of preparation. Thus, hydrolysis with sulfuric acid might be expected to yield surfaces that contain sulfate groups. The effect of surface charge density on the structuring of cellulose nanocrystal films was probed using quartz crystal microbalance with dissipation and atomic force microbalance measurements. Cellulose nanofibrils were prepared by mechanically disintegrating bleached sulfite pulp by a microfluidizer. Low charge density nanofibrils were pretreated by enzymatic hydrolysis and mechanical disintegration, whereas high charge density nanofibrils were carboxymethylated. The cellulose nanofibers were spin-coated on a silica wafer. Interestingly, the carboxymethylated anionically charged nanofibrils gave good homogeneous surface coverage (attributed to hydrogen-bonding) whereas the low charge density nanofibrils did not adhere readily to the silica surface.

Surface coverage was improved by treatment with polyvinylamine, titanium dioxide or 3-aminopropyltrimethoxysilane, implying that these low charge density nanofibrils carry a negative charge. Quartz crystal microbalance measurements in aqueous media showed that low charge density nanofibril films were relatively insensitive to changes in electrolyte concentration and pH but high change density nanofibril films swelled and de-swelled dramatically under the influence of such changes.

Electrolyte addition caused the films to imbibe water; much more for the high charge density nanofibers. This enhanced swelling was attributed to a Donnan effect; increased electrolyte concentration causes cm increase in the pH inside the film, leading to dissociation of more carboxyl groups that in turn cause polyelectrolyte swelling. At high electrolyte concentrations, the water uptake decreases again and this can be explained by electrochemical attraction of counter ions to the nanofibrils being favored over the chemical potential-driven diffusion of counterions into the surrounding aqueous environment. The resulting proximity of the counterions shields the nanofibril charges and causes de-swelling of the film.

Atomic force microscope measurements of the interfibril interaction were conducted by attaching a cellulose sphere to the tip of the probe and then carefully measuring force as a function of distance between the nanofibril film and the cellulose sphere. These measurements in water at pH 8 indicated the presence of electrical double layer repulsion, consistent with DLVO theory. However, when the ionic strength was increased, the forces did not decay to the extent expected by double layer repulsion. This indicates that there is steric repulsion, for both low charge density and high charge density nanofibrils and this may also indicate the presence of anchored soluble polymers, presumably hemicelluloses, at their surface.

Impurities in polysaccharides often diffuse to the surface, making it difficult to measure the true surface energy. Chitosan and cellulose fall under same class of materials but they differ chemically since OH groups in the cellulose are replaced by NH_2 groups. The dispersive components of the surface energy are comparable within the two polymers, but the polar component is higher in cellulose than chitosan.[40-42]

In one study, chitosan surface energies were compared with N-acetyl-D-glucosamine (GlcNAc) before and after purification and extraction processes. These processes removed nonpolar impurities present in chitosan; then samples in the form of pellets and films were obtained. Before purification chitosan showed low values of the polar component of surface free energy compared to GlcNAc but after purification there was a dramatic increase. For the purified pellets, increase in the polar component confirmed that nonpolar impurities caused the decrease in the polar component of chitosan. The polar component was independent of degree of deacetylation (DDA). For films, the polar component was lower compared to GlcNAc, as the residual impurities in films migrated to the surface and caused a decrease in the surface energy. Scratching the film surface spontaneously increased the surface energy. Thus, the impurities present in the commercially available chitosan were responsible for low polar component of surface energies.[43]

These latest findings indicate that the industry's understanding of the interactions between nanofibrils is far from complete and more fundamental studies could yield rich rewards in the design of new, improved rheology modifiers and nanofiber composites.

Published June 2008 Cosmetics and Toiletries magazine

References

1. C Vogel, E Wessel and HW Siesler, FT-IR imaging spectroscopy of phase separation in blends of poly(3-hydroxybutyrate) with poly(L-lactic acid) and poly(E-caprolactone), Biomacromolecules 9 523 (2008)
2. T Karbowiak, F Debeaufort, D Champion and A Voilley, Wetting properties at the surface of iota-carrageenan-based edible films, *J Colloid Interface Sci* 294 400 (2006)
3. A Hambleton, F Debeaufort, T Karbowiak and A Voilley, Protection of active aroma compound against moisture and oxygen by encapsulation in biopolymeric emulsion-based edible films, *Biomacromolecules ASAP*, published on the Internet (Feb 8, 2008)
4. SD McConaughy, PA Stroud, B Boudreaux, RD Hester and CL McCormick, Structural characterization and solution properties of a galacturonate polysaccharide derived from aloe vera capable of in situ gelation, *Biomacro molecules*, 9 472 (2008)
5. M Gidley, ER Morris, EJ Murray, DA Powell and DA Rees, *Chem Commun* 990–991 (1979)
6. DA Rees, Carbohydr Polym 2 254–263 (1982)
7. DA Powell, ER Morris, MJ Gidley and DA Rees, *J Mol Biol* 155 517–531 (1982)
8. R Langer, JP Vacanti, Tissue engineering, *Science* 260 920–926 (1993)
9. L Huang et al, Synthesis of biodegradable and electroactive multiblock polylactide and aniline pentamer copolymer for tissue engineering applications, *Biomacromolecules ASAP*, published on the Internet (Feb 9, 2008)
10. CH Lee, A Singla and Y Lee, Biomedical applications of collagen, Int J Pharmaceutics 221 (2001)
11. W Friess, H Uludag, S Foskett, R Biron and C Sargeant, Characterization of absorbable collagen sponges as rh BMP.2 carriers, *Int J Pharmaceutics* 187 91 (1999)
12. S Yunoki, N Nagai, S Suzuki and M Munekata, Novel biomaterial from reinforced salmon collagen gel prepared by fibril formation and cross-linking, *J Biosci Bioeng* 98 40 (2004)
13. S Yunoki and T Matsuda, Simultaneous processing of fibril formation and cross-linking improves mechanical properties of collagen, *Biomacromolecules ASAP*, published on the Internet (Feb 9, 2008)
14. KY Lee and DJ Mooney, Hydrogels for tissue engineering, *Chem Rev* 101 1869 (2001)
15. AS Hoffman, Hydrogels for biomedical applications, *Advanced Drug Delivery Reviews* 54 3 (2002)
16. LG Griffith and MA Swartz, Capturing complex 3D tissue physiology in vitro, Nature Reviews Molecular Cell Biology 7, 211 (2006)
17. D-Q Wu, Y-X Sun, X-D Xu, SX Cheng, Xi-Z Zhang and R-X Zhuo, Biodegradable and pH-sensitive hydrogels for cell encapsulation and controlled drug release, *Biomacromolecules ASAP*, published on the Internet (Feb 29, 2008)
18. TP Richardson, MC Peters, AB Ennett and DJ Mooney, Polymeric system for dual growth factor delivery, *Nature Biotechnology* 19 1029 (2001)
19. KC Wood, HF Chuang, RD Batten, DM Lynn and PT Hammond, Controlling interlayer diffusion to achieve sustained, multiagent delivery from layer-by-layer thin films, *Proc Nat Acad Sci* 103 10207 (2006)
20. C Picart et al, Molecular basis for the explanation of the exponential growth of polyelectrolyte multilayers, *Proc Natl Acad Sci* 99 12531–12535 (2002)
21. K Kamburova, V Milkova, I Petkanchin and T Radeva, Effect of Pectin Charge Density on Formation of Multilayer Films with Chitosan, *Biomacromolecules*, published on Internet (Feb 22, 2008)
22. NA Peppas and SL Wright; Drug diffusion and binding in ionizable interpenetrating networks from poly(vinyl alcohol) and poly(acrylic acid); *European J Pharm Biopharm* 46 15 (1998)

23. C-C Lin and AT Metters, Bifunctional monolithic affinity hydrogels for dual-protein delivery, *Biomacromolecules ASAP*, published on the Internet (Feb 8, 2008)
24. YM Chen, N Shiraishi, H Satokawa, A Kakugo, T Narita and JP Gong, Cultivation of endothelial cells on adhesive protein-free synthetic polymer gels, *Biomaterials* 26 4588 (2005)
25. SE Kirkland, RM Hensarling, SD McConaughy, Y Guo, WJ Jarrett and CL McCormick, Thermoreversible hydrogels from RAFT-synthesized BAB triblock copolymers: steps toward biomimetic matrices for tissue regeneration, *Biomacromolecules* 9 681 (2008)
26. DS Jones, BCO Muldoon, AD Woolfson, GP Andrews and FD Sanderson, Physiochemical characterization of bioactive polyacrylic acid organogels as potential antimicrobial implants for the buccal cavity, *Biomacromolecules* 9 624 (2008)
27. D Paolino, D Cosco, M Licciardi, G Giammona, M Fresta and G Cavallaro, Polyapastylhydrazide copolymer based supramolecular vesicular aggregates as delving devices for anticancer drugs, *Biomacromolecules ASAP*, published on Internet (Feb 29, 2008)
28. J Ouimet and M Lafleur, Hydrophobic match between cholesterol and saturated fatty acid is required for the formation of lamellar liquid ordered phases, *Langmuir* 20 7474 (2004)
29. J Zhang, H Cao and SL Regen, Cholesterol-phospholipid complexation in fluid bilayers as evidenced by nearest-neighbor recognition measurements, *Langmuir* 23 405 (2007)
30. K Chandrasekar, R Vijay and G Baskar, Ionic polymeric amphiphiles with cholesterol mesogen: Adsorption and organization characteristics at the air/water interface, from *Langmuir Film Balance Studies*, *Biomacromolecules ASAP*, published on the Internet (Feb 29, 2008)
31. W Yinsong, L Lingrong, W Jian and Q Zhang, Preparation and characterization of self-aggregated nanoparticles of cholesterol-modified O-carboxymethyl chitosan conjugates, *Carbohydrate Polymers* 69 597 (2007)
32. J Kisiday et al, Self-assembling peptide hydrogel fosters chondrocyte extracellular matrix production and cell division: Implications for cartilage tissue repair, *Proc Natl Acad Sci* 99 9996 (2002)
33. RG Ellis-Behnke et al, Nano neuro knitting: Peptide nanofiber scaffold for brain repair and axon regeneration with functional return of vision, *Proc Natl Acad Sci* 103 5054 (2006)
34. DA Salick, JK Kretsinger, DJ Pochan and JP Schneider, Inherent antibacterial activity of a peptide-based β-hairpin hydrogel, *J Am Chem Soc* 129 14793 (2007)
35. C Valéry et al, Biomimetic organization: Octapeptide self-assembly into nanotubes of viral capsid-like dimension, *Proc Natl Acad Sci* 100 10258 (2003)
36. MG Ryadnov and DN Woolfson, MaP peptides: Programming the self-assembly of peptide-based mesoscopic matrices, *J Am Chem Soc* 127 12407 (2005)
37. M Zhou, D Bentley and I Ghosh; Helical supramolecules and fibers utilizing leucine zipper-displaying dendrimers, *J Am Chem Soc* 126 734 (2004)
38. K Murasato, K Matsuura and N Kimizuka, Self-assembly of nanofiber with uniform width from wheel-type trigonal-sheet-forming peptide, *Biomacromolecules ASAP*, published on the Internet (Feb 21, 2008)
39. S Ahola, J Salmi, L-S Johansson, J Laine and M. Österberg, Model films from native cellulose nanofibrils. Preparation, swelling and surface interactions, *Biomacromolecules ASAP*, published on the Internet (Feb 29, 2008)
40. A Gandini and MN Belgacem, *Cellulose Fibre Reinforced Polymer Composites*, Old City Publishing: Philadelphia, PA, ch 3 (2007)
41. H Angellier, S Molina-Boisseau, MN Belgacem and A Dufresne, *Langmuir* 21 2425 (2005)
42. MN Belgacem, A Blayo and AJ Gandini, *J Colloid Interface Sci* 182 431 (1996)
43. A Cunha, S Fernandes, C Freire, A Silvestre, C Neto and A Gandini, What is the real value of chitosan's surface energy?, *Biomacromolecules* 9 610 (2008)

CHAPTER 3

Fluid Gels Based on Natural Polymers for Cosmetic Applications

Peter A. Williams and Martina Hickey
Centre for Water Soluble Polymers, North East Wales Institute, Wrexham UK
David Mitchell
Chesham Chemicals Ltd, Harrow UK

KEY WORDS: *polymers, fluid gels, xanthan gum, konjac mannan, rheology*

ABSTRACT: *Varying the concentration of two polymers – xanthan gum and konjac mannan – mixed in solution and subjected to shear while cooling yields fluid gels whose viscosity can vary from a pourable solution to a spreadable gel.*

Water-soluble polymers are widely used as thickeners and gelling agents in a broad range of cosmetic and personal care products today. Examples include shampoos and conditioners, hair and body gels, skin creams, liquid and cream foundations, toothpaste, sunscreen lotions and sprays. Numerous polymers are available commercially and these include both natural and synthetic polymers.

The natural polymers are mainly polysaccharides and their chemical derivatives. Polysaccharide thickeners include guar gum plus its derivatives (hydroxypropyl-, carboxymethyl- and hydroxypropyltrimonium-), locust bean gum, cellulosics (carboxymethyl-, methyl-, methylhydroxypropyl-, hydroxyethyl-, cationic hydroxyethyl- and others) and xanthan gum. Gelling agents include alginate, carrageenan, pectin and gellan gum.

The synthetic polymers used are largely acrylate-based and may be crosslinked or in alkali-soluble or swellable forms.

There is an increasing trend, which is driven by environmental concerns and consumer awareness, for the use of natural materials in cosmetic formulations. This chapter reports on the development of a novel thickening system with unique rheological characteristics and natural ingredients. The system consists of a combination of two naturally occurring polymers, namely xanthan gum and konjac mannan. The two polymers interact synergistically and will form "fluid gels" under the appropriate processing conditions.

Xanthan Gum

Xanthan gum was discovered in the 1950s and was introduced into the food sector in the 1970s. It is now finding extensive application in a wide range of industrial areas because of its characteristic rheological properties.[1-3]

Xanthan gum is a bacterial polysaccharide obtained from the genus *Xanthomonas*, notably *X. campestris*, by aerobic fermentation. The xanthan molecules have a cellulosic backbone consisting of β1,4-linked glucose residues. They also have a trisaccharide side-chain on every other glucose linked through the C3 position (**Figure 1**). The side-chain consists of two mannose units linked on either side to a glucuronic acid. The inner mannose residue connected to the backbone may be acetylated while the terminal mannose residue may be pyruvated.

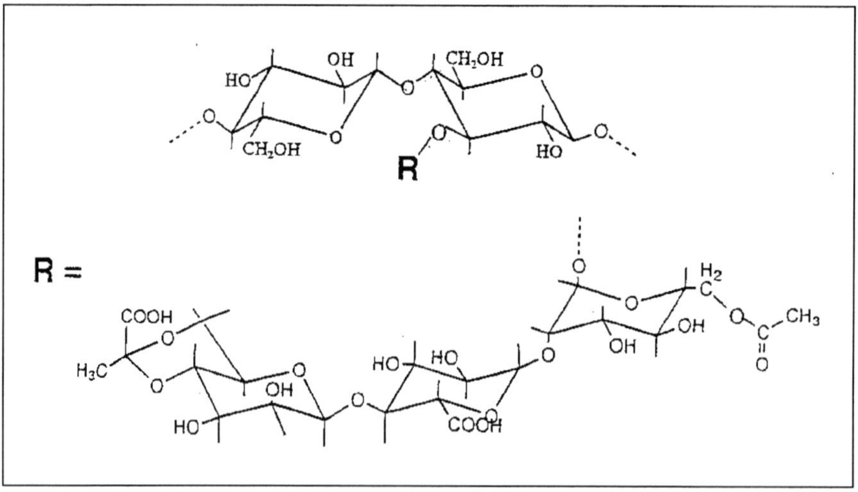

Figure 1. Repeating structure of xanthan gum

The molecular mass of the xanthan molecules is very high (>3x10^6) and the gum dissolves in water to yield highly viscous solutions.

The xanthan molecules undergo a thermoreversible coil-helix transition in solution. At high temperatures, where the molecules are in the disordered coil form, the side-chains are envisaged as protruding away from the cellulosic backbone into solution. At low temperatures, where the molecules are in the ordered form, they adopt a stiff helical structure with the side-chains folded in and associated with the backbone.

Acetyl groups promote helix formation because they can facilitate side-chain interaction with the backbone by hydrogen bonding. Pyruvate groups, however, inhibit helix formation because there is greater electrostatic repulsion between these groups in the ordered form, due to their closer proximity. The transition shifts to higher temperatures by the addition of electrolyte.

The stiffness of the xanthan molecules gives rise to unique rheological properties. Solutions have a very high viscosity at low shear and possess an apparent yield stress that enables the polymer to prevent the sedimentation or creaming of particles, oil droplets or bubbles. The solutions are also highly pseudoplastic and on the application of shear, the viscosity decreases rapidly and the solutions readily flow. In addition, unlike other charged polymers, the viscosity of xanthan solutions can actually increase rather than decrease when electrolyte is added or when pH is low because these conditions will promote helix formation and self association.

Konjac Mannan

Konjac mannan is a polysaccharide obtained from the tuber of the konjac plant, notably the *Amorphophallus konjac* species that grows in Southeast Asia, particularly in Japan, China and Indonesia.[4,5]

Konjac is a perennial plant and the tuber grows in size each year. Three- to five-year-old plants produce purplish-red flowers. In Japan the young tubers are planted in spring and removed from the soil in winter and stored in heated warehouses. They are replanted the following spring and harvested in the late autumn.

The main component of the tuber is glucomannan, which is present in egg shaped cells that can be up to 650 microns in size. The glucomannan is extracted by first washing the tubers and then cutting them into thin slices. These are dried and pulverized to produce so-called konjac flour, which may be further purified by alcohol washing.

Konjac mannan is a high molecular mass (>106) polysaccharide consisting of linear chains of glucose and mannose units linked b1,4 (**Figure 2**). At approximately every 10 sugar units on average, the chains have branches of up to 16 sugar units linked to the C3 position of the mannose and glucose, which are in a ratio of 1.6:1. It is believed that there are no block sequences of glucose or mannose along the chain. Possible structures for the repeating unit are:

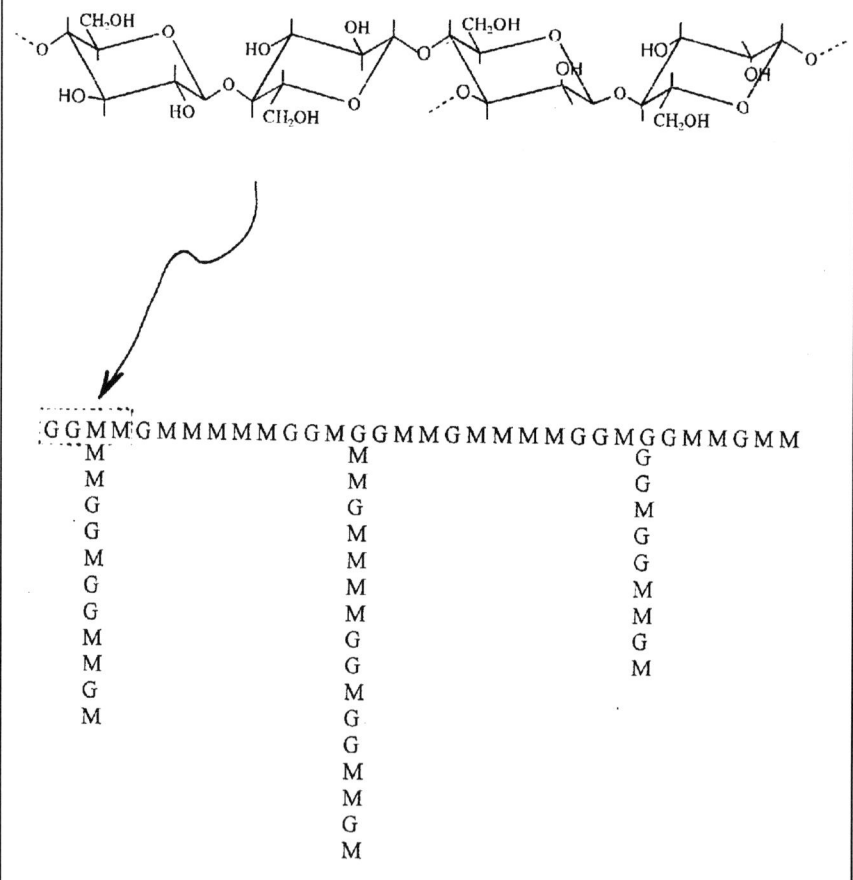

Figure 2. Repeating structure of konjac mannan

(G-G-M-M) M-M-G-M
and
G-G-M-G-M-M-M-M

Konjac mannan dissolves in water to form highly viscous solutions. It is acetylated (~1 acetyl group for every 19 sugar residues) and in the presence of alkali, deacetylation occurs and thermally irreversible gels are produced. Konjac gel is a popular food in Japan and has now been approved as a food additive in the United States and Europe.

Synergistic Interaction

Neither xanthan gum nor konjac mannan forms gels independently in neutral solution. However, it is well known that when these materials are mixed together, a strong, optically clear gel can be produced.[6] Gelation can also occur with xanthan gum and locust bean gum but the gels formed are not as strong as with konjac mannan.[7]

The gel is formed by initially mixing solutions of the polymers at high temperature (~90°C) and cooling. In water alone, gelation starts to occur at ~60°C, while in the presence of electrolyte, gelation will occur at ~40°C. The gels formed are thermoreversible and on heating to just above the gelation temperature they will melt to form viscous solutions. Gelation will not occur when the solutions are mixed cold.

The strength of the gel is greater in water alone than in the presence of electrolyte and varies with the xanthan:konjac mannan mixing ratio.[7] The optimum mixing ratio in water is ~1:1 and in the presence of sodium chloride (~0.25%) it is ~2:1. This is illustrated in **Figure 3**,

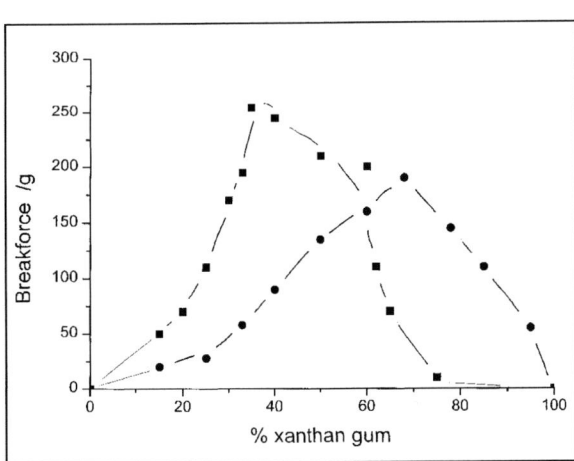

Figure 3. Breakforce of gels of xanthan gum and konjac mannan mixed at varying ratios in water (■) and 0.25% sodium chloride (●) (adapted from reference 7)

which shows measurements[a] of the breakforce of the gel prepared at varying mixing ratios while holding the total polymer concentration constant at 1.2%.[7]

Numerous studies have been undertaken to elucidate the mechanism of gelation using a variety of techniques including rheometry, differential scanning calorimetry and electron spin resonance spectroscopy.[3,8-10] It has been concluded that the gel is formed by associative interaction between the ordered xanthan helices and the konjac mannan chains.

On cooling solutions in water alone, the association and gelation occurs as soon as the xanthan molecules start to form the stiff helical structure (~60°C). In the presence of very low levels of electrolyte (~0.05% sodium chloride), however, the xanthan molecules order at much higher temperatures (>80°C) but the association and gelation process does not occur until the system is cooled to ~40°C.

Fluid Gels

We have recently been investigating the formation of novel fluid gels based on patented mixtures of xanthan gum and konjac mannan.[11] For the purposes of this chapter, we'll use the term XK sheared gels to identify these patented mixtures. XK sheared gels are produced by subjecting the mixed polymer solutions to shear while cooling. Depending on the concentration of the polymers used, the product can vary from a pourable viscous solution to a spreadable gel.

In one set of experiments, sheared and non-sheared gels were produced by dissolving 0.25 g xanthan gum and 0.25 g konjac mannan prepared as a powder blend in 100 ml water by heating to 90°C with stirring. One sample was allowed to cool to room temperature without shearing. The other was cooled while applying shear using a mechanical stirrer fitted with a four-bladed propeller set at a speed of 550 rpm. The influence of shear on the characteristics of the gel is clearly illustrated in **Figure 4**. The non-sheared gel is strong and free standing, while the sheared gel is fluid and can be readily spread by hand.

The mechanical spectra of sheared gels containing either 0.5% or 0.25% xanthan gum and konjac mannan (1:1) were determined by controlled stress rheometry. **Figure 5** presents

---
[a]Stevens Texture Analyser, Stevens, Dunmow, Essex, UK

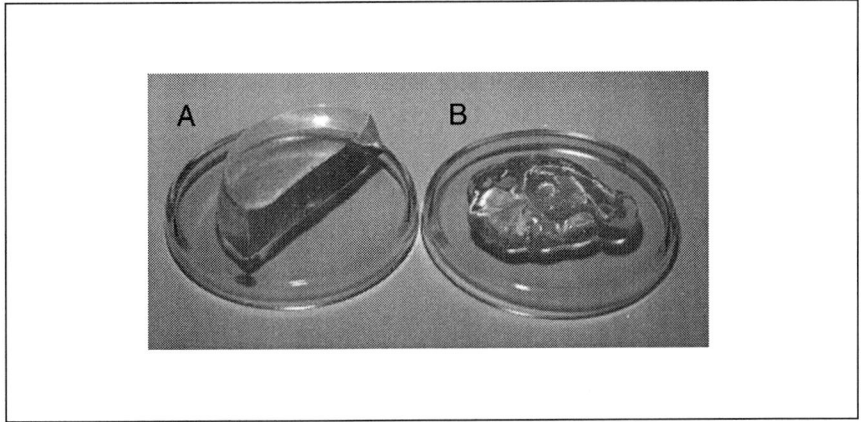

Figure 4. Comparison of gels formed without (left) and with (right) stirring during the cooling phase

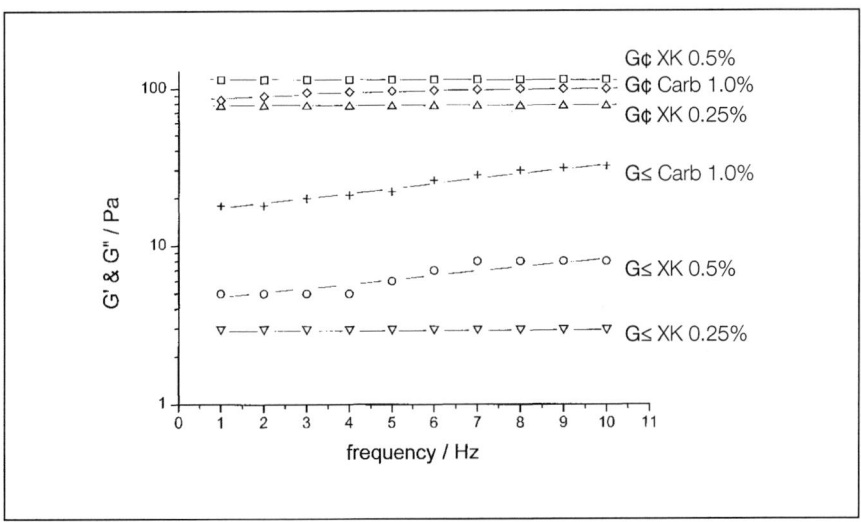

Figure 5. G′ and G″ respectively as a function of frequency for XK sheared gels at 0.5% (O, 0) and 0.25% (Δ, —) total polymer concentration (1:1 ratio) and 1% Carbopol 981 at pH 7.4 (‡, +)

the storage (G′) and loss (G″) moduli, which correspond to the elastic and viscous components of the system, respectively, as a function of the frequency of oscillation. The spectra show that G′ is greater than G″ over the frequency range studied and that both are independent of frequency. This is indicative of a three-dimensional gel structure. The 0.25% fluid gel has similar G′ values to that of a 1% solution of crosslinked polyacrylate[b], a commonly used carbomer shown in **Figure 5** for comparison. The G″ values for the sheared gel are significantly lower than for the carbomer, indicating stronger gel characteristics.

The preparation temperature is an important factor in controlling the characteristics of the gel. As a general rule, the mixed polymer solutions should be heated to a temperature above the gelation temperature prior to cooling and shearing. This is illustrated in **Figure 6**, which gives G¢ as a function of frequency for a 0.5% XK sheared gel (1:1) in the absence of electrolyte for preparation temperatures of 90°C, 70°C and 50°C. This system gels at ~60°C and it is evident that G' values obtained for mixtures prepared at 90°C and 70°C (meaning, above the gelation temperature) are identical, while G¢ values obtained for mixtures prepared at 50°C (meaning, below the gelation temperature) are much lower.

The presence of co-solutes has also been investigated. It has been found that for 0.5% XK sheared gel at a 1:1 ratio, G¢ is

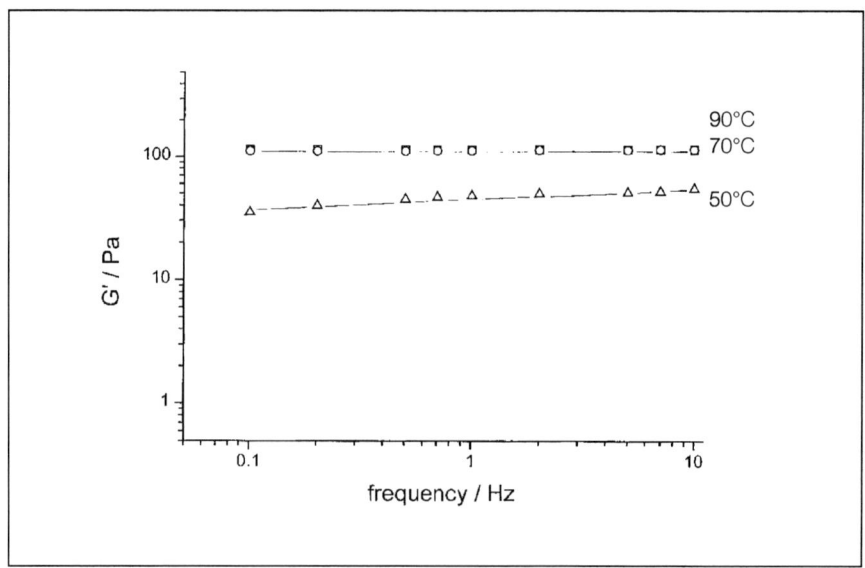

Figure 6. G¢ as a function of frequency for XK sheared gels (0.5% total polymer and at a 1:1 mixing ratio) having been prepared and cooled from 90°C (□), 70°C (★) and 50°C (✢) (Note: The data for 70°C and 90°C are identical.)

---

[b]Carbopol 981, a product of Noveon, Brecksville, Ohio USA.

reduced in the presence of 0.25% sodium chloride (as expected from Figure 3), but a slight increase is observed in the presence of 20% methanol (**Figure 7**).

The pH of the solution during preparation is also important, as illustrated in **Figure 8**. It is seen that G¢ values are relatively constant for XK sheared gels prepared at neutral pH and above, but when prepared at low pH (pH 2), very weak gels are formed. This is explained by the fact that at low pH the uronic acid groups on the xanthan side-chains will be largely undissociated, and intermolecular charge repulsions between xanthan molecules will be dramatically reduced. This promotes self-aggregation of the xanthan molecules and reduces xanthan-konjac mannan interaction. Stronger gels can be formed at low pH by preparing initially at high pH – so that the xanthan-konjac mannan interaction can occur — and then adding acid.

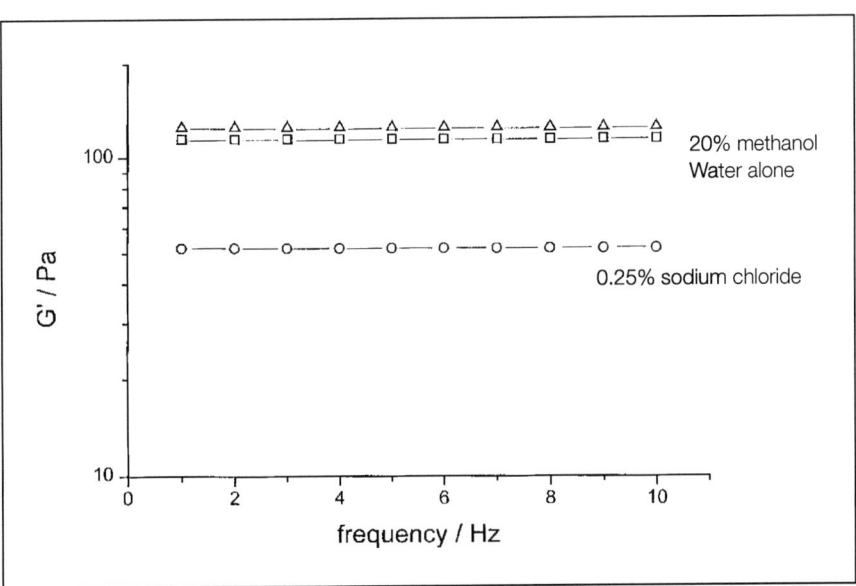

Figure 7. G¢ as a function of frequency for XK sheared gels (0.5% total polymer and at a 1:1 mixing ratio) prepared at 90°C in the presence of water alone (□), 0.25% sodium chloride (★) and 20% methanol (✤)

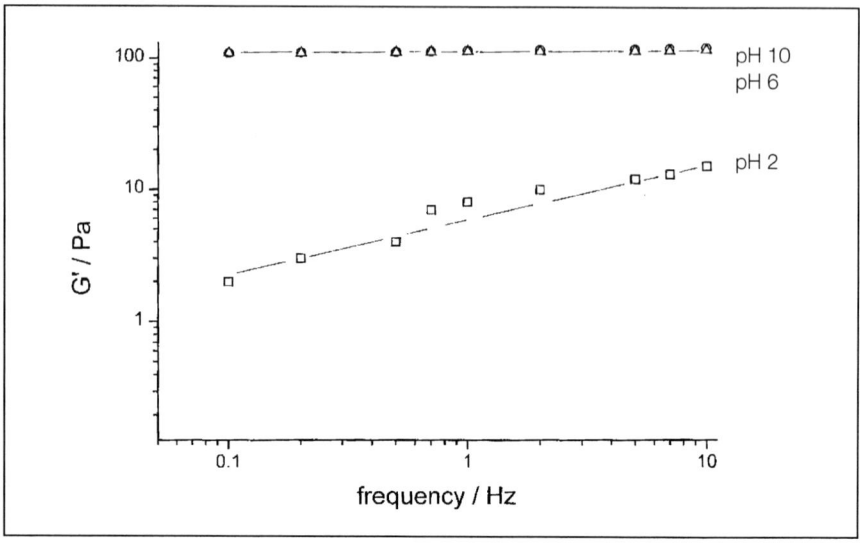

Figure 8. G′ as a function of frequency for XK sheared gels (0.5% total polymer and at a 1:1 mixing ratio) prepared at pH 2 (□), pH 6 (✤) and pH 10(★)

Application in Cosmetic Formulations

The XK sheared gels have been screened for application in a broad range of cosmetic applications.[11] Some examples are given here.

Shampoo: A typical shampoo formulation incorporating the XK sheared gel is given in **Formula 1**.

Formula 1
Shampoo incorporating xantham gum and konjac mannan

Water (*aqua*)	100.00% w/w
Sodium lauryl sulphate	7.80
Sodium chloride	0.75
Cocamidopropyl betaine	0.75
Glycol distearate	0.80
Laureth-3	2.00
Mannan (and) xanthan gum (Glucovis, Chesham)	0.20
Preservative	qs
Fragrance (*parfum*)	qs

The shampoo was prepared by adding the components to water with stirring in the following order: sodium lauryl sulfate, sodium chloride, laureth-3, cocamidopropyl betaine and XK sheared gel. The bulk was then heated to 80°C with continued stirring and the glycol distearate added. Once uniform, the bulk was cooled with constant stirring to below 35°C. The preservative and fragrance were added and the product made to weight with purified water. The product was stirred until cool and uniform and the pearl had set up.

Adding the XK sheared gel had several effects. It provided a stable and reproducible viscosity build. It improved pouring and eliminated drips. It provided a soft and conditioned hair feel effect, and it acted as a pearl stabilizer.

Body lotion: A body lotion was prepared using **Formula 2**.

Formula 2
Body lotion incorporating xantham gum and konjac mannan

Water (*aqua*)	qs 100.00% w/w
Sodium hydroxide	0.028
Glycerine	5.000
Glyceryl monostearate and polyoxyethylene	4.000
Stearate fatty acid ester	2.000
Paraffinum liquidum (mineral) oil	15.000
Cholesterol	5.000
Oleyl alcohol	2.000
Tetrasodium EDTA	0.050
Mannan (and) xanthan gum (Glucovis, Chesham)	0.300
Preservative	qs

The EDTA was dissolved in the water and the XK sheared gel added with stirring. The glycerin was added until the system was homogeneous and it was then heated to 80°C. The paraffin oil was heated to 70°C until it had melted and was added to the aqueous phase. An emulsion was formed by homogenizing under high shear for 10 min. Sodium hydroxide was added and shear maintained for a further 5 min. The emulsion was allowed to cool to 35°C with continued stirring and the preservative added. The XK sheared gel enhanced the rheological properties and provided emulsion stability. It facilitated a conditioned end feel, a skin conditioning effect and improved textural properties. It also helped create a stable and reproducible viscosity build.

Hair gel: A hair gel was produced using **Formula 3**.

Formula 3
Hair gel incorporating xanthum gum and konjac mannan

Water (*aqua*)	qs 100.00% w/w
Mannan (and) xanthan gum (Glucovis, Chesham)	0.35
Glycerin	0.50
Tetrasodium EDTA	0.05
Potassium hydroxide	0.06
Preservative	qs

The EDTA was dissolved in water and the XK sheared gel was added with stirring. Glycerol was added and the mixture heated to 80°C with stirring and then allowed to cool to 35°C with continued stirring. The preservative was then added. The XK sheared gel acted as a rheological modifier, gave a stable and reproducible viscosity build, and provided a hair conditioning effect. It also enabled hair styling and hold, improved the textural properties, and facilitated a conditioned end feel.

Sun lotion: A sun lotion is given in **Formula 4**.

The EDTA and glycerin were added to water with stirring followed by the XK sheared gel. The mixture was heated to 80°C with continued stirring. The oil phase (including the sunscreens) was heated separately to 80°C and added to the aqueous phase under high shear using a homogenizer for 10 min. The emulsion formed was cooled to 30°C with stirring and the tocopheryl acetate, ethanol, preservative and fragrance were added.

Formula 4
Sun lotion incorporating xanthum gum and konjac mannan

Water (*aqua*)	qs 100.00% w/w
Ethanol	10.00
Octyldodecanol	8.00
Glycerin	5.00
Hydrogenated cocoglycerides	3.00
Drometrizole trisiloxane	3.00
Terephthatylidene dicamphor sulphonic acid	3.00
4-Methylbenzylidene camphor	1.00
C12-15 Alcohols bezoate	1.00
Coco-glucoside	1.00
Theobromo cacao	0.50
Tocopheryl acetate	0.20
Tetrsodium EDTA	0.05
Mannan (and) xanthan gum (Glucovis, Chesham)	0.35
Preservative	qs
Fragrance (*parfum*)	qs

The addition of XK sheared gel provided a stable and reproducible viscosity build. It also enhanced the SFP efficacy and improved the textural properties.

Conclusions

Xanthan gum and konjac mannan interact synergistically through molecular association leading to the formation of strong thermoreversible gels. Fluid gels can be prepared by applying shear to the system during cooling and they can vary in characteristics from highly viscous fluids to spreadable gels. The strength of the gel is influenced by the xanthan gum to konjac mannan mixing ratio, the preparation temperature, the presence of electrolyte and the solution pH. The gels formed are optically clear, have excellent skin feel and offer a "natural" route to enhancing the properties of cosmetic formulations.

Published August 2003 Cosmetics and Toiletries magazine

References

1. G Sworn, in *Handbook of Hydrocolloids*, GO Phillips and PA Williams, eds, Cambridge, UK: Woodhead Publishing Ltd (2000) p 103
2. KS Kang and DJ Petitt, in *Industrial Gums*, RL Whistler and JN BeMiller, eds, San Diego: Academic Press (1993) p 341
3. A Nussinovitch, in *Hydrocolloid Applications*, A Nussinovitch, ed, London: Blackie Academic and Professional (1997) p 154
4. K Nishinari, in *Novel Macromolecules in Food Systems*, G Doxastakis and V Kiosseoglou, eds, Amsterdam: Elsevier Science BV (2000) p 309
5. S Takigami, in *Handbook of Hydrocolloids*, GO Phillips and PA Williams, eds, Cambridge, UK: Woodhead Publishing Ltd (2000) p 413
6. PA Williams and GO Phillips, in *Food Polysaccharides*, AM Stephen, ed, New York: Marcel Dekker (1995) p 463
7. PA Williams, DH Day, MJ Langdon, GO Phillips and K Nishinari, *Food Hydrocolloids* 4 489 (1991)
8. PA Williams, SM Clegg, DH Day, GO Phillips and K Nishinari, in *Food Polymers*, Gels and Colloids, E Dickinson, ed, RSC Special Publication no 82 (1991) p 339
9. P Annable, PA Williams and K Nishinari, *Macromolecules* 27 4204 (1994)
10. C Gomes, MP Goncalves and PA Williams, in *Gums and Stabilizers for the Food Industry*, PA Williams and GO Phillips, eds, Cambridge: RSC (1998) p 239
11. Intl Pat Ap PCT/GB01/02637, Polysaccharide based gel, assigned to Chesham Chemicals Ltd (Dec 20, 2001)

CHAPTER 4

A Surfactant/Biopolymer Stabilizer for Emulsions

Tharwat Tadros
Wokingham, Berkshire UK

Sandra Leonard and Marie-Claire Taelman
Uniqema Personal Care, Wilton Redcar UK

KEY WORDS: *nonionic surfactant, biopolymer system, emulsion, viscosity, rheological measurements, steric stabilization, hydrocolloids*

ABSTRACT: *An emulsifier/biopolymer system using a mixture of nonionic surfactants and 2 biopolymers was developed. The surfactants provide effective steric stabilization against coalescence, whereas the biopolymers provide a high residual viscosity and yield value, thus providing stability against creaming. The mechanism of stabilization is discussed in terms of the synergy between the 2 biopolymers.*

Introduction

Oil-in-Water (O/W) emulsions that are commonly used in many personal care formulations need to be stabilized against creaming or sedimentation, flocculation, Ostwald ripening, coalescence, and phase inversion.[1,2] To achieve these objectives, hydrocolloids (i.e., Konjac mannan (K) and Xanthan (X) gums [KX]) have been proven as excellent stabililizers for O/W emulsions against any coalescence and creaming. K is a β-1,4–linked glucomannan with branches consisting of about 16 sugar units linked to C-3 of the glucose and mannose at approximately every 10 residues along the chain.[3] Native K is acetylated and does not gel in water. On deacetylation in the presence of alkali, however, a thermally reversible gel is produced.[4] Xanthan gum is a charged polysaccharide consisting of a β-1,4–linked glucopyranose backbone with a trisaccharide side chain–linked to every second glucose residue. The side chain consists of 2 mannose units separated by a glucoronic acid residue. Xanthan gum does not gel at any concentration but it undergoes a temperature-induced conformational transition from an ordered helical structure to a disordered structure. Mixtures of KX form reversible gels, which most workers agree is attributable to molecular association.[6-9]

In this paper, we will demonstrate the synergy between the 2 hydrocolloids using rheological measurements. A robust "gel" is produced that prevents any creaming or sedimentation. In addition, the possible adsorption of the gums at the O/W interface enhances stabilization against coalescence. This was demonstrated by preparing emulsions containing the surfactant/biopolymer mixtures.

Experiment

Materials: The oil used for preparation of the emulsions was a mixture of 4 components: isohexadecane[a] 55.5% W/W, caprylic/capric triglyceride[b] 22.3%, *Persea gratissima* (avocado) oil[c] 11.1%, and *Helianthus annus* (sunflower) seed oil[d] 11.1%. The thickener systems consist of a mixture of KX. Two emulsifier/thickener systems were used:

- steareth-100 (and) steareth-2 (and) glyceryl stearate citrate (and) sucrose (and) mannan (and) xanthan gums[e] (which we will refer to as S100/S2 emulsifier/thickener)
- sucrose palmitate (and) glyceryl stearate (and) glyceryl stearate citrate (and) sucrose (and) mannan (and) xanthan gums[f] (which we will refer to as SP emulsifier/thickener)

A preservative blend is used in all solutions, based on phenoxyethanol (and) methylparaben (and) propylparaben (and) 2-bromo-2-nitropropane-1,3 diol[g].

Preparation of Powder Dispersions

Dispersions of KX were prepared by adding the powder slowly to water at 20°C, while stirring at 600 rpm[h] until all the powder was dispersed. The preservative was then added while stirring and

---

[a]Arlamol HD is a product of Uniqema.
[b]Estasan 3575 is a product of Uniqema.
[c]The Persea gratissima (avocado) oil used in this experiment is a product of Mosselman.
[d]Florasun 90 is a product of Floratech.

homogenized at 9500 rpm[i] to produce the gel. Stirring was continued for at least 5 minutes at 600 rpm until a smooth dispersion was obtained.

Preparation of the Emulsions

Both powders[e,f] were dispersed at 20°C and oil was then added while stirring at 600 rpm, followed by homogenization for 2 minutes at 9500 rpm. Alternatively, the powder was dispersed in water at 20°C, followed by heating to 80°C, and the oil that was kept at 20°C was added followed by homogenization at 9500 rpm. Emulsions with an oil volume fraction of 0.2 could be prepared using 0.5% S100/S2 emulsifier/thickener[e] or 0.5% SP emulsifier/thickener[f]. When the emulsion oil volume fraction was increased to 0.6, the emulsifier system concentration was increased to 2%. This concentrated emulsion could be diluted with water to give an oil volume fraction of 0.2. Both emulsions were of the same quality as assessed by droplet size analysis.

Rheological Measurements

A spectrometer[j] was used for all rheological measurements. Two types of measurements were carried out—constant stress (creep) and oscillatory methods. A plate-plate geometry with a 1 mm gap was used, and the temperature was controlled using a Peltier plate and a solvent trap (to avoid evaporation). In the creep measurements, a constant stress was applied on the system and the deformation (strain) was followed as function of time for 2 minutes. The slope of the linear portion of the creep curve (strain over time) gives the shear rate.

The viscosity at any applied stress is simply the ratio of the stress to the shear rate. The viscosity of any viscoelastic system increases with decrease of applied stress and, ultimately, it reaches a limiting (high value) below a critical stress (referred to as the yield stress).

---

[e]Arlatone V-100 is a product of Uniqema.
[f]Arlatone V-175 is a product of Uniqema.
[g]Nipaguard BPX is a product of Clariant.
[h]RW 20 IKA-werk is a product of Janke and Kunkel.
[i]Ultra Turrex mixer is a product of IKA.
[j]Universal Dynamic Spectrometer, Physica UDS, Anton Paar Physica.

This limiting viscosity is the residual or zero shear viscosity. The compliance J is simply the strain divided by the applied stress (Pa^{-1}). After 2 minutes, the stress was removed and the strain (which reversed sign) was followed for another 2 minutes to obtain the elastic recovery of the system. In the oscillatory technique, 2 types of measurements were carried out:

- (i) Amplitude sweep at constant frequency of 1 Hz. This allows one to obtain the linear viscoelastic region where the moduli are independent of the applied strain.
- (ii) Frequency sweep, whereby the strain is kept constant at a value in the linear viscoelastic region, whereas the frequency is changed from 10 to 0.01 Hz. From the amplitudes of the stress and strain and the phase angle shift one cloud, obtain the following viscoelastic parameters: the complex modulus G^*, the storage modulus G' (the elastic component of the complex modulus), and the loss modulus G'' (the viscous component of the complex modulus).

Results

Comparison of Xanthan gum and KX Solutions: **Figure 1a** shows a plot of low shear (residual) viscosity versus xanthan gum concentration (0.5%-1%), whereas **Figure 1b** shows the results for KX solutions (0.05%-0.1%). It can be clearly shown that the residual viscosity of KX solutions is one order of a magnitude higher than that of xanthan gum, even though the concentration of KX is one order of a magnitude lower. The results for G and G also showed the same trend.

Indeed G for 0.1% KX is close to that of 0.9% xanthan gum (10 Pa). In addition, the KX solutions have a relatively higher elastic to viscous components (G/G) when compared with the solutions of xanthan gum alone. This clearly demonstrates the synergy between KX gums.

Rheological Investigations of Stabilizing Systems: Figure 2 shows typical creep curves for a 1.0% SP emulsifier/thickener system[f] using the cold procedures (**Figure 2a**) and cold/hot (**Figure 2b**) procedures.

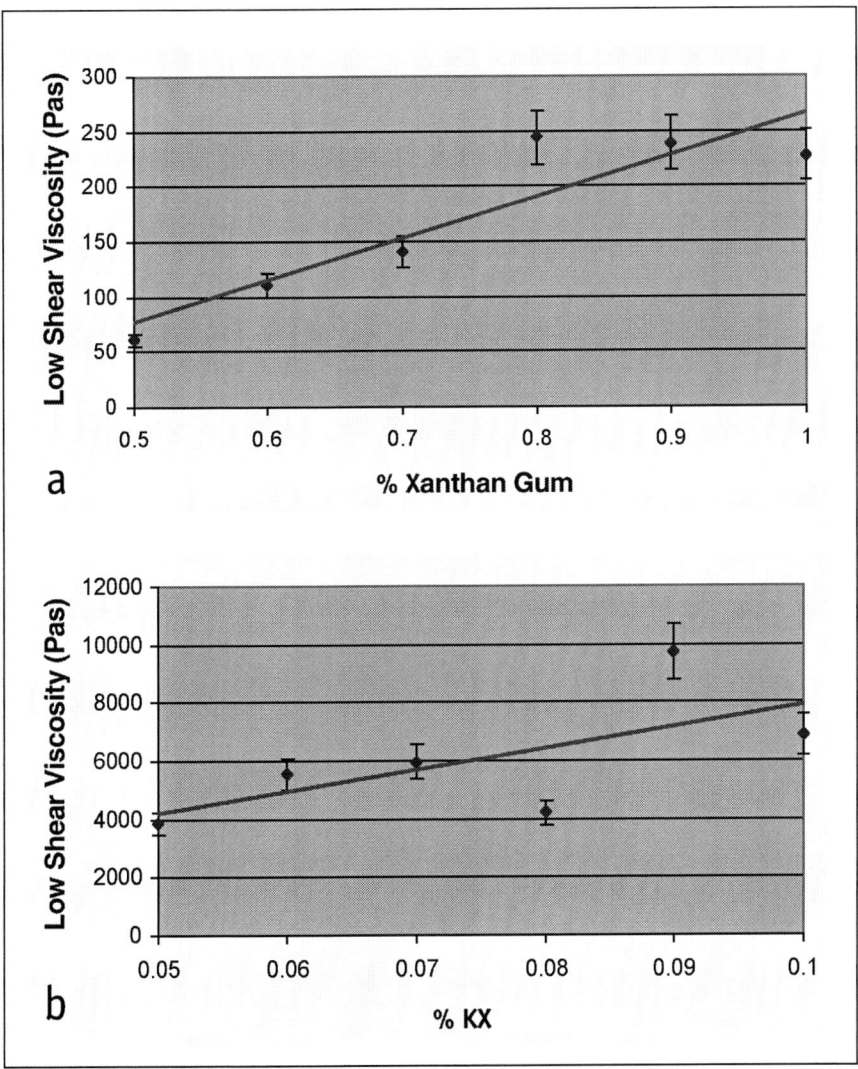

Figure 1. Low shear rate viscosity for xanthan gum (above) and KX (below) solutions

Similar results were obtained for the S100/S2 emulsifier/thickener system[e] and KX solutions. In all cases, the strain increases very slowly with time when the stress is below a certain critical value. When the stress is removed, appreciable recovery of the strain is obtained. Above this critical stress the strain shows a rapid increase with time, and when the stress is removed only partial recovery of the strain is observed. The results show that the stabilizer

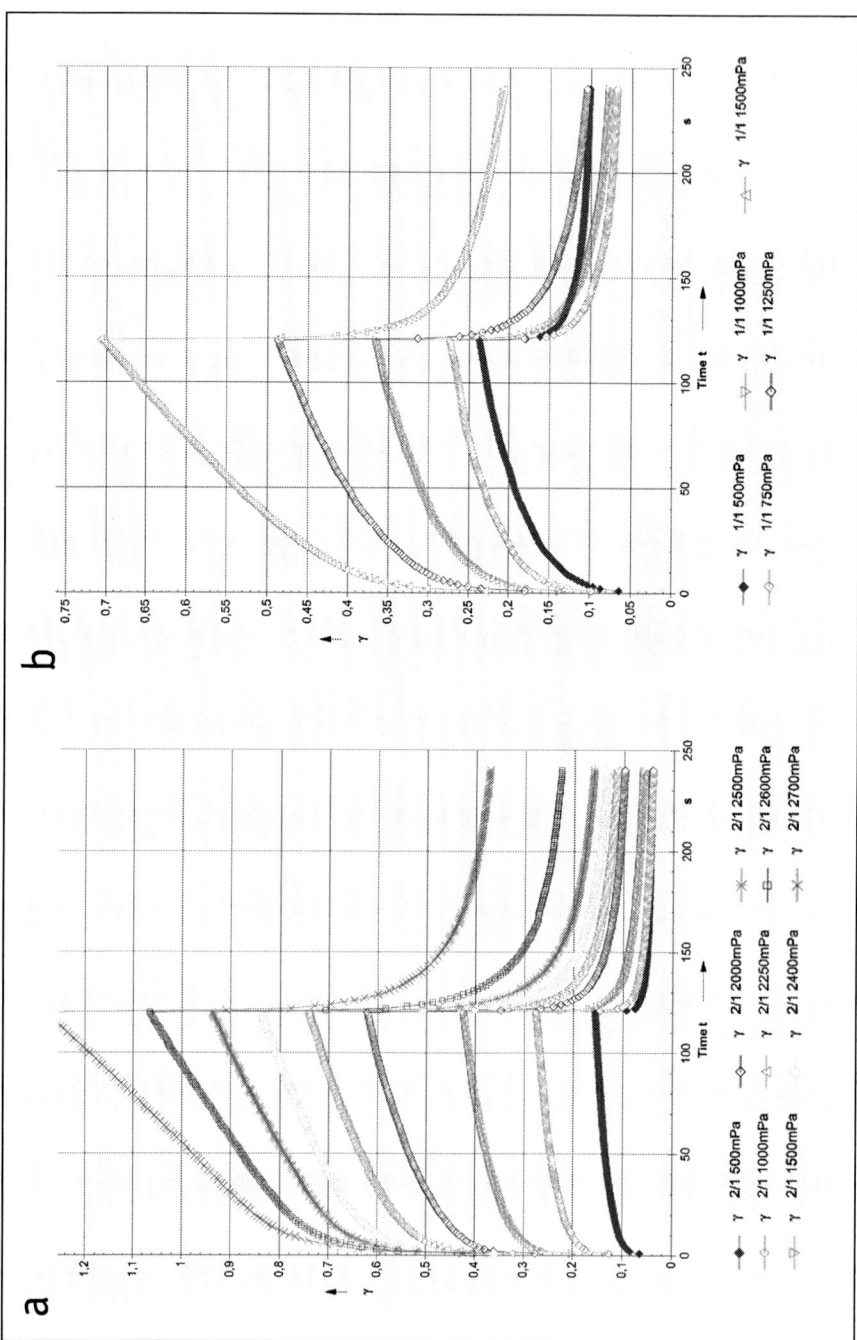

Figure 2. Typical creep curves for 1% SP emulsifier/thickener system[f] (a) prepared by cold process, (b) prepared by cold/hot process

system prepared using the cold procedure gives higher stress when compared with that obtained using the cold/hot procedure. The residual (zero shear viscosity) is also higher for the cold process. The opposite, however, was obtained with the S100/S2 emulsifier/thickener system,[e] in which case the values of the residual viscosity were higher for the cold/hot procedure. Frequency sweep results (**Figure 3**) for the 1% SP emulsifier/thickener system[f] also shows much higher G' than G'' in the frequency range 10-0.01 Hz. This is typical of a system that is more elastic than viscous.

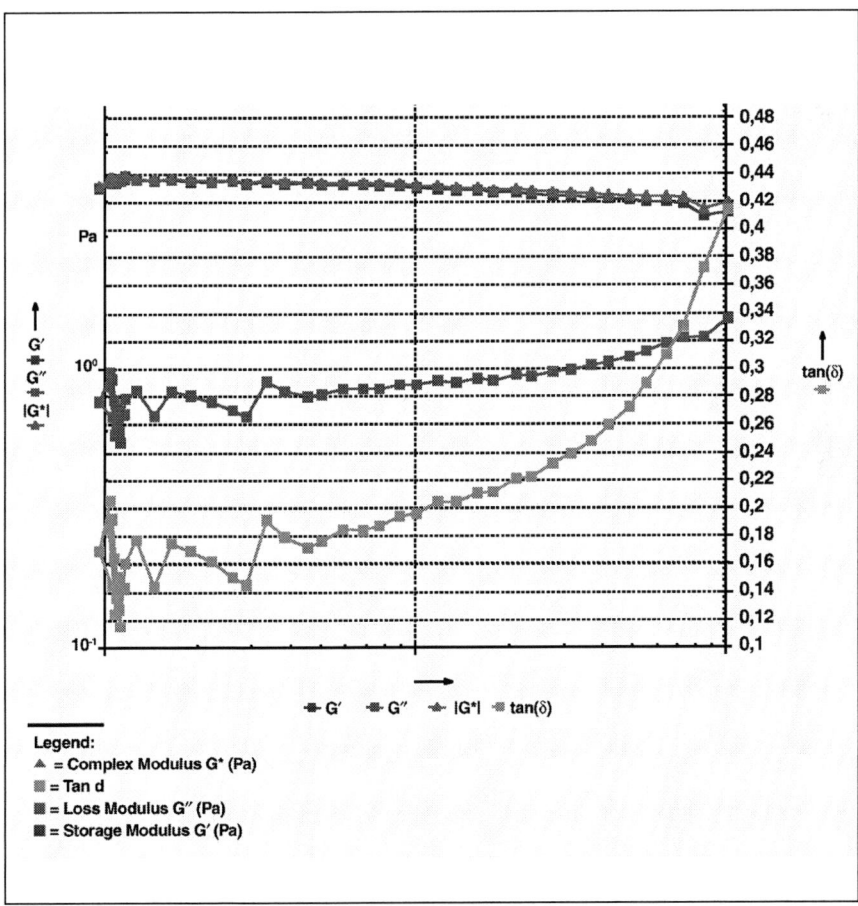

Figure 3. Frequency sweep results for 1% SP emulsifier system[f] dispersion measured at 50°C

Rheological Investigations of Emulsions: The results for an O/W emulsion with a volume fraction of 0.2 as a function of an S100/S2 emulsifier/thickener[e] concentration (0.5%-1.0%) are summarized in **Tables 1 and 2**. These results show, in general, an increase in the low shear viscosity and critical stress with increases in stabilizer concentration. In some cases, however, such a trend is not always followed, and the results sometimes show an increase followed by a decrease as the stabilizer concentration is increased.

Table 1
Creep measurements for emulsions (Ø = 0.2) stabilised with S100/S2 emulsifier/thickener systeme as a function of stabiliser concentration and storage time

% S100/S2 Emulsifier/Thickener System[e]	Low shear viscosity (Pas) Shear Rate~ $10^{-3}s^{-1}$			Critical Stress (Pa)		
	1 day	1 month	2 months	1 day	1 month	2 months
0.5	907	806	830	1.1	0.9	1.1
0.6	1347	863	853	1.3	0.9	0.9
0.7	1675	1460	613	1.7	2.0	1.1
0.8	1500	1413	1314	2.0	2.2	1.6
0.9	1855	1265	1243	2.5	1.9	1.75
1.0	2494	1415	1947	2.5	2.25	2.25

The storage time results did not always show a regular trend, although in some cases, particularly with the S100/S2 emulsifier/thickener system[e] at stabilizer concentration above 0.8% there was an indication of an increase of rheological parameters with increase in storage time, which may indicate some flocculation of the samples on storage. Oscillatory measurements showed a critical strain value in the region of 1%-2%, and it did not show much change with stabilizer concentration and/or storage time. The values of the critical strain are reasonably high and they indicate a coherent viscoelastic structure of the emulsion that is stabilized with both emulsifier/thickener systems[e,f]. The results of the oscillatory measurements showed a regular trend of increase of

G' and G" with increase in stabilizer concentration. On storage, these moduli did not show significant change for up to 2 months. The only exceptions are the results for the SP emulsifier/thickener system[f] ≥ 0.8%, which showed an increase on storage, indicating some flocculation of the emulsion.

Table 2
Creep measurements for emulsions (∅ = 0.2) stabilised with SP emulsifier/thickener systemf as a function of stabiliser concentration and storage time

% S100/S2 Emulsifier/Thickener System[e]	Low shear viscosity (Pas) Shear Rate~ $10^{-3} s^{-1}$			Critical Stress (Pa)		
	1 day	1 month	2 months	1 day	1 month	2 months
0.5	1899	806	830	1.1	0.9	1.1
0.6	1272	863	853	1.3	0.9	0.9
0.7	1333	1460	613	1.7	2.0	1.1
0.8	1584	1413	1314	2.0	2.2	1.6
0.9	1584	1265	1243	2.5	1.9	1.75
1.0	1168	1415	1947	2.5	2.25	2.25

Influence of temperature on the rheology: The influence of temperature on the rheology of KX, both emulsifier/thickener systems,[e,f] and the emulsions using the stabilizers was measured. For 0.1% KX, G' showed a slow increase with an increase in temperature to 35°C, above which G' decreased with a further increase in temperature up to 50°C. G", however, seemed to decrease when the temperature of the thickener was increased above 30°C. With a 1% S100/S2 emulsifier/thickener system,[e] G' and G" remained virtually constant up to 35°C, after which it showed a gradual reduction with a further increase of temperature. The 1% SP emulsifier/thickener system[f] showed a rapid reduction in G' and G" when the temperature was increased from 25°C to 30°C, after which no change in G' was obtained in the temperature range 30°C-50°C. In contrast, G" showed a gradual decrease with an increase of temperature in this range.

In contrast to the results with KX and the stabilizers, the O/W emulsion (with a volume fraction of 0.2) prepared using either emulsifier/thickener system[e,f] showed a remarkable independence of G' in temperature within the range 25°C-50°C for both emulsions. This is illustrated in **Figure 4**, which shows the variation of G' and G" with temperature for both emulsion systems. G" shows a small reduction when the temperature is increased above 30°C. These results clearly illustrate the high physical stability of the emulsions based on the surfactant/biopolymer systems.

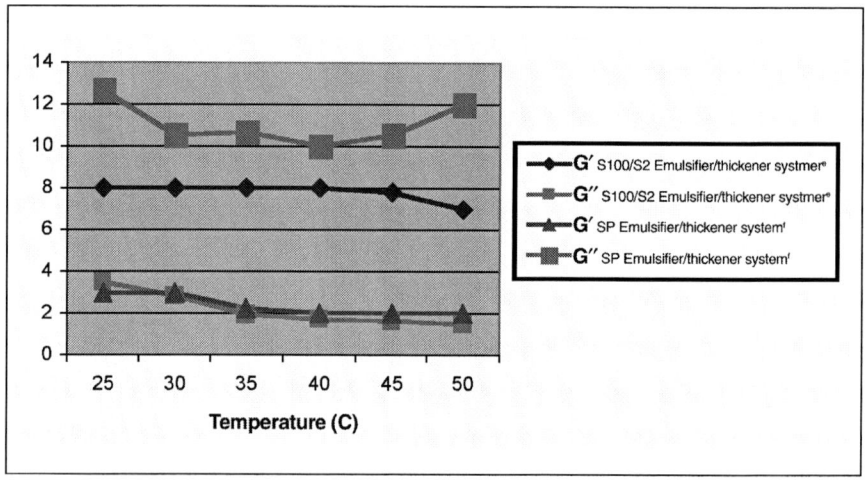

Figure 4. Variation of G' and G" for emulsions (volume fraction 0.2) prepared using 1% emulsifier/thickener systemse,f

Discussion

The emulsifier/stabilizer system used in the current study shows a number of interesting features. The emulsifiers[e,f] are both nonionic and they are commonly used in many personal care formulations. Both emulsifiers are expected to significantly lower the interfacial tension between the oil and water, thus aiding the emulsification process. For an O/W emulsion with an oil volume fraction Ø of 0.2 the optimum concentration of the emulsifier/stabilizer system is 0.8%. This amount is sufficient to completely cover the interface with emulsifier molecules, thus reducing the interfacial tension to a minimum, and this helps the emulsification process. This low stabiliser concentration (against creaming) must be attributable to the synergy obtained when using the 2 gums. Using either of the 2 gums at such low concentration would certainly be insufficient for reduction of creaming and/or separation. There is ample evidence in the literature concerning the interaction between the 2 polysaccharide molecules. A summary of the arguments presented is given in the sidebar.

From the literature discussed, it is clear that KX should result in synergy in the rheological behaviour, when compared with the 2 gums alone. This is clearly demonstrated by the results shown in Figure 1. For example, the low shear viscosity of 0.1% KX is 6149 Pas, whereas that of 1% xanthan gum, which is an order of magnitude higher in concentration is 228 Pas (i.e., more than one order of magnitude lower). This very high viscosity at low shear rates—sometimes referred to as residual or zero shear viscosity—ç(o) explains the absence of creaming of emulsions stabilised with the 2 emulsifier/thickener systems[e,f], when the concentration of KX in the continuous phase is only 0.1%.

It should be mentioned that addition of surfactants to KX (i.e., when using emulsifier/thickener systems[e,f]) resulted in the reduction of the viscosity of KX. This seems to be owing to the interaction of the surfactants with the gums, resulting in reduction of their interaction.

The above-stated reduction in creaming rate with an increase in η(o) has been discussed recently in detail.[15] One should consider the stress exerted by a droplet σ_p in the continuous phase, which is simply the ratio of the gravity force exerted on the droplet to the area of the droplet (i.e., where R is the droplet radius, $\Delta \rho$ is the density difference between oil and continuous phase and g is the acceleration owing to gravity).

For a droplet with R = 10, μm and density difference of 0.2 g cm^{-3}, σ_p is equal to 6.5 X 10^{-3} Pa. This means that the viscosity of the emulsion needs to be measured at low stresses or low shear rates (i.e., the residual or zero shear viscosity η(o)) to predict the creaming and separation of the emulsion. The results using KX have shown that η (o) at low shear rates (of the order of 6 X 10^{-4} s^{-1}) is > 6000 Pas. Emulsifier/thickener systems[e,f] prepared also gave values of η (o) > 1000 Pas. These high residual viscosities are sufficient to eliminate any creaming of the emulsions, as found experimentally over long periods (i.e., several months of storage).

The interaction between K and Xanthan gums

As mentioned in the introduction, Konjac mannan gum (K) is essentially a noncharged polysaccharide, whereas xanthan gum (X) is a charged polysaccharide. The mixture forms thermally reversible gels, which most workers agree to be because of molecular association.[6,7] However, the nature of the interaction has been a matter of great debate.[9,10] As mentioned in the introduction, Dea et al.[8] proposed that association occurs between the ordered xanthan helix and unsubstituted regions of the galactomannan backbone. McCleary,[11] however, modified this model and suggested that interaction could occur between the ordered xanthan chains and sequences along the mannan backbone where the galactose residues are positioned only on one side. X-ray diffraction studies[12] confirmed the molecular binding. However, since gels are only formed at temperatures above that expected for the xanthan conformational changes, one may conclude that the xanthan interaction must occur in the disordered form. Williams et al.[13,14] proposed that KX interaction could occur with xanthan both in the ordered and disordered form depending on the ionic strength of the solution.

Using spin label technique (ESR) Annable et al.[9] could follow the molecular motion of the polymer chains in solution, which enabled them to follow the conformational change and K association as a function of temperature, and they correlated these processes with gelation. From these results, Annable et al.[9] could propose a model for the interaction between K and xanthan gums. On cooling, the xanthan molecules are thermodynamically driven to adopt a predominantly ordered structure. The side chains that are directed away from the xanthan cellulosic main chain of the disordered xanthan molecules (single coils or expanded dimers) begin to associate with the backbone, thus reducing polymer-solvent contacts, and they give rise to chain stiffening. In the absence of K, this leads to either double helix formation or xanthan self association. In the presence of K, ordered or disordered sequences within the xanthan molecules prefer to interact with K chains rather than other xanthan chains. One of the main reasons for this interaction is the uncharged chain of K when compared with xanthan chains, which are highly charged.

It should be mentioned that the emulsifier/thickener systems prepared[e,f] give a different consistency when compared with emulsions prepared using other thickeners. The critical stress obtained when using 0.1% KX was significantly higher than that obtained at the same concentration when using, for example, carbomer[k] (5.9 Pa vs. 0.5 Pa, respectively).

This high critical stress indicates that the "gels" that are produced when using KX are more "coherent" than those used with carbomer[k]. This may have some implication on the long-term physical stability, as well as the skin feel of the emulsions prepared using the current system.

Another important stabilising mechanism when using the emulsifier/thickener systems[e,f] is the absence of coalescence, as detected using optical microscopy. The lack of coalescence in these emulsions is owing to 2 main effects:

- (i) Steric stabilisation produced when using mixtures of nonionic surfactants[16]
- (ii) Possible adsorption of the gums at the O/W interface, thus producing a viscoelastic film at the interface, which prevents any thinning and disruption of the aqueous film between emulsion droplets

Conclusions

Using a combination of nonionic surfactants and 2 polysaccharides, namely Konjac mannan and Xanthan gums (referred as KX), one can produce very stable emulsions against any creaming or coalescence. The stabilising mechanism of KX is owing to the interaction between Konjac mannan and Xanthan gums, thus resulting in a synergistic effect. The residual or zero shear viscosity of KX is much higher than that of Xanthan gum alone, and this explains the absence of creaming. Emulsions prepared using emulsifier/thickener systems[e,f] also show a residual or zero shear viscosity >1000 Pas, which is sufficient to eliminate any creaming and coalescence of the emulsion. Any flocculation of the emulsion on storage is quite weak, and the samples can be simply redispersed by gentle shaking. The mixture of surfactants and KX eliminate

---

[k]Carbopol is a product of Noveon, Inc.

coalescence by effective steric repulsion produced by the nonionic surfactants, as well as the possible co-adsorption of the gums at the interface producing a viscoelastic film, thus preventing any thinning and disruption of the liquid film between the droplets.

Published August 2005 Cosmetics and Toiletries magazine

References

1. TF Tadros and B Vincent, Encyclopedia of Emulsion Technology, vol 1, P Becher, ed, Marcel Dekker (1983)
2. BP Binks, Modern Aspects of Emulsion Science, Cambridge, Royal Society of Chemistry Publication (1998)
3. K Nishinari et al, Food hydrocolloids 6 199 (1992)
4. K Maekaji, Agric Biol Chem, 38 315 (1974)
5. G Holzwarth, Carbohydrate Res, 66 173 (1978)
6. KP Shatwell et al, Carbohydr Polym, 14 (29) 131 (1991)
7. FM Goycoolea et al, in Gums and Stabilisers for the Food Industry, GO Phillips, PA Williams and DJ Wedlock eds, Oxford University Press, pp 333-344 (1994)
8. ICM Dea et al, Carbohyd Res, 57 249 (1977)
9. P Annable et al, Macromolecules, 27 4204 (1994)
10. PA Williams et al, Cosmetics and Toiletries, 118 51 (2003)
11. BV McCleary, Carbohydr Res, 71 205 (1979)
12. GJ Brownsey et al, Carbohydr Res, 176 329 (1988)
13. PA Williams et al, Food hydrocolloids 4 4891 (1991)
14. PA Williams et al, in Food Polymers, Gels and Colloids, E Dickinson ed, RSC Publication no 82, Royal Society of Chemistry, Herts, U.K. p 339 (1991)
15. TF Tadros, Advances Colloid and Interface Sci, 108-109 227 (2004)
16. DH Napper, Polymeric Stabilisation of Colloidal Dispersions, London: Academic Press (1983)

CHAPTER 5

Castor Polyesters for Personal Care

Anthony J. O'Lenick Jr.
Siltech LLC, Dacula, Georgia USA

Carter LaVay
Zenitech LLC, Old Greenwich, Connecticut USA

KEY WORDS: *Castor oil, polymers, polyesters*

ABSTRACT: *Naturally occurring castor oil and succinic acid can be reacted to make a polyester (such as castor succinate) and then functionalized to provide benefits in cosmetic formulations.*

This chapter describes a series of polymers based on the naturally occurring castor oil and succinic acid, reacted to make a polyester (such as castor succinate) and then functionalized to provide benefits in cosmetic formulations. Several formulations are provided to demonstrate the use of the various castor succinate polyester compounds.

Castor Oil

Castor oil is a unique triglyceride derived from Ricinus communis L.[1] The castor plant grows wild in many subtropical and tropical areas. Today Brazil, China and India provide more than 90% of the oil.

Castor oil contains a large content of hydroxy-containing compounds that are unsaturated (**Table 1**). It is a high purity oil in terms of carbon chain distribution as provided by nature. This makes castor oil both compositionally pure and natural.

This versatile material is a clear, viscous, light-colored, freely flowing fluid that is nondrying and quite stable. The purity of composition of castor oil occurs with remarkable uniformity.

Regardless of country of origin or season in which it is grown, the composition and chemical properties (**Table 1**) remain within a very narrow range. Castor oil has broad compatibility with oils, waxes, natural resins and gums.

Table 1
Carbon distribution

Component	Typical % Weight
C16:0	1
C18:0	1
C18:1-OH	89
C18:1	3
C18:2	6

ICAS Number: 8001-79-4
EINECS Number: 232-293-8
Titer Point: 2°C

Castor oil also has an outstanding oxidative stability, in spite of its unsaturation. We can demonstrate this by looking at color formation at 200°C. Refined oils were held at this temperature and color change was monitored.[3] The results are shown in **Figure 1**.

Chemical Structure

The unique chemical structure of castor oil, shown in **Figure 2**, is key to its functionality.

The OH is a hydroxyl group, the CH=CH is an alkene, and the C(O)-O is an ester.

The castor polyesters of interest use the three-hydroxyl groups to make the polymer and to incorporate functional groups onto the polymer. Castor oil is a polar oil by virtue of the presence of the hydroxyl group. It also can be considered a branched oil because of the location of the hydroxyl group (at the 12 position). This is made more rigid by the presence of the double bond in the molecule. The polarity of the castor oil is seen in the fact that it is insoluble in many other more traditional oils such as soybean oil.

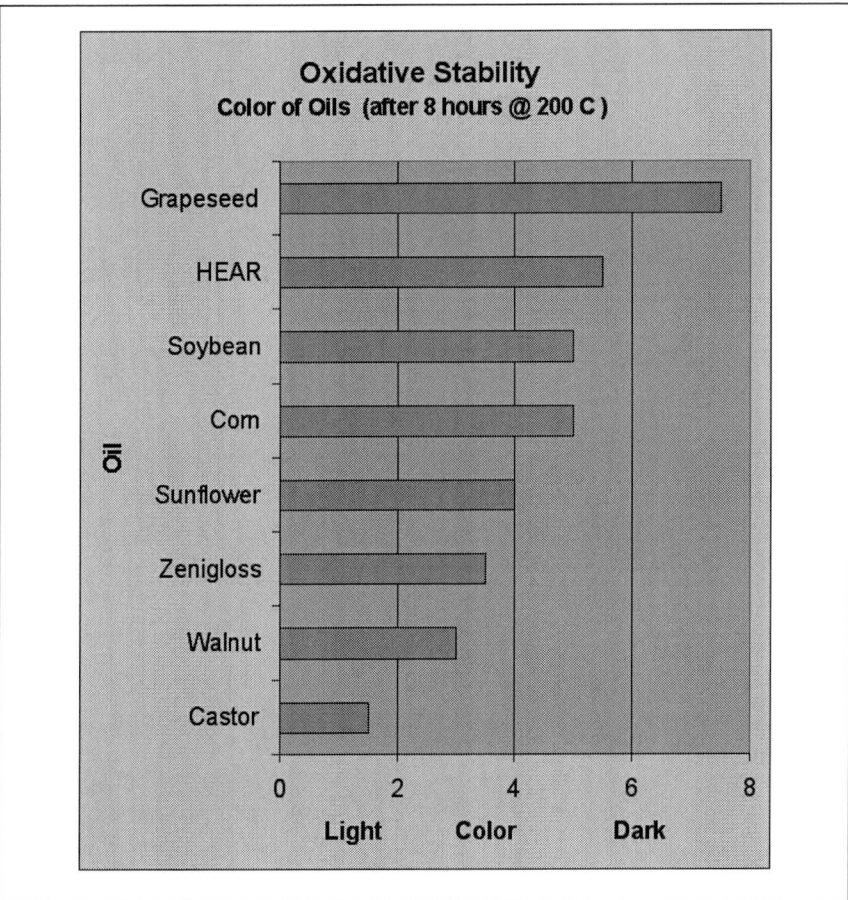

Figure 1. Oxidative stability

$$CH_3\text{-}(CH_2)_5\text{-}\underset{\underset{OH}{|}}{C}HCH_2CH=CH(CH_2)_7\text{-}C(O)\text{-}O\text{-}CH_2$$

$$H\text{-}C\text{-}O\text{-}C(O)\text{-}(CH_2)_7CH=CHCH_2CH\text{-}(CH_2)_5\text{-}CH_3$$

$$CH_3\text{-}(CH_2)_5\text{-}\underset{\underset{OH}{|}}{C}HCH_2CH=CH(CH_2)_7\text{-}C(O)\text{-}O\text{-}CH_2 \qquad OH$$

Figure 2. Chemical Structure of Castor Oil

Polymers

Many polymeric materials are made by the free radical polymerization of vinyl-containing monomers to form high molecular weight polymers. These polymers have desirable properties, but also contain residual unreacted monomer. This residual monomer is undesirable and is avoided by many formulators. This has forced chemists to look at new raw materials, processes and reaction parameters in an attempt to make a suitable cosmetically acceptable product, by reducing free monomer levels. This approach, while viable, is only one approach.

Another approach is to make polymers that do not make use of vinyl-containing monomers as raw materials to conduct the polymerization. Products from this route contain no free vinyl monomers! One series of polymers is based upon the naturally occurring castor oil and succinic acid, reacted to make a polyester. The polymers can be made to varying molecular weights, allowing for the custom selection of viscosity, playtime on the skin and penetration through the skin. Finally, by placing functional groups on the polymer, a variety of properties like gloss, conditioning and hardness can be affected.

Polyesters

Castor polyesters contain a number of castor oil groups linked together through an ester bond. In order to make polymers, there must be at least two raw materials that contain multiple reactive groups.[4] In this case the poly hydroxyl group is provided by castor oil and the poly acid is succinic acid.

Castor succinate polyester is the backbone for a series of functional polymers. The reaction of castor (having three-hydroxyl groups) with succinic acid (having two-hydroxyl groups) is the first step in the creation of the polyester. **Figure 3** shows the reaction. The first step is reaction of one carboxyl group with one hydroxyl group.

The product has no free vinyl monomer. There is simply none used in the reaction. The monomers are castor oil and succinic acid. This carboxylated castor oil still has a free carboxylic group, which reacts in turn with another hydroxyl group on another castor oil to make a diester as shown in **Figure 4**.

If only one succinic acid is added per castor, given the correct catalyst and process conditions, the product shown in **Figure 4** results. The diester product has no free acid groups and four free hydroxyl groups. The degree of polymerization (otherwise known as "dp") is 2. The molecular weight of the material has more than doubled, and the polarity has decreased compared to castor oil.

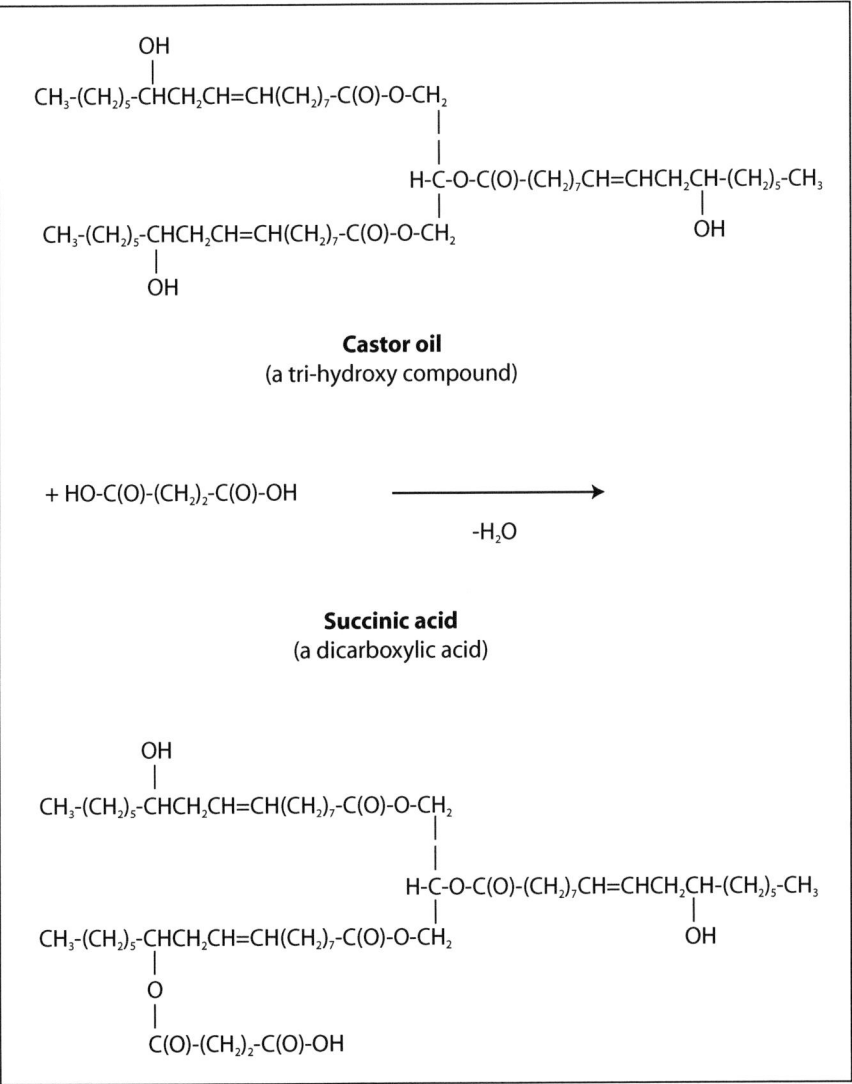

Figure 3. Caster succinate half-ester

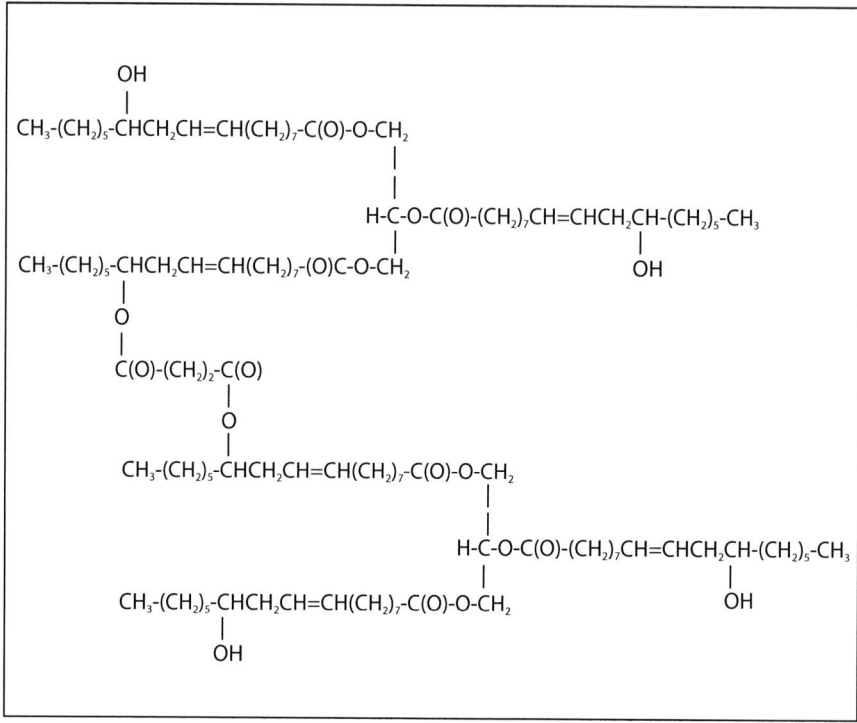

Figure 4. Castor Succinate diester

The lowest molecular weight polyester has a dp of 3, has three castor oils linked together and has five remaining hydroxyl groups, having started with nine.

As one continues to increase the amount of succinic relative to castor, the polymer grows (**Figure 5**), the dp increases and more of the center castor groups are added. In addition, for each new castor added the amount of hydroxyl functionality present decreases (**Table 2**). This results in a less polar polyester.

It is quite interesting that the polymer will become so different in terms of polarity as to become insoluble in castor oil, the majority raw material!

As the dp of the polymer increases, several desirable properties also occur:
- Increased molecular weight;
- Increased viscosity;
- Increased play time on the skin;

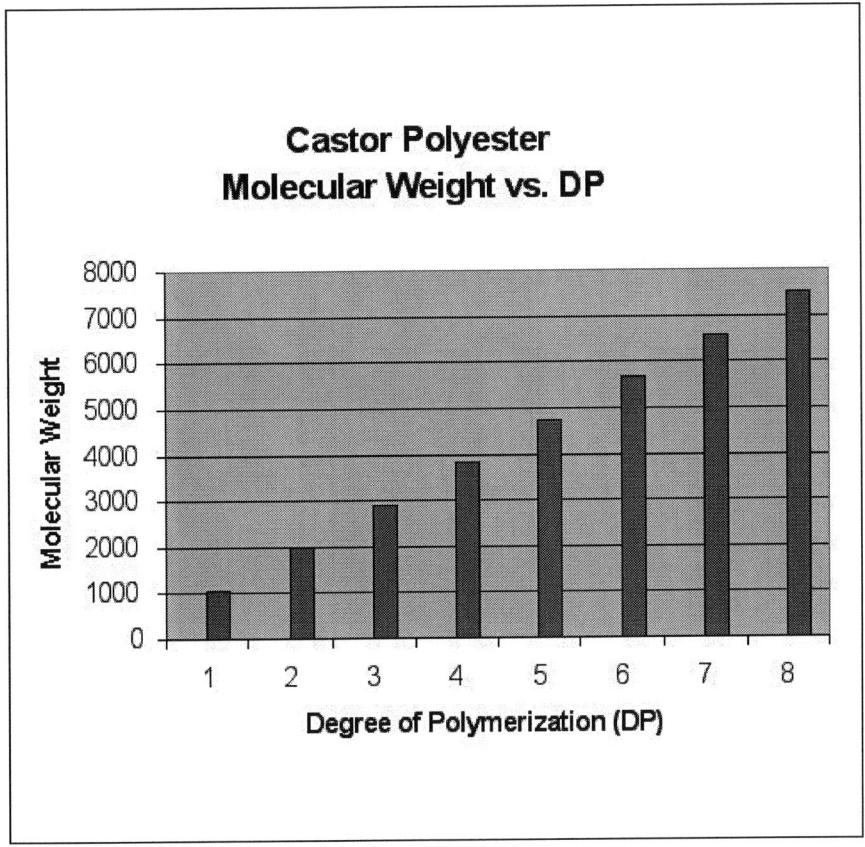

Figure 5. Castor polyester molecular weight vs. dp

Table 2.
Polarity of castor oil polyester versus dp

DP	Total Hydroxyl	Reacted Hydroxyl	Free Hydroxyl	% Free Hydroxyl
Castor oil	3	0	3	100
2	6	2	4	66.6
5	15	8	7	46.6
10	30	18	12	40.0

- Decreased skin penetration;
- Solubility changes (due to polarity change).

This allows the formulator to choose a product that provides the desired attributes for a given formulation.

Polymer Functionalization

The introduction of functionalized capping groups into the polyester is accomplished by "reacting in" the proper mono-hydroxy compound. One such capping group is ricinoleylamidopropyl trimethyl ammonium chloride, shown in **Figure 6**.

If the proper ratio and reaction conditions are employed, the simple polyester shown in **Figure 7** results.

The resulting terminal cationic polymer has two cationic sites and provides substantive conditioning and gloss to hair (**Table 3**). The material is also useful in stabilizing water-in-oil emulsions.

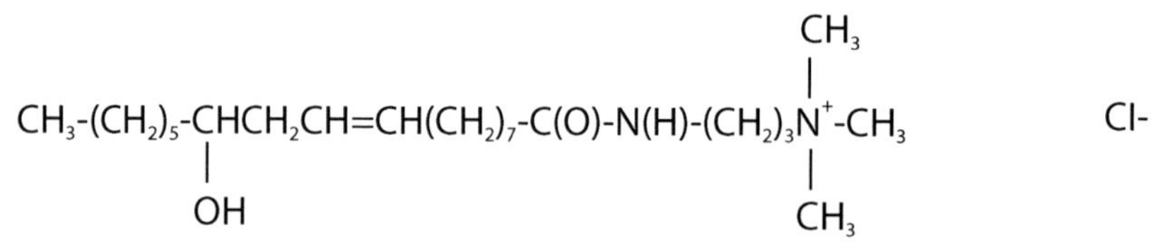

$$CH_3\text{-}(CH_2)_5\text{-}CHCH_2CH=CH(CH_2)_7\text{-}C(O)\text{-}N(H)\text{-}(CH_2)_3\overset{+}{N}(CH_3)_3 \quad Cl^-$$
$$|$$
$$OH$$

Figure 6. Ricinoleylamidopropyl trimethyl ammonium chloride

Functionalization of the Backbone

If the free hydroxyl groups on the polyester are esterified with fatty acid, all hydroxyl groups react. This reaction results in a non-polar compound that provides outstanding gloss when applied to hair and skin. The exact properties of the compound, such as gloss, playtime and viscosity, are determined by the dp of the particular polyester. A higher dp will yield a compound with higher molecular weight, higher viscosity, higher playtime and lower penetration. If the acid used to cap is saturated and has 18

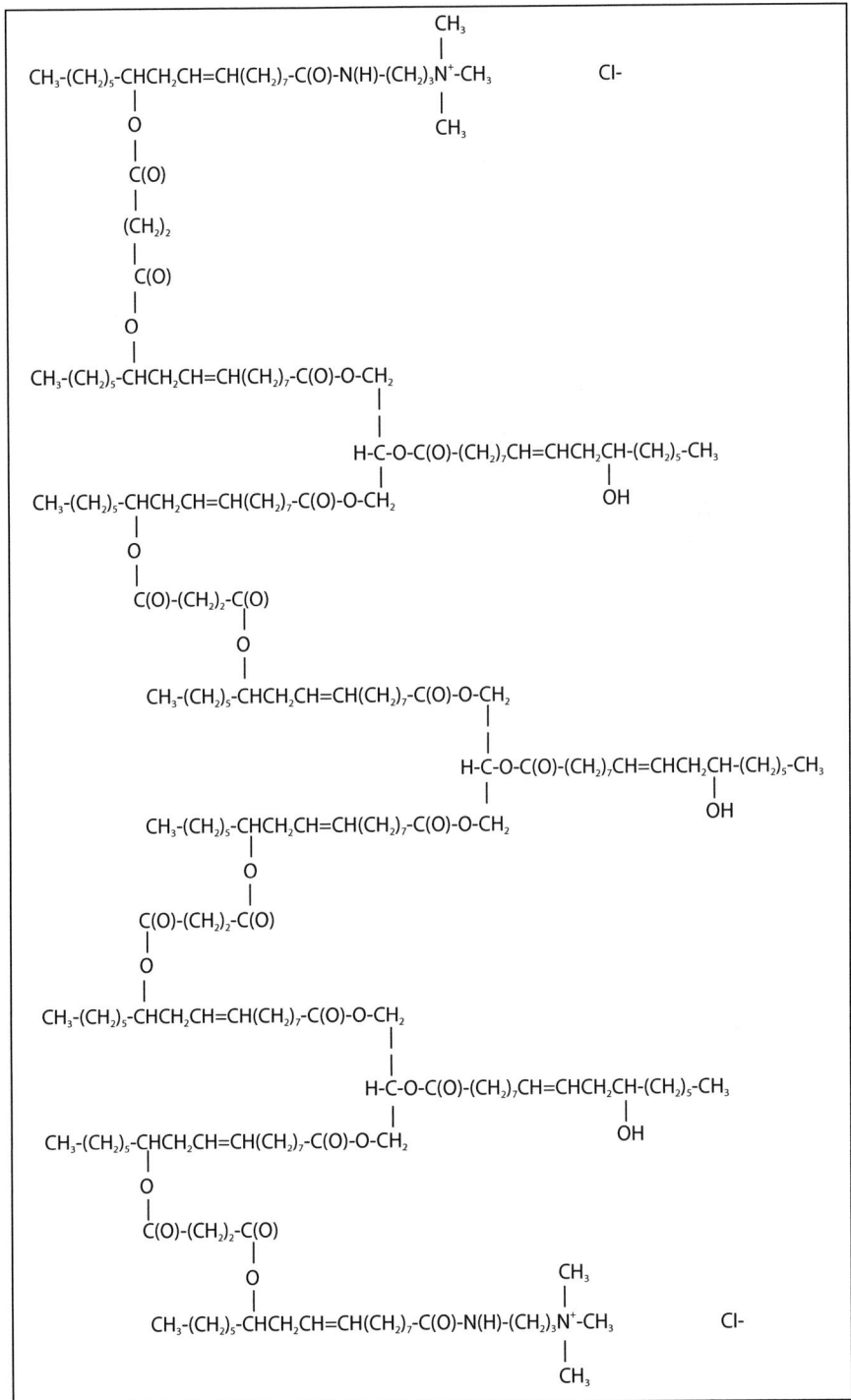

Figure 7. Cationic Polyester

or more carbon atoms, a solid polyester will result. The specific fatty acid chosen will determine the melting point and hardness of the polyester.

Table 3.
Features and benefits of castor polyesters

100% active	High total performance product. Fully functional.
Pigment wetter	Improves color brightness.
Versatile	Hair, skin, sun and color applications.
Natural organic ingredients	No petroleum base or phenyl groups. Biodegradable.
High molecular weight	Gives high substantivity and gloss. Little penetration of skin.
High oxidative solubility	Retards dicoloration in finished formula.
Known ingredient*	Easy to formulate product.

* castor oil and succinic acid

Formulations

Combining the compounds with the properly chosen emulsifier will result in a clear product. When added to water, this clear anhydrous product will bloom into a stable oil-in-water emulsion. The technology can be applied to numerous product types.

Formulations for a hair spray (**Formula 1**), a hair conditioners (**Formula 2**), a lip gloss stick (**Formula 3**) and a sunscreen emulsion (**Formula 4**) demonstrate the use of the various castor succinate polyester compounds in personal care applications.

Published June 2002 Cosmetics and Toiletries magazine

References

1. Oils and Fats Manual, A Karleskind, ed, Paris, France Intercept Ltd (1996) p 212
2. AJ O'Lenick, D Steinberg and K Klein, Primary Ingredients, Carol Stream, Illinois: Allured Publishing (1998); available for download on www.zenitech.com
3. Zenitech Technical Bulletin, No 2001-5 (2001) p 4
4. AJ O'Lenick, Surfactants Chemistry and Properties, Carol Stream, Illinois: Allured Publishing (1999)

Formula 1
Sheen Spray with Gloss

A. Diethylhexyl sebacate	38.0% wt
Cyclomethicone	40.0
Octyl methoxycinnamate	1.0
Melaleuca alternifolia (Tea Tree) leaf oil	0.2
B. Castor isostearate succinate	20.0
Tocopheryl acetate	0.1
Retinyl palmitate	0.1
Ascorbyl palmitate	0.1
Fragrance (*parfum*)	0.5
	100.0

Procedure: Combine A and B at RT. Add B to A. Package.

Formula 2
Hair Conditioner

A. Water (*aqua*)	79.9% wt
Glycereth-26	2.0
Dicetylmonium	2.0
B. Peg-40 stearate	0.5
Cyclomethicone	5.0
Cetearyl alcohol	2.0
Cetearyl alcohol, ceteareth-20	2.0
Castor isostearate succinate	3.0
Behentrimonium methosulfate, cetearyl alcohol	3.0
C. Fragrance (*parfum*)	0.4
DMDM hydantoin	0.2
D. Sodium hydroxide	qs

Procedure: Heat A to 75oC. Heat B to 75oC. Add B to A while maintaining temperature 70 – 75oC. Cool to 40C and add C. Adjust pH to 5.0.

Formula 3:
Lip Gloss Stick

A. Silica dimethyl silylate/castor oil	2.0% wt
B. Castor Oil	28.7
C. Carnauba	2.0
Candelilla	7.5
Ceresin	3.5
Triisostearin	20.0
Octyldodecanol	6.0
Castor Isostearate succinate beeswaxate	25.0
Polyglyceryl-3 diisostearate	5.0
Methylparaben	0.2
Propylparaben	0.1
	100.0

Procedure: Prewet A in B. Mill until homogenous using a three-roll mill. Combine C with AB. Heat to 85 – 90oC with stirring until clear. Stir and allow to cool to 70 – 72oC and fill.

Formula 4:
Sunscreen Emulsion

A. Water (*aqua*)	53.65 % wt
Disodium EDTA	0.10
Propylene glycol	2.50
Keltrol T, 2%	15.00
B. Octyl methoxycinnamate	7.50
Oxybenzone	3.00
Cetearyl alcohol	2.00
Octyl salicylate	5.00
Octyldodecanol	5.00
Cyclomethicone	2.00
Castor isostearate succinate, PEG ricinoleate	3.00
Vitamin E acetate	0.25
C. Diazolidinyl urea, methylparaben, propylene glycol, propylparaben	1.00
	100.00

Procedure: Combine A at 75oC. Combine B at 75oC. Add B to A. Cool to 40oC and add C.

CHAPTER 6

Rhizobium Gum: A Novel Cosmetic Ingredient from Soil to the Skin

Anthony Bresin, Ghislain Sanhaji and Romain Reynaud
ARD/Soliance, Pomacle, France.

KEY WORDS: *Patches, polysaccharide, gelling agent, fermentation, sensation of freshness, rhizobium gum*

ABSTRACT: *A new polysaccharide, produced by fermentation of a Rhizobium sp. strain, is introduced as a typical example of how technology can create new properties and new applications from a "basic" natural ingredient.*

Whereas many products used by cosmetic customers come from natural molecules extracted and purified from various sources, most of them are modified by technical steps in order to give new functionalities. An example of this is rhizobium gum, a new polysaccharide[a] produced by fermentation of a Rhizobium sp strain. It is a typical example of what technology can design to create new properties and new applications from a "basic" natural ingredient. In this chapter, we look at its origin, evolution and properties.

Origin

The soil is a complex biotope with many interactions occurring between plants and microorganisms. These interactions, such as symbiotism, commensalism or parasitism, are based on evolution and the necessity for each microorganism to position itself in the alimentary chain.

---

[a] Soligel is a product of Soliance, Pomacle, France

Our study focuses on a symbiotic interaction between a bacterium and a plant that is advantageous for both parts. For instance, rhizobium strains are well known to transform the inorganic nitrogen (gas) from the atmosphere into nitrogen usable by the plant (ions); and to counterbalance, the bacteria use the organic molecules synthesized by plants and released near the roots to grow and to maintain their metabolism.

The strength of microorganisms such as bacteria is the diversity and various skills of their species. During a screening program, in collaboration with the Centre National de la Recherche Scientifique (CNRS) – the National Council for Scientific Research – a new strain of rhizobium bacteria was isolated. Identified as a Rhizobium sp., this new species demonstrates the ability to produce a polymer near the roots of sunflowers.[1]

In soil, during dry conditions or drought, this strain synthesizes the polymer[2,3] in order to modify the structure of the soil near the roots of the sunflower to enhance the aggregation of root-adhering soil.[4,5] The bacteria create a thin layer of polymer in contact with the roots system (**Figure 1**).[6] This polymer maintains a high water supply near the roots that is usable by the plant in severe drought. The strain finds nutrients near the roots resulting from the roots system leaking metabolites.

Thus, a symbiotic relationship exists between the plant and the bacteria: the polymer keeps the moisture near the roots of the plant and the bacteria uses nutrients lost by the plant.[1,7,8]

The particular ability of the polymer to maintain a high water supply is useful for the cosmetic industry. Indeed, such a polymer can be used as a vector for hydrophilic actives molecules without using woven matrix as usually used for cosmetic patches. Moreover, used at 0.3 up to 0.5% in creams, it brings a slipping sensation and so the polymer can be used as a texturing agent.

But before having a usable product, many technical operations are needed.

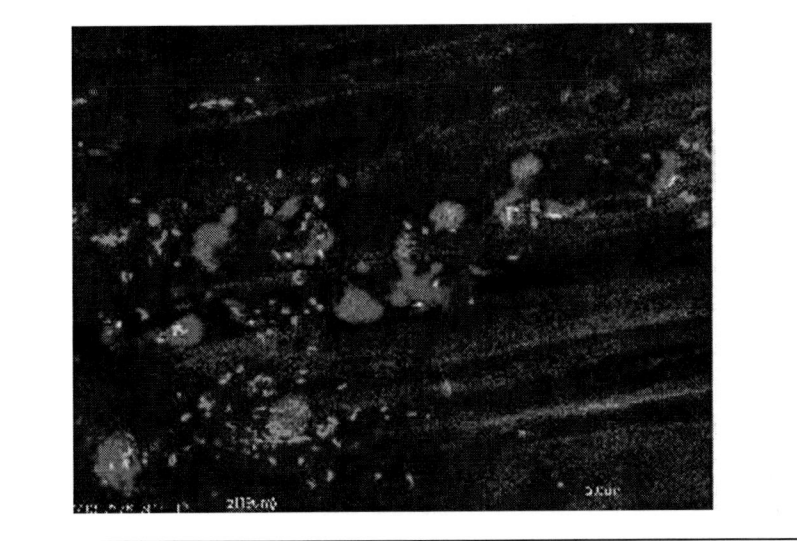

Figure 1. Rhizobium sp and polymer localization near a root (Green spots: bacteria labeled by GFP probe; Red spots: polymer labeled by concanavaline Alexa 660) LEMIR 2002

Development

The Rhizobium sp. strain, which is non-pathogenic towards man, was isolated from the rhizoplane (the soil near the roots) of sunflowers in a French field. Screening experiments were carried out in collaboration with the Labratoire d'Ecologie Microbienne de la Rhizosph re (LEMIR-CNRS-CEA). Rhizobium sp. was selected from many strains because of its capacity to synthesize great quantities of extracellular polysaccharides, also known as exopolysaccharides (EPS).

To improve its ability to produce EPS, a drastic selection has been carried out between all the bacteria isolated from the soil sample. The strain is a Gram-negative bacterium mobile, which takes the appearance of small mobile sticks forming colonies in the rhizoplane. ARD/Soliance developed an original fermentation[9,10] and purification process to produce EPS. The EPS is produced during a stationary phase, meaning when the bacterium is under stress such as nutrient deficiency, to insure carbohydrate and nutrient storage.

EPS production occurs under aerobic conditions, i.e. maintaining a high oxygen content by supplying air in a 40,000–liter fermentor with controlled and monitored parameters. When the glucose content of the fermentation broth reached 0.5 g/L, the fermentation broth was stabilized by direct steam injection in a jet cooker and cells were removed by continuous centrifugation. The supernatant was then purified by sterilized filtration (0.22 µm).

The heat treatment has several functions. First of all by heat disruption, cells are lysed. The product is thus sterilized and totally free of any living microorganisms, but the main purpose of the heat treatment is to modify the structure of the polymer to improve its rheological properties.

The conformational form of polymer synthesized by the Rhizobium sp. is a double helix.[11,12] The native form of the polymer does not show any special properties; it is a poor viscous ingredient and it does not form a gel. During the heat treatment, the double helix of rhizobium gum (RG) is partially denatured and forms a random coil.[13,14] The viscosity of the fermentation broth decreases, allowing the separation of the cells by centrifugation.

During the cooling of the supernatant, a rearrangement of the RG molecules occurs. Some chains of the polymer form a new organization that leads to the creation of a network structure.

Thus, the native polymer which does not show any special properties becomes a new gelling agent by the modification of the 3D structure of each RG molecule.

The primary structure of this exopolysaccharide has been identified by nuclear magnetic resonance (NMR) and the molecular weight of the molecule by gel permeation chromatography.

The polymer (**Figure 2**) is a branched polysaccharide composed of a series of monomer units made of 6 neutral sugars in the main chain (3 molecules of glucose and 3 molecules of galactose) in the shape of pyranose, 1 glucuronic acid, and with 1 pyruvyl substituent. Some acetyl groups also occur in the macromolecular chain with an average of 1.9 groups per repetitive unit. The occurrence of the pyruvyl and acid sugar charges make it a polyelectrolyte.

The molecular weight of the native molecule (in the fermentation broth) is around 1,500,000 Daltons.

```
→ 4)– GlcA– (1→ 4) - β - Glcp - (1→ 4) - β - Glcp– (1→ 6) - α -Glcp - (1→ 4) - α - Galp– (1→
                                                6
                                                1
              β - Galp - (1→ 3) - β - Galp
                      ╱ ╲
                     4   6
                      ╲ ╱
                       C
                      ╱ ╲
                   H₃C   COOH
```

Figure 2. Structure of Rhizobium gum

Properties

The acetyl groups (not well localized along the main chain and side chain) are involved in the interactions between polymer chains and the 3D conformation of the network; thus, the rheological properties are affected. The viscosity of a solution at 10 g/L of RG decreases with the increases in pH (**Figure 3**) because of the removal of acetyl groups at a high pH level (pH>8). Thus, the order of the polymer is no longer maintained, leading to the formation of flexible chains with lower interactions between themselves.

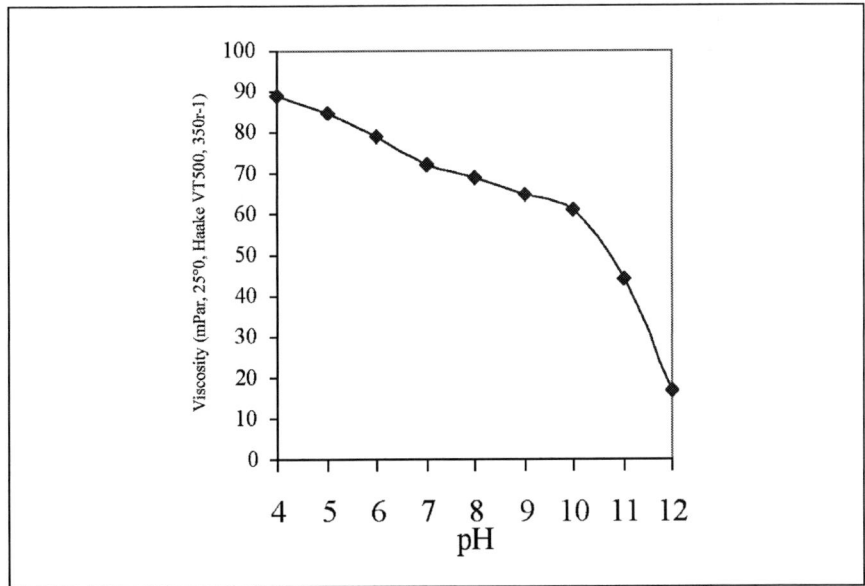

Figure 3. Evolution of the viscosity of a solution of 10 g/L depending on the pH of the solution

Due to the presence of two carboxylic groups and depending on the pH of the solution, the polymer is potentially negatively charged. The poly-anionic properties of the polymer allow interactions between the polymer and cationic ions. These ions enhance the organization of the network and so increase the viscosity of a solution with RG. The sodium form of the polymer shows gelling properties whereas a solution with acid form is close to the properties of a viscous solution rather than a gel (**Figure 4**). These behavior modifications of the molecule are due to the organization of the polymer chains in the presence of cationic ions. The interactions between chains and ions lead to an increase in the organization order of the network and so create gelling properties.

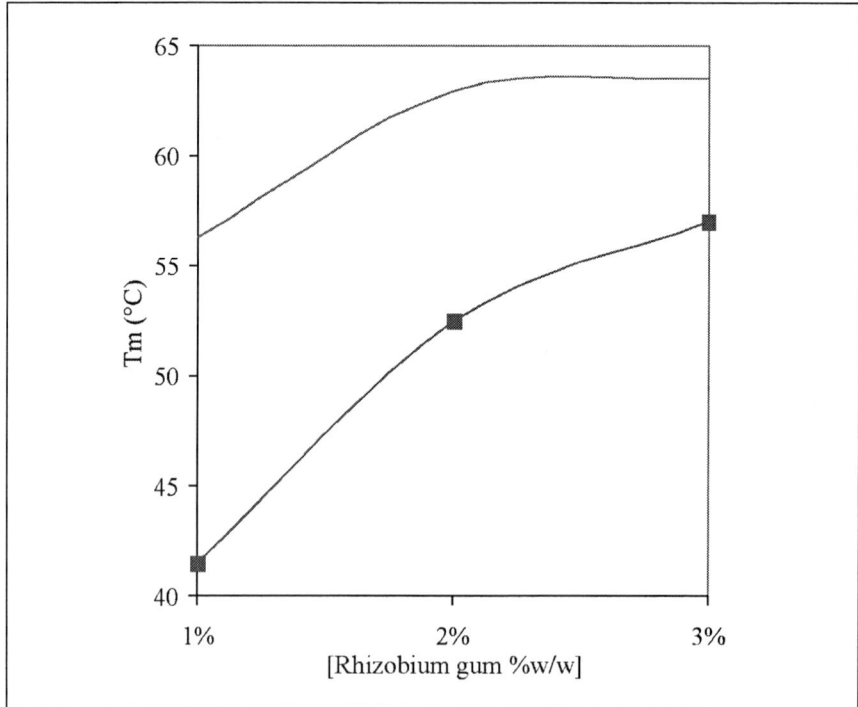

Figure 4. Relation between "melting point" and concentration of Rhizobium gum with (—) or without NaCl (■)

At low concentration (around 0.02 mol/L), the use of divalent cation rather than monovalent cation provides a stronger gel by enhancing the interactions between the polymer chains. The carboxylic groups of pyruvyl substituent and glucuronic acid along

RG chains interact with themselves and as a result, the maximum strength of the gel is reached very quickly. From a concentration of 0.04 mol/L, the difference between monovalent and divalent cations is very low and the gel strength is stabilized at 60 N/m².

Concerning the RG sodium form, when the concentration reaches 0.1 mol/L, the gel strength becomes independent of the sodium chloride concentration (**Figure 5**).

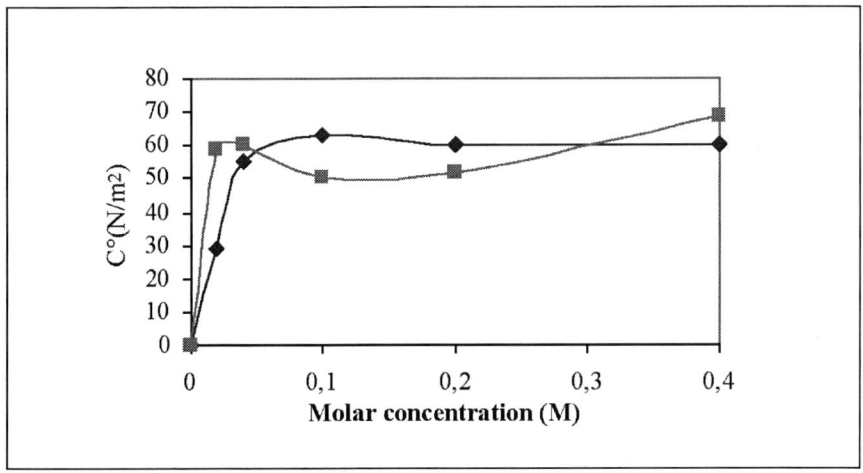

Figure 5. Relationship between ion concentration and elasticity of a 1% w/w Rhizobium gum gel (pH 5.5) NaCl (◆) CaCl$_2$ (■)

Rhizobium gum can provide many applications because of its complex structure. It can be used to stabilize emulsions at a low concentration by creating complex networks between water/oil/air interfaces,[14] or it can be used as a texturing agent by its specific gliding sensation in emulsions or lotions. One of its main applications is for its original purpose in the soil: its ability to be an exchanger of water and water-soluble molecules.

At a high concentration (around 20 g/L) and with sodium chloride (0.1 M), the RG forms a strong and elastic gel that can be used as a vector for active molecules.[15] The conformation modification provided by the heat treatment during the production process enhances the natural skill of the polymer to pump and release water and molecules. These properties depend on the nature of the surface in contact with the polymer.

A 2% w/w RG gel is an ideal raw material to create a patch composed of only RG and 0.1 M sodium chloride (**Figure 6**). This semi final product can be used as a vector to deliver an active molecule to its target.

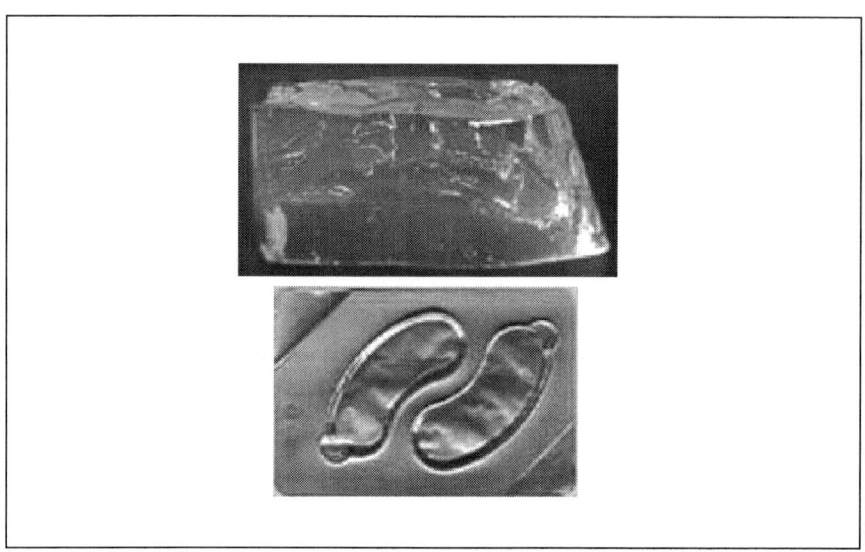

Figure 6. The patch, from the raw material to semi final product

A Sensation of Freshness

An unexpected property of an RG gel is its amazing sensation of freshness on skin when the patch is applied. To compare the sensation provided by the patch to a common cucumber disk used under the eyes, sensorial tests were carried out to evaluate the impact of the patch on the feelings of potential customers.

A patch composed of 20 g/L (2%) of RG with 0.1 mol/L of sodium chloride with or without menthol was compared to the same patch composed of carrageenan[b], with or without menthol in a study on 28 volunteers. When asked, "Which did you feel had the most sensation of freshness?" 82% of the volunteers chose the RG patch with menthol versus 14% for the carrageenan patch with menthol (4% were undecided). For the non-mentholated patch, results were similar: 79% chose the RG patch versus 14% for the carrageenan patch (with 7% finding no difference).

---

[b] Gelcarin SA 911 is a product of FMC Biopolymer, Philadelphia, PA, USA.

To compare the fresh effect of both polysaccharide gels and cucumber, a 3 mm thickness gel of both RG gel and kappa carrageenan gel was applied on a surface of volunteers' arms. The temperature of the skin was checked every 10 seconds under controlled atmosphere with 20ºC±1ºC and 60%±2% humidity. This data was compared to the measurements obtained previously from the application of a 3 mm thickness cucumber disc, under same conditions and on the same skin area (the internal surface of the right arm). Each patch or cucumber disk had been stored overnight at room temperature (20ºC) and its temperatures had been checked before application (19.8ºC±0.9ºC).

Consistent with the sensorial results, the RG patch also demonstrates the best control of temperature decrease. Compared to both cucumber, which shows a linear decrease of the temperature with time, and kappa carrageenan patch, the RG patch provides a fresh sensation by decreasing the surface temperature very quickly and by keeping it constant during the test (**Figure 7**). Even the menthol added to the k-carrageenan patch cannot reach the results of the RG powder alone in a sodium chloride solution.

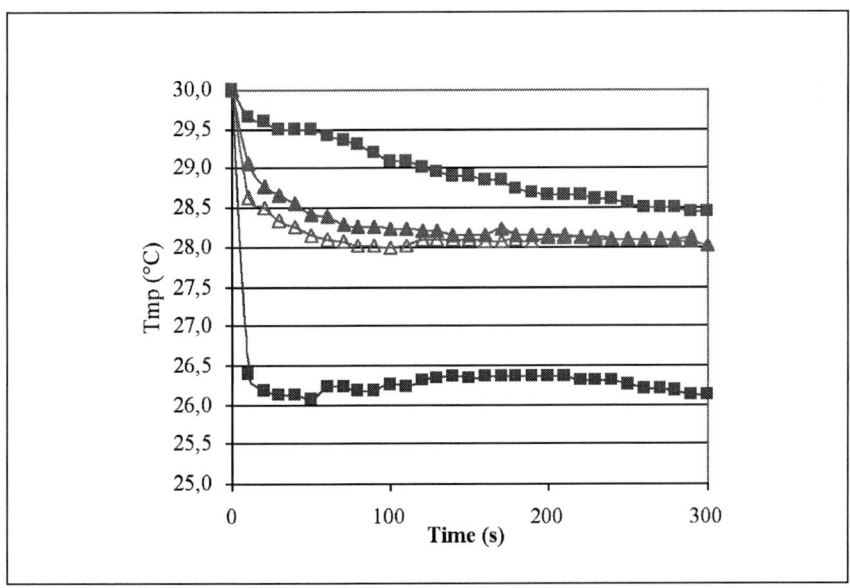

Figure 7. Freshening effect of Rhizobium gum (■) on the skin compared to k-carrageenan gel with menthol (▲) or without menthol (△) and cucumber (■)

The cucumber used to keep hydratation and fresh sensation around the eyes is now superseded by a biotechnological cucumber. The development of the patch application is a result of fruitful collaboration between fundamental research and industrial needs for the cosmetic.

Conclusion

To conclude, the water exchange properties and the molecule supply, the primary purposes of the polysaccharide, are used and provide a wide range of applications to the cosmetic industry. The original rheological properties of the molecule and the transparency of a 20 g/L patch made of RG are a great molecule to create patches for many active cosmetic ingredients. The freshness sensation on skin when the patch is applied is also an expected property providing a pure relaxing sensation. Consequently, we recommend the use of polymer as a principal component of patches with hydrophilic actives molecules dedicated for the face. Moreover, at a low concentration between 0.2 and 0.5, the sensory properties of emulsions or milks are modified by the addition of a unique slipping feeling allowing the use of this molecule as a texturing agent.

Published April 2004 Cosmetics and Toiletries magazine

References

1. Y Alami, W Achouak, C Marol and T Heulin, Rhizosphere soil aggregation and plant-growth promotion of sunflower by an EPS-producing Rhizobium sp. strain isolated from sunflower roots, Appl Environ Microbiol 66(8) 3393-3398 (2000)
2. PG Hartel and M Alexandre, Role of extracellular polysaccharide production and clays in the desiccation tolerance of cowpea Bradyrhizobia, Soil Sci Soc Am J 50 1193-1198 (1986)
3. EB Roberson and M Firestone, Relationship between dessication and exopolysaccharide production in a soil Pseudomonas sp., Appl Environ Microbiol 58 1284-1291 (1992)
4. M Watt, ME McCully and CE Jeffree, Plant and bacterial mucilages of the maize rhisosphere: Comparison of their soil binding properties and histochemistry in a model system, Plant Soil 151 151-165 (1993)
5. N Amellal, G Burtin, F Bartoli and T Heulin, Colonization of wheat roots by EPS-producing Pantoea agglomerans and its effect on rhizosphere soil aggregation, Appl Environ Microbiol 64 3740-3747 (1998)
6. C Chenu and EB Roberson, Diffusion of glucose in microbial extracellular polysaccharide as effected by water potential, Soil Biol Bio-chem 28 877-884 (1996)
7. R Chabot, H Antaoun and MP Cecas, Growth promotion of maize and lettuce by phosphate-solubilizing Rhizobium leguminesarum biovar phaseoli, Plant Soil 184 311-321 (1996)

8. Y Alami, L Champolivier, A Merrien and T Heulin, R le de Rhizobium sp., rhizobact rie productrice d'exopolysaccharide dans l'agr gation du sol rhizosph rique du tournesol: Cons quences sur la croissance de la plante et sa r sistance ˆ la contrainte hydrique, Ol Corps Gras Lip 6(6) 524-528 (2000)
9. WO 985993, EP 0960132, FR 9800269, Polysaccharide, micro-organism and method for obtaining same, composition containing it and application, R Baynast de, T Heulin, A Heyraud, M Milas, A Villain, Y Alami (Nov 2, 1997)
10. JM Crompin, Extraction industrielle de la production et de la purification d'un nouveau polysaccharide bact rien issu de la rhizosph re des plantes, PhD dissertation, University of Reims (2000)
11. A Villain-Simmonet, M Milas and R Rinaudo, A new bacterial polysaccharide (YAS34), I. Caracterization of the conformations and conformational transition, Int Journal of Biological Macromolecules 65 75 (2000)
12. A Villain-Simonnet, M Milas and M Rinaudo, A new bacterial exopolysaccharide (YAS34), II: Influence of thermal treatments on the conformation and structure, Relation with gelation ability, Int J Biol Macromol 27 77-87 (2000)
13. A Villain-Simonnet, Nouveaux polysaccharide d'origine bact rienne Strucutres et propri t s, PhD dissertation, University Joseph Fourier, Grenoble (1999)
14. F Dargelas, Structure et propri t s d'un nouveau polysaccharide bact rien, Nouvelles applications, PhD dissertation, University Joseph Fourier, Grenoble (2002)
15. WO 03038069A1, FR 0213095, Milieu de culture solide pour microorganisme et cellules eucaryotes ainsi que son proc d d'obtention, R Baynast de, A Belarbi and A Bresin (2002)

CHAPTER 7

Recent Polymer Technologies for Hair Care

Bernice Ridley *(Ciba Specialty Chemicals)* • **Colleen M. Rocafort** *(Ciba Specialty Chemicals Corporation)* • **Julie Shlepr, with Julie Castner and Dale Willis** *(Noveon Inc.)* • **M. Creamer, A. Keenan, M. Merlau Johnson, A. Kar, A. Nakatani, D. Routzahn, C. Schwartz, M. Wang and F. Zeng** *(Rohm and Haas Company)* • **J. Jachowicz, J.C. Chuang, T. Winkler, R. McMullen, S. Chen and D. Streuli** *(International Specialty Products)* • **Tom Burns** *(Interpolymer Corporation)* • **Jennifer Lee** *(Croda Inc.)* • **Bethany K. Johnson** *(Dow Corning Corporation)* **and Erik Gyzen** *(Dow Corning Australia)*

KEY WORDS: *Hair and hair care, polymers, resins, styling, conditioning, rheology*

ABSTRACT: *More than 20 polymers from seven companies are reviewed in this survey of recent polymer technologies for hair care. A variety of new functions and multifunctionalities are seen in these products launched within the past two years.*

Today's hair care polymers offer a range of functionalities, such as color enhancement, hair strengthening, antiaging, sun protection, color retention and moisturization. It is hard to beat the old standbys: styling, conditioning and rheology modification.

In this roundup of recent polymer technologies for hair care, seven companies and more than a score of authors report on the claims, tests and functionalities of two dozen polymers. Full-length versions of these roundup reports can be accessed at *www.cosmeticsandtoiletries.com*. *Cosmetics & Toiletries* magazine thanks these contributors and hopes this roundup will help you identify new possibilities from polymers.

A Rheology Modifier from Ciba

The polymer: Acrylates/beheneth-25 methacrylate copolymer[a] is a new associative rheology modifier manufactured by Ciba Specialty Chemicals Corp. designed to give effective thickening in crystal-clear gel systems over a wide pH range. It is a hydrophobically modified (long C-22 alkyl chain) alkali-activated aqueous emulsion, with an acrylate backbone modified to allow thickening at pH>6 while maintaining the solids content at 30% active polymer.

Acrylates/beheneth-25 methacrylate copolymer is supplied as a 30% active aqueous emulsion. The development of viscosity in aqueous solutions of this copolymer occurs on the addition of a suitable base. The acid groups present in the alkyl backbone become ionized and structuring occurs by electrostatic repulsion. The presence of the hydrophobically modified associative group enhances the rheology modification by the formation of inter- and intra-molecular micelles that provide extremely high apparent viscosities at very low shear rates. The presence of such groups also allows association with other hydrophobic moieties that may be present in personal care formulations.

The combination of the optimized acrylic backbone, hydrophobic associative monomer and the level of cross-linking in the polymer results in a shear-thinning nonthixotropic rheology modifier with excellent yield value and suspension characteristics. Acrylates/beheneth-25 methacrylate copolymer provides good thickening over a pH range of 6.0–12.5. It provides excellent, cost-effective viscosity development along with the easy handling properties of a liquid. For optimum thickening efficiency, solutions of this polymer need to be adjusted to greater than pH 6.0 using common neutralizing bases.

Clarity: One of the best differentiating features of acrylates/beheneth-25 methacrylate copolymer is that it can be used to produce crystal-clear gel systems, with gel clarity exceeding any that can be obtained with competitive products (lower value for nephelometric turbidity units (NTU) means better clarity). **Figure 1**

---

[a]Tinovis GTC (INCI: Acrylates/beheneth-25 methacrylate copolymer) is a product of Ciba Specialty Chemicals.

illustrates the clarity measurement of acrylates/beheneth-25 methacrylate copolymer versus two commercial rheology modifiers in the marketplace at pH 6.0 and 7.0. The picture to the right of the graph illustrates the visual differences of this new copolymer versus polymer C in deionized water. The jar on the left contains the copolymer in water at pH 6.0, and the jar to the right contains polymer C in water at pH 6.0. The acrylates/beheneth-25 methacrylate copolymer produces a crystal-clear gel.

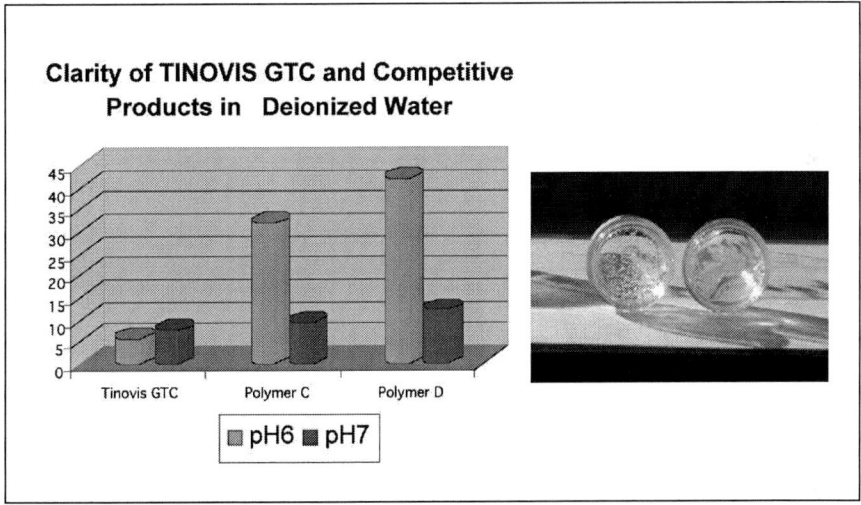

Figure 1. Clarity of acrylates/beheneth-25 methacrylate copolymer and competitive products in deionized water (from Ciba)

Stability: The second differentiating feature is its stability profile, especially in clear packaging. Acrylates/beheneth-25 methacrylate copolymer, tested at 1% active polymer in deionized water at pH 6.5, passed five freeze/thaw cycles without a significant loss in viscosity, separation or sedimentation. The copolymer tested in clear packaging is stable at room temperature (RT), 45°C, and after exposure to ultraviolet (UV) light. Gel formulations with traditional carbomer-type thickeners (polymers C and D) were shown to lose viscosity quite significantly after only four weeks when exposed to daylight. Formulations with acrylates/beheneth-25 methacrylate copolymer remained stable even when exposed to daylight. **Figure 2** illustrates the percent change of viscosity over a four-week period.

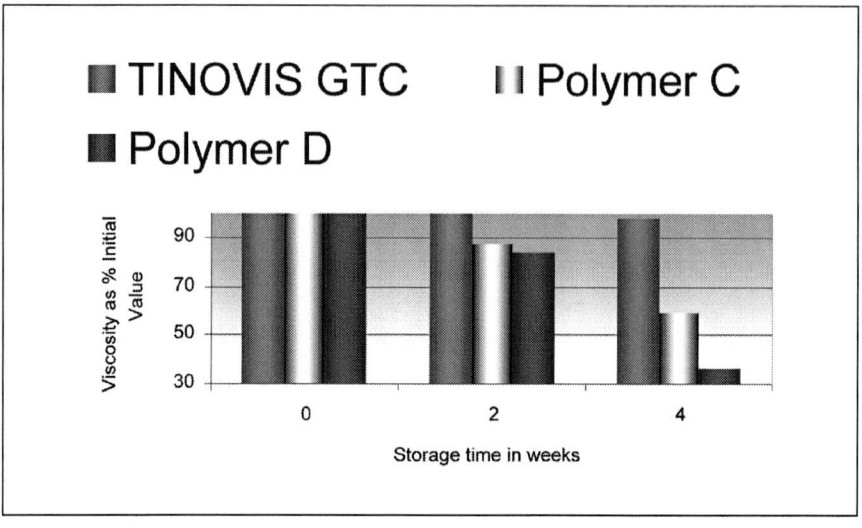

Figure 2. Stability results of gel formulations containing acrylates/beheneth-25 methacrylate copolymer or traditional carbomer-type thickeners (from Ciba)

Summary: Acrylates/Beheneth-25 methacrylate copolymer provides these benefits in clear gel systems:

- It is an effective alternative to carbomer-type rheology modifiers in clear gel systems, providing crystal-clear gels.
- It provides good thickening over a pH range of 6.0–12.5.
- It provides a shear-thinning nonthixotropic rheology modifier with excellent yield value and suspension characteristics.
- It offers the advantage of being supplied in an easy-to-use liquid form that can alleviate the formulation problems and lengthy processing times commonly encountered with carbomer-type rheology modifiers.
- It offers a better stability profile than carbomer-type rheology modifiers.

A Rheology Modifier from Noveon

There can be no doubt that aesthetic properties are some of the most important features in personal care products. While almost any shampoos can cleanse the hair, those with more attractive shelf-appeal and a better sensory experience during use are the ones that ultimately win the battle for market share. Thus, the need to enhance the sensory experience, rather than focus solely on product functionality, is a critical challenge facing formulators. This is why, for example, surfactants are not used solely for cleansing, but also to deliver richer, more billowy lather while minimizing the risk of irritation.

Similarly, rheology-control agents are not used solely for thickening. Today's rheology modifiers must offer not only the functional aspects of thickening, suspension and stabilization, but must also provide more enhanced appearance to the finished product, superior flow and pour properties; a pleasant after-feel, and a smooth, light, cushiony feel in use.

Noveon reports on three novel technologies specifically designed to surpass previous expectations for functionality as well as sensory attributes: acrylates copolymer for use in surfactant-cleansing systems, acrylates/C_{10-30} alkyl acrylate crosspolymer for use in surfactant-cleansing or aqueous-based systems, and polyacrylate-14 for use primarily in aqueous-based systems. Polyacrylate-14 will be discussed next as will two other technologies.

Polyacrylate-14: Polyacrylate-14[b] was designed specifically to improve hair style longevity while enhancing sensory and aesthetic properties, both in formulation and in use. Polyacrylate-14 is a unique, multifunctional polymer that delivers film-forming fixative and rheology-modifying properties in formulations. It is supplied as a milky white liquid with a viscosity of 15 mPa·s, active polymer 30% w/w and pH 3.0.

The patent-pending design of this alkali-swellable, associative polymer combines hard hydrophilic, soft hydrophobic and semi-hydrophobic components to deliver an optimized balance of properties. This novel combination leads to these performance advantages: excellent hold and good solubility; clear, uniform films with good adhesion; superior humidity resistance; and a smooth, natural feel on hair.

Traditional hydrophobic associative polymers, particularly those with long chain hydrophobes, can build very strong hydrophobic

---

[b]Fixate PLUS polymer (INCI: Polyacrylate-14) is a trademarked product of Noveon, Inc., a wholly owned subsidiary of The Lubrizol Corporation. The trademark is owned by The Lubrizol Corporation.

associations in solution. The resulting gels can be highly thixotropic, with poor texture and appearance in the presence of shear stress. In contrast, the semi-hydrophobic pendants in the structure of polyacrylate-14 enable *controlled* hydrophobic association. Thus, this uniquely designed polymer enables improved thickening efficiency while maintaining the smooth, buttery feel and classic shear-thinning rheology characteristic of gels formulated with carbomer[c] polymers.

When neutralized with a base, the polymer opens and develops viscosity with high clarity at approximately pH 6.5. At 1.0% active polymer, viscosity reaches 7,000 mPa·s, with viscosity increasing rapidly as concentration is increased, while maintaining high clarity (**Figure 3**).[6]

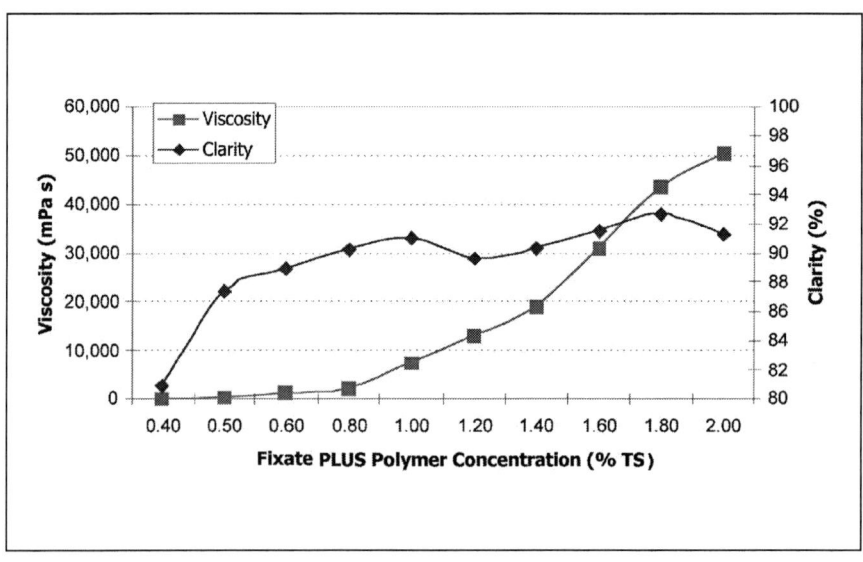

Figure 3. Viscosity and clarity of polyacrylate-14 at selected concentrations (from Noveon)

Due to its hydrophobic modification, polyacrylate-14 offers exceptional efficiency with hydrophobically-modified carbomer copolymers (such as acrylates/C_{10-30} alkyl acrylate crosspolymer) due to association between the hydrophobic groups. Again, clarity in formulations is very high.

---

[c]Carbopol is a registered trademark of The Lubrizol Corporation.

As noted, polyacrylate-14 is a multifunctional polymer. Even at low use levels, it provides fixative properties with exceptional high-humidity curl retention (HHCR), whether used alone (**Figure 4**) or when used in combination with leading rheology modifiers.

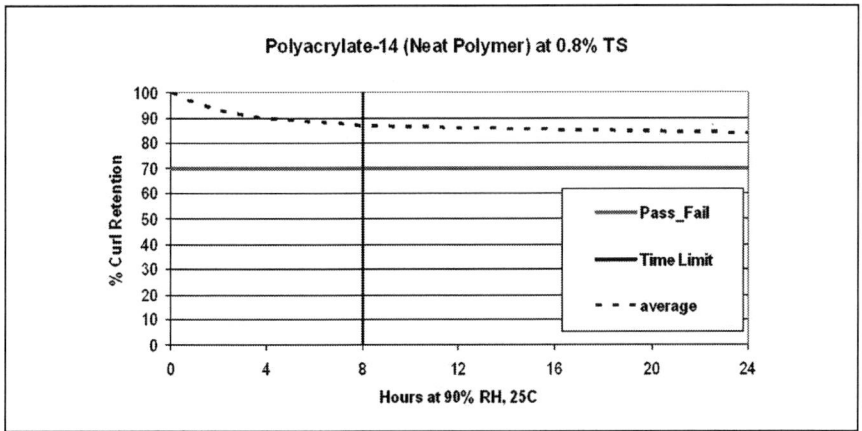

Figure 4. High-humidity curl retention of neat polyacrylate-14 at 0.8% TS (from Noveon)

In laboratory evaluations, styling gels formulated with just 1.0% w/w total solids (0.5% w/w polyacrylate-14 with 0.5% w/w acrylates/C_{10-30} alkyl acrylate crosspolymer[d]) demonstrated greater than 90% curl retention after 24 hours (h) at 90% relative humidity (RH), 25°C.

In qualitative salon tests, styling gels formulated with 0.8% w/w polyacrylate-14 and 0.2% w/w carbomer[7] were observed to impart greater fullness and body, without stickiness or heaviness, when compared to a commercial styling gel formulated with polyvinyl pyrolidone (PVP).

Other polymers from Noveon: Here are two additional Noveon polymers that enable versatility in formulation while providing efficiency essential to managing cost constraints.

Acrylates copolymer[e] is an alkali-swellable, lightly cross-linked acrylic emulsion polymer designed especially for use in high-surfactant-content (12–30% w/w) cleansing applications. Although not an associative polymer by chemistry, it does show some associative behavior

---

[d]Carbopol Ultrez 21 polymer (INCI: Acrylates/C10-30 alkyl acrylate crosspolymer) is a product of The Lubrizol Corporation.
[e]Carbopol Aqua SF1 polymer (INCI: Acrylates copolymer) is a trademarked product of Noveon, Inc., a wholly owned subsidiary of The Lubrizol Corporation. The trademark is owned by The Lubrizol Corporation.

and favors surfactant structuring. Thickening occurs via hydrodynamic volume expansion and through interaction of the hydrophobic portion of the polymer backbone with surfactant micelles. This three-dimensional structuring network builds viscosity and other rheological properties. In the presence of typical anionic and amphoteric surfactants, this copolymer displays the ability to "back acid thicken" while maintaining the inherent properties of the polymer.

Another benefit observed with acrylates copolymer is synergistic thickening with surfactants and salt. In the past, it proved difficult to produce a truly high clarity surfactant-based formulation with exceptional suspension properties. The three-dimensional structuring network provided by acrylates copolymer enables formulators to suspend beads, exfoliating agents and other insoluble agents without sacrificing the clarity of the formulation. Optimal clarity can be achieved at approximately pH 6.5.

Acrylates/C_{10-30} alkyl acrylate crosspolymer[f] is a hydrophobically modified, cross-linked polyacrylate polymer. As supplied, the polymer molecules are coiled and impart relatively little suspension and viscosity. Upon neutralization, the molecules ionize and expand due to charge repulsion, and provide suspending and thickening properties to the aqueous system in which they are present. In this hydrodynamic thickening mechanism, it is primarily the physical packing ("space-filling mechanism") of polymer molecules that is responsible for the development of viscosity and suspending capability. This is distinctly different from associative thickening. Acrylates/C_{10-30} alkyl acrylate crosspolymer provides the user with consistent dispersion viscosity and efficient thickening. The polymer features patented self-wetting technology, so it wets and disperses quickly, without requiring agitation.

A Styling Resin from Rohm and Haas

Rohm and Haas has introduced two new hair fixative resins within the last two years geared to formulators who want to create hair sprays, gels, mousses or pomades that deliver a durable hold, a novel texture and shine to the hair.

---

[f]Carbopol Ultrez 20 polymer (INCI: Acrylates/C10-30 alkyl acrylate crosspolymer) is a trademarked product of Noveon, Inc., a wholly owned subsidiary of The Lubrizol Corporation. The trademark is owned by The Lubrizol Corporation.

Acrylates/hydroxyesters acrylates copolymer: Conventional hair fixative resins meeting the limit of 55% volatile organic compounds (VOC) in sprays tend to be stiff and humidity resistant leaving an "acrylic" type of crunchiness to the hair. Acrylates/hydroxyesters acrylates copolymer[g] is a durable hold resin that goes beyond conventional resins to enable the formulator to create soft-to-strong-hold hair sprays where the style lasts longer, i.e., is more durable, than sprays formulated with the conventional acrylic fixative resins.

The difference is all the more remarkable when the formulator wants to enable a hairstyle that has a strong hold and a more natural movement to it; i.e., not the "helmet-head" artificial style. Three factors in the polymer design and mechanism make this possible.

- First, the polymer consists of a dispersion of interpenetrating hard and soft acrylic film-forming polymers that create tough spot welds that hold the hair style together. Because considerable stress is put on the spot welds that hold the hair style together during the day, tough spot welds help keep the hair style more durable because they do not break easily except when they are combed out.
- Second, the bimodality of the polymer tends to reduce the formulation viscosity relative to the same solids concentration of a conventional acrylic hair fixative resin. This results in a finer spray pattern for pump and aerosol sprays, leaving a less wet feel on the hair at a given stiffness. This also allows more resin to be optionally formulated into the pump or aerosol, as in 80% VOC formulations, to build hair stiffness without causing a wet feel to the hair.
- Third, the hydroxyester-type monomers on the polymer chain improve shampoo removability without reducing humidity resistance. This is because the polymer does not have a tendency to form tacky hydrates with water. The result is that this durable hold resin provides good humidity resistance (**Figure 5**), is easy to remove by shampoo and has a fast set time.

---

[g]Acudyne DHR Durable Hold Resin (INCI: Acrylates/hydroxyesters acrylates copolymer) is a product of the Rohm and Haas Company.

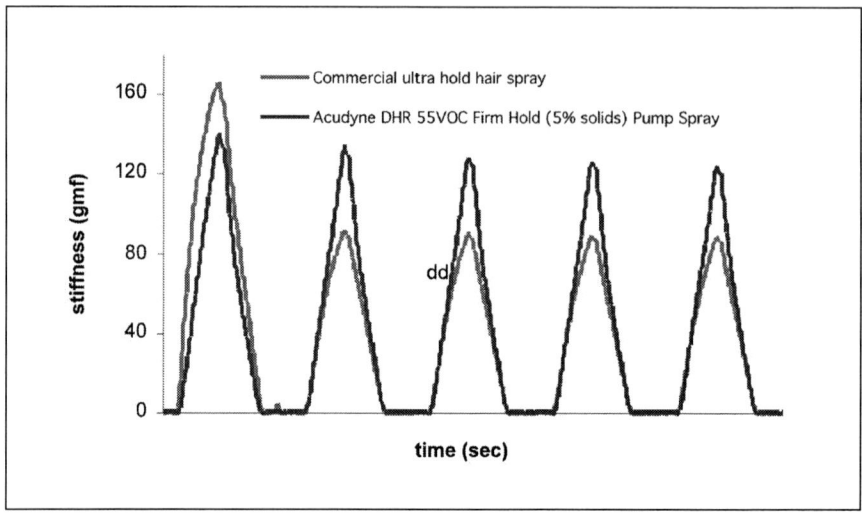

Figure 5. Dia-Stron durability testing. Curled tress was treated with hair fixative and compressed 5X in sequence. The work required to compress the curl is measured. The acrylates/hydroxyesters acrylates copolymer resin-treated tress maintained its stiffness after the compressions. (from Rohm and Haas)

Two other add-on benefits are the excellent film-forming properties of the resin, which when applied to the hair result in a slight shine benefit noticed in salon testing, and the ability to reform the film, enabling consumers to restyle their hair without adding more hairstyling product.

Other polymers from Rohm and Haas: Acrylamide/sodium acryloyl-dimethyltaurate/acrylic acid copolymer[h] is a water-soluble anionic terpolymer. This styling conditioning polymer enables the formulation of soft-to-medium-hold, humidity-resistant hair gels, pomades and mousses that provide a conditioned feel to the hair.

This polymer is also biphasic. The humidity resistance is engineered into the polymer design by having one phase of the polymer able to form hydrates with water at high humidity while the film is not plasticized. The second phase has similar humidity resistance to PVP. With this combination, the styling conditioning polymer provides a durable hold to the hair in high humidity. It is capable of forming clear, bubble-suspending gels with carbomer

---

[h]Acudyne SCP Styling Conditioning Polymer (INCI: Acrylamide/sodium acryloyldimethyltaurate/ acrylic acid copolymer) is a product of the Rohm and Haas Company.

types of rheology modifiers. The conditioning aspect to the hair is evident from salon evaluations and microscopy, which shows the smoothness of the hair shaft after treatment compared with conventional hair gel products.

A Styling Polymer from ISP

Copolymers of vinyl pyrrolidone and vinyl caprolactam find numerous applications in cosmetic technologies requiring water-soluble polymers with film-forming properties.[1] For hairstyling applications, one copolymer of this type is polyquaternium-69.

Polyquaternium-69 is a stiff-feel film former with long-lasting hold for clear formulations. It provides excellent high humidity curl retention as well as high shine and clarity. It also is compatible with carbomer, which allows for production of clear styling gels.

Polyquaternium-69 is sold as a 40% w/w colorless, low odor solution in water (48% w/w) and ethanol (12% w/w).

Polyquaternium-69 has been found to form clear, transparent films when cast on glass substrates. Similarly, clear films also are formed as fixative deposits on the surface of hair. Vigorous combing of polymer-treated hair does not lead to flaking as judged by fiber examination at low illumination angles and by taking high magnification images of hair with a flatbed scanner.

Polyquaternium-69 is characterized by high resistance to high humidity, which is reflected in the measured HHCR curves (**Figure 6**). This phenomenon primarily is due to the high vinyl caprolactam content in the structure of the polymer.

The films of polyquaternium-69 are characterized by high luster as indicated by visual observations of hair tresses as well as the quantitative results of image analysis (an increase in the maximum specular reflection intensity from 210±4 for untreated hair to 226±3 for the polymer-treated hair, **Figure 7a**).[2] Combination of styling and optical properties of polyquaternium-69 result in a significant improvement in reflectivity of frizzy and curly hair (elimination of frizziness and the appearance of high intensity reflection pattern, **Figure 7b**).[3]

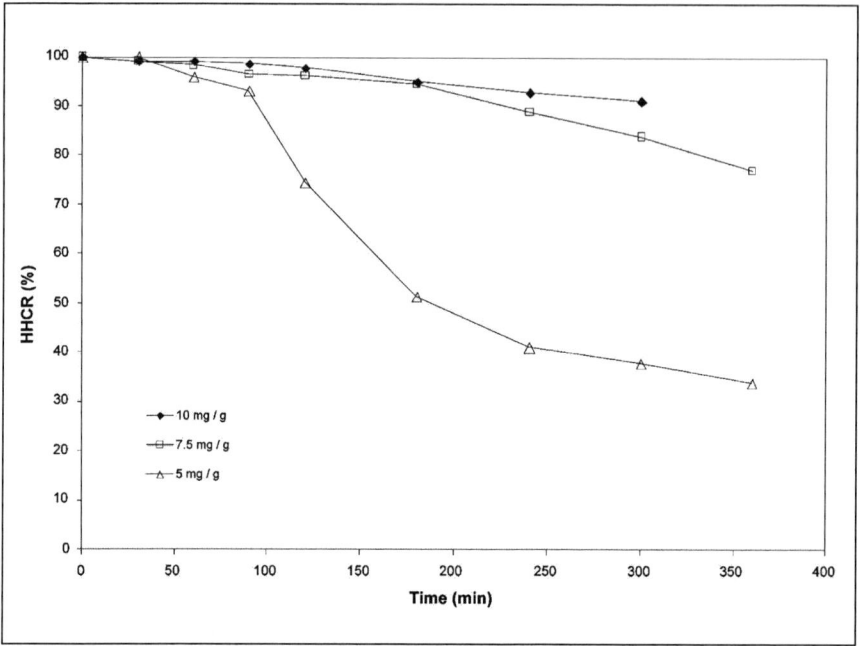

Figure 6. HHCR from polyquaternium-69 at 90% RH for the deposition amounts on hair of 5 mg/g, 7.5 mg/g and 10 mg/g. The test was carried out on very thick Chinese hair with a major elliptical axis of 110 μm. (from ISP)

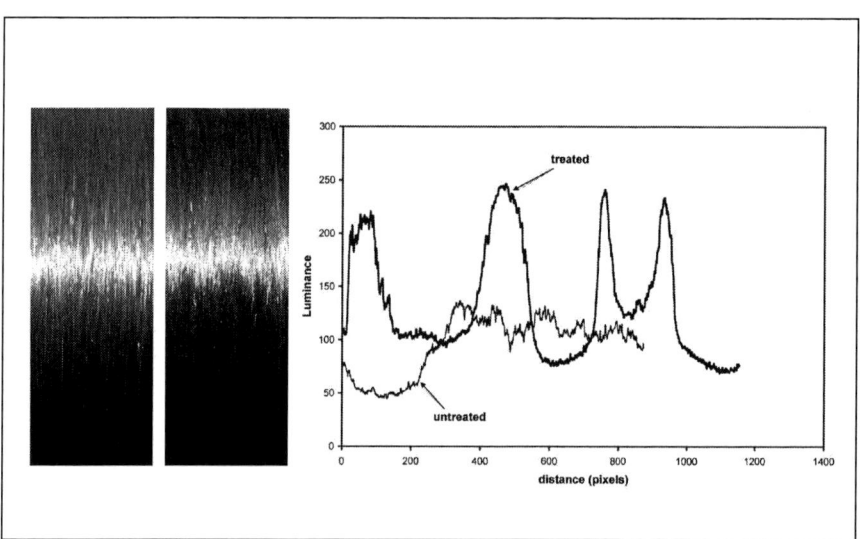

Figure 7. Specular and diffuse reflections (left) from untreated and polyquaternium-69 modified (with 1% aqueous solution) straight, dark brown hair. Light intensity plot (right) for free-hanging, untreated frizzy hair and the same hair treated with a 3% lotion based on polyquaternium-69. (from ISP)

The mechanical properties of hair treated with polyquaternium-69 have been characterized using stiffness parameters as well as the ratios of flexibility and plasticity; all were obtained experimentally using a texture analyzer.[4] The results suggest relatively high stiffness (F_1 = 473.3±14.8 G, stiffness ratio = 20.5 at the deposition of 22 mg/g), moderate flexibility (F_{10}/F_1 = 0.85, E_{10}/E_1 = 0.35) and low plasticity (H_{10}/H_1 = 0.89).

Thanks to its predominantly nonionic character (weakly cationic), polyquaternium-69 has broad compatibility with cosmetic ingredients, including other fixative resins and anionic polymers. Polyquaternium-69 can be used to prepare transparent gels by using a variety of thickeners such as carbomer, acrylates/C_{10-30} alkyl acrylate crosspolymer and PVM/MA decadiene crosspolymer. A typical product based on 0.5% carbomer and 3% polyquaternium-69 is characterized by a haze value of 10-20 NTU. This polymer also can be used to formulate hair mousses, lotions and shine products.

A Bimodal Styling Polymer from Interpolymer

Regulatory legislation and environmental consumer groups continue to challenge the personal care industry to reformulate aerosolized hair styling aids in an effort to lower levels of VOCs. The industry has contested that there may not be sufficient technology to permit the formulation of marketable aerosolized products that would deliver performance attributes economically, aesthetically and safely. A new polymer technology is ideally suited to bridging such gaps.

Consumers expect a number of often contradictory properties from hair styling sprays yet the ultimate goal is the same: the uniform application of a clear polymeric material to the hair to achieve certain improvements in appearance and manageability. The hairstyle must be held firmly in place under conditions of high temperature and humidity, yet the hair must not feel too stiff. The spray dispersion must be fine enough to avoid nozzle clogging and sputtering yet not a pose an acute inhalation risk. The formula must contain enough non-VOC components to meet regulatory requirements, yet even though it is an aqueous-based formula it must dry quickly after application. The resin solution must be able to flow along the hair shaft to help promote adherence to the adjacent hair fiber as the polymer dries, yet not create flakes during subsequent brushing or combing when either wet or dry. The hair must appear natural and glossy yet not feel tacky or sticky, even under conditions of high humidity. Finally, the fixative polymer must be long lasting yet readily removable from the hair during subsequent shampoo applications.

Acrylic copolymer technologies offer an alternative approach to traditional polymers such as PVP, PVP/VA and other high molecular weight copolymers. Interpolymer recently has developed an innovative technology identified as *bimodal*. This refers to its structure, which is composed of two different types of acrylic polymer molecules: one with anionic and the other one with cationic functionalities (patent pending). The unique bimodal technology was designed to enhance hairstyling products by improving hold performance in quick-setting low-VOC aqueous-based formulations.

Bimodal polymers: The bimodal technology is designed to enhance hairstyling products by improving "hold performance." These properties are accomplished through an innovative technology that uses a bimodal interpenetrating network that simultaneously delivers both cationic and anionic polymers to the hair shaft.

The result is a reversible, cross-linked polymer complex achieved by the ionic associations of the two oppositely charged polymer chains providing both excellent holding power and ease of removal. The anionic chain is designed to contribute to the polymer's removal properties while the cationic chain imparts strong hold and ease of styling. The ionic combination of the two oppositely charged polymer chains during drying allows the bimodal polymer to mimic the functions of higher molecular weight polymers.

This combination of lower molecular weight and high charge density allows the bimodal polymers to be easily sprayed and yield adequate hold when applied. The bimodal polymers have film formation temperatures that are balanced to give a pleasant feel without flaking.

A strong ionic association can be formed when two or more chains associate to form an interpenetrating network. The amino function is placed in an exposed position to interact with the acidic part of the anionic acrylic copolymer chain to form the interpenetrating network. Co-monomer selection and molecular weight control allow Interpolymer to optimize the steric hindrances and ionic interactions that result in specific setting and hold properties.

Polymer composition plays an important role in this geometrical and electrical interaction. The inclusion of strongly electropositive or electronegative groups on separate molecules causes an inductive shift of electrons. This shift affects the polymer's cohesive and adhesive properties. Because the bimodal polymers are composed of both electropositive and electronegative groups, there is a great potential for the polymer chains to exhibit this shift in electron density. At large distances, these polymer chains would behave like an electrically neutral system. However, as the ionic groups are brought into close proximity to their counterion during the drying process, strong secondary bond forces begin to exert their influence and give the bimodal polymers their unique characteristics.

This novel technology relies on the ability to produce stable dispersions and solutions containing polymer molecules with different ionic changes. During the drying process, the bimodal polymer will form an ionic complex, as already described, before the final film is completely dry and sets on the hair.

The resultant polymer complex prevents the formulation from migrating before the water or solvent has evaporated completely. This ability of the bimodal polymers to set quickly under high humidity conditions makes them a reliable alternative to current hair care polymers.

Bimodal polymers in very low VOC aerosols: Bimodal polymers were incorporated into aerosol sprays in an effort to determine if an aqueous-based 35% VOC formula could deliver comparable performance to existing branded 55% VOC hair sprays. An additional resin was incorporated into the control formula to assist with ancillary benefits such as gloss and luster. The bulk concentrate component of the control formula is shown in **Formula 1**.

For the final 35% VOC formulation, the ingredients were 50% w/w of the Formula 1 bulk concentrate and 50% w/w of hydrofluorocarbon 152A. For the final 55% VOC formulation, the ingredients were 63% of the bulk concentrate, 10.5% dimethyl ether, and 26.5% hydrofluorocarbon 152A w/w.

Formula 1
Low VOC aerosal bulk concentrate for a very low VOC aerosal (from Interpolymer)

A. Alcohol denatured	70.00% by wt
Aminomethyl propanol	0.50
PEG-12, dimethicone	0.10
PEG-45 Palm kernel glycerides	0.05
B. Polyacrylates-18 (and) polyacrylates-19	19.35
Ammonium acrylates copolymer	10.00
	100.00

Procedure: Add ingredients to appropriate vessel as listed. Stir between each addition until batch is clear and homogenous. Adjust pH to 8.4–8.8 with AMP-95 at end, stir until homogenous. Product is a slightly turbid solution.

A curl retention study was conducted to determine the efficacy of the bimodal technology in 35% and 55% low VOC aerosol hair spray formulations. Materials chosen for this evaluation were the polyacrylate 18 (and) polyacrylate 19 bimodal and the ammonium acrylate copolymer as stipulated in the control formula in Formula 1. A major brand with flexible hold, labeled as containing no chlorinated fluoro carbons (CFCs) but no mention of CAS compliance, also was evalutated.

Two swatches for each spray were prepared by washing with a commercial shampoo per manufacturer's instructions and blown dry using a standard consumer-grade, hand-held hair dryer set on a low setting. To insure that the swatches were dry, they were placed in a 38°C circulating air oven for 10 minutes before styling. The swatches then were cooled before styling with a consumer-grade curling iron set on its highest setting. Curls were held in the iron for 45 seconds to set the curl. When the swatch was removed, it was set immediately on its side while the second curl for the same test spray was prepared.

After both swatches were prepared and still lying on their sides, the test spray was applied by spraying each swatch with approximately a one-second burst of hair spray. The swatches were then flipped and then sprayed again on the opposite side. This was done for each spray. The swatches were allowed to dry for five minutes before moving into a vertical position for measurement. Before the tresses were measured, they each received another one-second application of spray while in the vertical position and allowed to dry.

The swatches were divided into the test groups and hung for evaluation. Ambient conditions were 74°F and 45% RH. Humidity conditions were 84°F and 95% RH.

Curl length was determined as a function of time. The percent curl retention (PCR) was calculated by means of the following equation:

$$PCR = 100 \times [(L - L_t) / (L - L_0)]$$

where
L = length of hair fully extended (before curling),
L_0 = length of curled hair before exposure, and
L_t = length of curled hair after exposure as a function of time.

Table 1 shows the results of the measurements of curl length and PCR under ambient conditions and high humidity conditions for periods of four hours.

Conclusion: This novel bimodal polymer technology is based on unique, interpenetrating polymer networks. By incorporating both cationic and anionic functionalities, the bimodal polymers offer a formulator the opportunity to create alternative very low or low VOC aqueous-based hair sprays.

The test data indicates that bimodal polymers can provide good high-humidity curl retention and can set quickly. Furthermore, due to the molecular weight of these polymers, formulators can deliver excellent dispersion patterns and particle size distributions (data not shown). And finally, the polymers exhibit good aesthetic characteristics when evaluated on wet and dried hair. This versatility makes them a reliable alternative to current hair care polymers and for the next generation of lower VOC hairstyling products.

Table 1
High-humidity curl retention of hair swatches curled and sprayed with 35% and 55% low VOC aerosol hair sprays containing bimodial polymer or with a major brand flexible hold spray without bimodial polymer (from Interpolymer)

Condition and Sample	Curl (and Percent Curl Retention) at Hourly Intervals				
	Start	Hour 1	Hour 2	Hour 3	Hour 4
Ambient Conditions					
35% Control	14.5	15.5 (69.7)	15.0 (84.8)	15.0 (84.8)	15.3 (75.8)
55% Control	14.0	15.0 (73.7)	14.5 (86.8)	14.5 (86.8)	14.5 (86.8)
Major Brand	12.5	14.0 (71.7)	13.5 (81.1)	13.5 (81.1)	13.8 (75.5)
High Humidity Conditions					
35% Control	14.0	15.0 (73.7)	15.9 (50.0)	15.7 (55.3)	16.0 (47.4)
55% Control	13.5	14.5 (76.7)	15.0 (65.1)	15.0 (65.1)	15.5 (53.5)
Major Brand	12.5	14.0 (71.7)	14.7 (58.5)	14.7 (58.5)	14.7 (58.5)

A Conditioning Polymer from Croda

Croda strives to provide quality raw materials with proven efficacy that help personal care companies create innovative products. With this goal in mind, five new raw materials for hair care were launched in the past year. These raw materials are used in numerous types of hair care applications and provide a range of claims from enhanced color uptake to cuticle smoothing. All of these materials were developed in one of Croda's core technology areas: esters, phosphate esters, proteins and quaternary compounds.

The polymer: Utilizing years of work in protein chemistry, Croda has entered the styling polymer market with hydroxypropyltrimonium hydrolyzed maize starch[i], a trimethyl quaternized hydrolyzed maize starch with an average molecular weight of 250,000 d. This high molecular weight compound is able to provide excellent style retention properties and has been proven to reduce static flyaway, provide antifrizz properties from both leave-on and rinse-off products, and retain style even in high humidities (**Figure 8**).

---

[i] MiruStyle MFP (INCI: Hydroxypropyltrimonium hydrolyzed maize starch) is a product of Croda Inc.

Hydroxypropyltrimonium hydrolyzed maize starch (5% inclusion level) helps maintain a controlled sleek look. The tresses in **Figure 9** were treated with a retail product and a cream form of the Croda polymer. The naturally curly hair then was exposed to 85% RH for 15 minutes.

Hydroxypropyltrimonium hydrolyzed maize starch was evaluated at 10% inclusion in a Croda conditioner concentrate to be described later. This combination showed excellent antifrizz benefits (not presented here) demonstrating that hydroxypropyltrimonium hydrolyzed maize starch is effective from a rinse-off system.

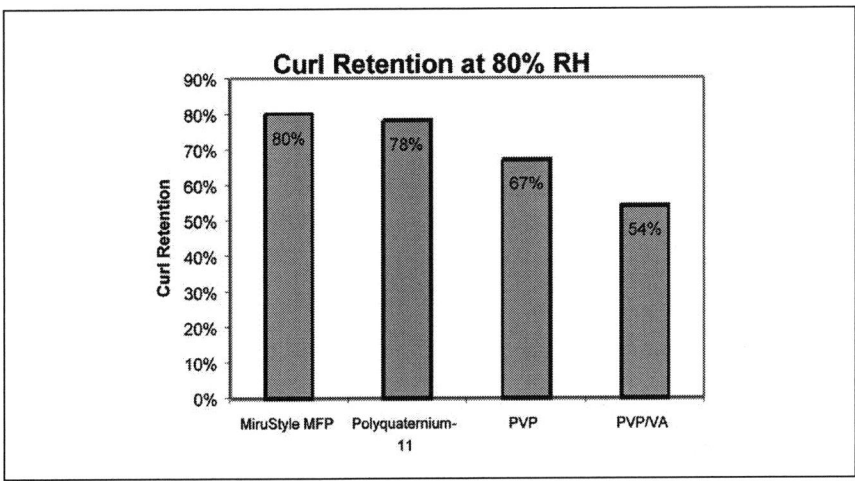

Figure 8. Curl retention studies show hydroxypropyltrimonium hydrolyzed maize starch is able to preserve style better even at high RH. (from Croda)

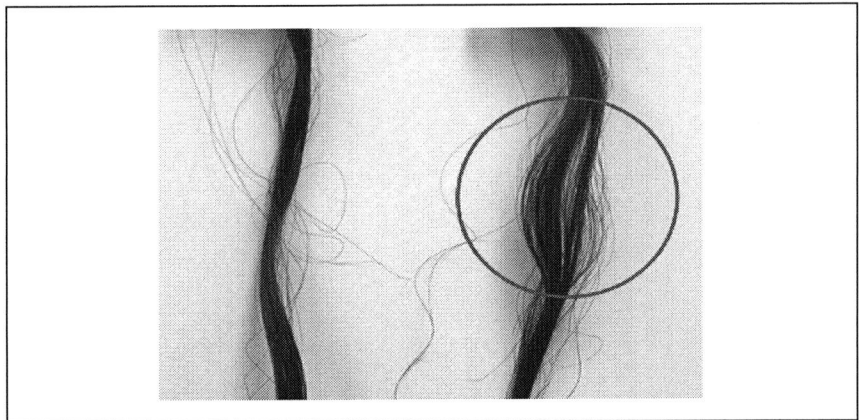

Figure 9. The antifrizz effect of hydroxypropyltrimonium hydrolyzed maize starch (left) at 5% versus a commercial conditioner (right) (from Croda)

Other polymers: A second protein launched this year and based on keratin was designed to moisturize and condition the hair. This keratin hydrolysate[j] is extracted from wool keratin fibers. It contains an unusually high level of cystine (~4%), the highest proportion of which (~65%) is S-sulfo cystine, occurring as a Bunte salt. This Bunte salt is charged inherently, giving it semireactivity in oxidative/reductive-type environments. As a result, this keratin hydrolysate is the ideal protein of choice for use in hair color, bleaching or permanent wave systems, and is suitable for pre- and post-treatment products.

As the winner of the 2004 Frost and Sullivan Excellence in Technology award in the field of fatty ester technology, Croda builds on this distinction with the introduction of an oligo ester[k] derived from sebacic acid and hydrogenated castor oil. This product was engineered specifically to seal down hair cuticles that have been damaged through coloring, bleaching, perming or thermal straightening. It adheres to the lifted cuticles, cementing them together and smoothing out the hair fiber. Its high refractive index, in combination with its smoothing action, contributes to shiny, glossy hair, and its substantivity will maintain this look even through multiple shampooings. It is recommended for use in deep conditioners, after-salon treatments or any other product designed for damaged hair.

Croda's work in phosphate ester technology has resulted in a color enhancer for hair dyes that also functions as an emulsifier in the tint. This complex mixture[l] of mono- and di-phosphate esters displays rheological behavior that slows down the initial oxidation rate in the emulsion and then promotes faster release of the oil-based dye active inside the hair. The smaller hair dye and coupler molecules are able to penetrate and react within the hair cortex, which allows more color to develop inside the hair fiber. This yields more vibrant color and better shampoo durability for long-lasting color.

---

[j]Keratec Pep (INCI: Water (aqua) (and) hydrolyzed keratin) is a product of Croda Inc.
[k]Crodabond CSA (INCI: Hydrogenated castor oil / sebacic acid copolymer) is a product of Croda Inc.
[l]Crodafos HCE (INCI: Oleth-5 phosphate (and) dioleyl phosphate) is a product of Croda Inc.

In addition to the functional raw materials that Croda launched this year, the company also has released a conditioner concentrate[m] designed for the salon hair care market. As the superior blend selected from a scientific screening process of 30 different prototypes, this concentrate is an optimized blend of conditioning agents, emulsifiers and stabilizers designed to create an elegant daily conditioner or intensive treatment. It is proven to deliver premium quality performance by adding only water and fragrance. This proprietary blend has been evaluated at 9% in a conditioner for wet comb benefits and tested for salon performance against a premium salon conditioner, where it performed as well as the commercial product. This provides a means for a formulator to create a high performance, salon-tested product with little development time and expense. As a conditioning base, the conditioner concentrate also provides for the creation of a range of products by the simple addition of carefully selected actives. A new dimension in functionality is provided by each variant.

A hair-strengthening protein[n] from Croda is composed of a copolymer of hydrolyzed vegetable protein and silicone. It is able to penetrate the cortex to bind moisture as well as form a protective film on the hair fiber to lubricate and reinforce the cuticle. It was evaluated at 1% inclusion in Croda's conditioner concentrate[q] by the flexabrasion fatigue lifetime method that evaluates the hair's resistance to breakage (strength). The addition of the protein to the conditioner increased the hair's flexabrasion lifetime by 68% over the conditioner alone and increased the strength of untreated bleached hair by 125% (data not shown).

An age-defying hair complex[o] has been derived from smaller molecular weight peptides and the higher molecular weight intermediate filament protein. Operating through sacrificial degradation and antioxidant mechanisms, this complex shields the hair from the aging and damaging effects of the environment (in particular, UV light and pollution). Evaluating tryptophan degradation as a marker for damage, the inclusion of 1% of this

---

[m]KeraMax+ is a proprietary blend from Croda Inc.
[n]Keravis (INCI: Hydrolyzed vegetable protein BG-propyl silanetriol) is a product of Croda Inc.
[o]Keratec IFP (INCI: Water (aqua) (and) keratin (and) hydrolyzed keratin) is a product of Croda Inc.

complex in Croda's conditioner complex[m] gave 100% protection of the hair from tryptophan damage caused by UV irradiation, thus providing an antiaging claim.

A polyester, polyquaternized UV absorber[p] has been designed to protect hair from the sun's UV rays. Previous studies demonstrated that it could preserve hair fiber tensile strength, hydrophobicity, combing properties and natural color. A conditioner comprised of 9% of Croda's conditioner concentrate[m] plus 2% of this UV absorber showed a 99.5% protection of the hair's tryptophan content (data not shown), implying complete UVB and total hair protein protection.

A hydrolyzed vegetable protein[q] capable of penetrating the hair's cortex brings moisture into the hair shaft. Studies show that addition of 4% of this protein to the Croda's conditioner complex[q] significantly improves its moisture regulating ability, showing a 37% improvement in the hydration protection index (data not shown).

A Conditioning Polymer from Dow Corning

Silicones have a long history of use in hair care, where they are recognized for providing conditioning, shine, manageability, improved combing and reduced flyaway. These versatile raw materials also offer heat and color protection, aid detangling, provide body, enhance straightening, or impart flexible styling properties. Here some novel properties and traditional conditioning functions of recently introduced silicone materials for hair care applications are reviewed.

Multifunctional silicone emulsions: Efficient formulating can be aided by silicones delivered in emulsion form, an approach that facilitates incorporation of potentially incompatible ingredients. It also allows simple pouring and mixing, as part of cold processes or with the addition of heat. Several recently introduced silicone emulsions offer processing advantages along with multifunctional properties in formulations.

Divinyldimethicone/dimethicone copolymer (and) C12-C13 pareth-3/C12-C13 pareth-23 is an emulsion[r] of ultra high

[p]Crodasorb UV-HPP (INCI: Butylene glycol (and) polyquaternium-59) is a product of Croda Inc.
[q]Hydrosolanum (INCI: Hydrolyzed vegetable protein) is a product of Croda Inc.
[r]HMW 2220 Nonionic Emulsion (INCI: Divinyldimethicone/dimethicone copolymer (and) C12-C13 pareth-3/C12-C13 pareth-23) is a product of Dow Corning Corp.

molecular weight silicone for use in shampoos, rinse-off and leave-on conditioners and styling products to meet several objectives. Among these objectives are increased fragrance intensity, extended fragrance release and prolonged hair color retention without loss of conditioning performance. The material is a 60% nonionic emulsion of very high viscosity (>120x10^6 mm^2/s at 0.01 Hz) polydimethicone/vinyl copolymer. It is dispersed easily in water and is suitable for cold processing. Researchers at Takasago International Corp. showed that presence of the silicone emulsion in a test shampoo resulted in greater perceived fragrance intensity of hair during the in-use phases of lathering, rinsing, blow drying and six hours after blow drying, when compared to the results of the same formulation without the silicone emulsion.[5]

Silicone quaternium-16 (and) undeceth-11 (and) butyloctanol (and) undeceth-5 microemulsion[s] performs multiple functions without sacrificing conditioning. The patented quaternary silicone polymer also has demonstrated protection from heat, improved permanent color retention, and enhanced body and volume. For still greater versatility, this silicone quat microemulsion can be used to create opaque and clear formulations.

An antifrizz silicone emulsion: Silicone quaternium-16/glycidoxy dimethicone crosspolymer (and) trideceth-12 emulsion[t] is modified by amine and elastomer technologies, resulting in an all-in-one solution for styling aids and fixatives. The effect in formulations is a soft feel combined with flexible hold.

This multifunctional ingredient protects hair from heat styling by helping to retain its moisture. It improves wet and dry combing, protects from heat, aids curl retention, adds shine, controls frizz and imparts superior aesthetics. The material also can be used in rinse-off products such as shampoos and conditioners. Its emulsion form simplifies formulation, particularly because the material is compatible with many other hair care ingredients.

Figure 10 illustrates how silicone quaternium-16/glycidoxy dimethicone crosspolymer (and) trideceth-12 controls frizz, which

---

[s]Dow Corning 5-7113 Silicone Quat Microemulsion (INCI: Silicone quaternium-16 (and) undeceth-11 (and) butyloctanol (and) undeceth-5) is a product of Dow Corning Corp.
[t]Dow Corning 5-7070 Si Amino Elastomer Emulsion (INCI: Silicone quaternium-16/glycidoxy dimethicone crosspolymer (and) trideceth-12) is a product of Dow Corning Corp.

is measured by the expansion of hair over time at 90% relative humidity. The material shows a marked improvement in frizz control over a silicone gum, cyclic and elastomer blend[u] and a commercial benchmark hair serum.

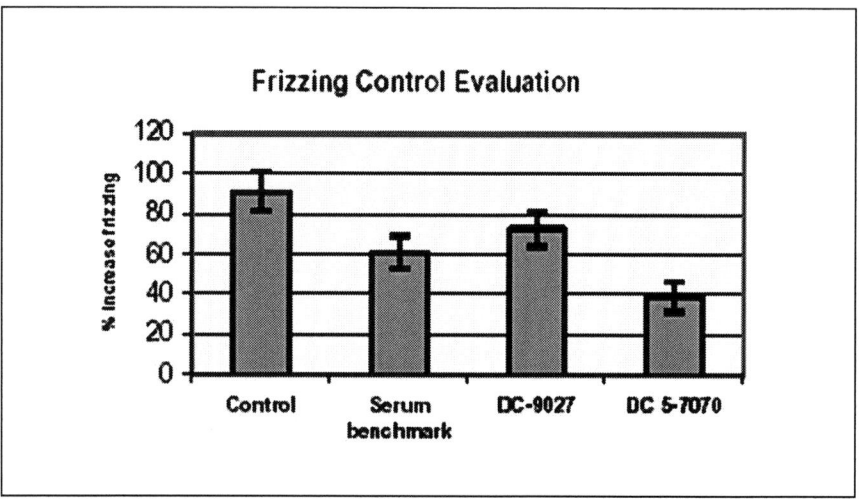

Figure 10. Silicone quaternium-16/glycidoxy dimethicone crosspolymer (and) trideceth-12 emulsion reduces the hair expansion associated with frizz after 2 h and 90% RH. (from Dow Corning)

Multifunctional silicone fluids: In addition to silicone emulsions, a number of silicone fluids have multifunctional properties in hair care formulations. These materials range from polyether- and amino-based fluids to silicone resins.

PEG/PPG-15/15 dimethicone[v] is a silicone polyether polymer that can be incorporated into clear and opaque product forms, where it imparts ultra shine with light-to-medium conditioning. The result is improved wet and dry detangling and a smooth feel, without weighing down the hair. In rinse-off conditioners, the silicone fluid helps control flyaway hair. The water-soluble material allows easy formulation for cold and hot processes, without the need for pre-emulsification, solubilizers or suspending agents.

---

[u]Dow Corning 2-9027 Styling Aid (INCI: Cyclopentasiloxane (and) dimethiconol (and) dimethicone crosspolymer) is a product of Dow Corning Corp.
[v]Dow Corning 5330 Fluid (INCI: PEG/PPG-15/15 dimethicone) is a product of Dow Corning Corp.

Bis (C_{13-15} alkoxy) PG amodimethicone[w] is an amino-functional silicone polymer. It was designed for clear and opaque conditioning shampoos, semipermanent and permanent colorants, and leave-in conditioning treatments such as detanglers, cuticle coats, hot oils, hair masks and mousses. It can be used in anhydrous as well as water-based systems for superior conditioning, excellent wet and dry detangling, a smooth feel and color retention. Formulators may choose cold or hot processing, and the silicone can be added at any stage. The material requires no solubilizers or suspending agents and is easy to emulsify.

Aminopropyl phenyl trimethicone[x] is a silicone resin that contains both amino- and phenyl-functional groups. Amino-functional silicones are known in the hair care industry for their ability to improve deposition on negatively charged hair.[6] The phenyl group imparts shine due to its high refractive index, and the liquid nature of the resin provides good film-forming capabilities to help ensure efficacy and uniformity once it is delivered onto the hair. Furthermore, because it is able to withstand a high pH environment, the silicone resin can be incorporated into relaxers and permanent wave formulations.

Conclusion

Consumer demand for hair care products goes beyond traditional washing and conditioning. Today's hair care marketplace is a competitive arena of highly differentiated products that offer a range of functions, including ease of combing, softness and manageability, easy styling, body and elasticity, and color retention. Fragrance is an enhanced part of the sensory experience, and consumers increasingly select products based on scent as well as performance. Multifunctional materials provide a route to innovative product forms, allowing formulators to capitalize on efficient product development and ease of processing.

Published November 2005 Cosmetics and Toiletries magazine

---

[w]Dow Corning 8500 Conditioning Agent (INCI: Bis (C13-15 alkoxy) PG amodimethicone) is a product of Dow Corning Corp.
[x]Dow Corning 2-2078 Fluid (INCI: Aminopropyl phenyl trimethicone) is a product of Dow Corning Corp.

References

1. *International Cosmetic Ingredient Dictionary and Handbook*, Washington, DC: Cosmetic, Toiletry, and Fragrance Association (1997)
2. R McMullen and J Jachowicz, Optical properties of hair – Effect of treatments on luster as quantified by image analysis, *J Cosmet Sci* 54 335 (2003)
3. R McMullen and J Jachowicz, Optical Properties of Hair – Detailed examination of specular reflection patterns in various hair types, *J Cosmet Sci* 55 29–47 (2004)
4. J Jachowicz and R McMullen, Mechanical analysis of elasticity and flexibility of virgin and polymer-treated hair fiber assemblies, *J Cosmet Sci* 53 345 (2002)
5. A Vagts et al, An emulsion of ultra high molecular weight silicone for enhanced hair care with fragrance delivery, presented at Personal Care Ingredients Asia (PCIA), Manila, March 5–7, 2003
6. CA Hoag, Evaluating silicone emulsions for global hair care applications, *GCI* 44–55 (Apr 1999)

Deposition from Conditioning Shampoo: Optimizing Coacervate Formation

Robert Y. Lochhead, Lisa R. Huisinga and Tara Waller
The Institute for Formulation Science, The University of Southern Mississippi, Hattiesburg, Miss., USA

KEY WORDS: deposition, coacervate, polymers, hair conditioning, shampoos

ABSTRACT: *New techniques are being offered to produce formulations faster and more cost effectively than ever before. Researchers at the Institute for Formulation Science have addressed this challenge by developing robotic combinatorial techniques for the preparation and investigation of complex mixtures.*

Most conditioning shampoos depend on deposition of a polymer-surfactant coacervate to confer good wet-combing and manageability. Complex coacervate formation is crucially dependent on the molecular characteristics of the polymer and surfactant species, and it is significantly affected by the presence of other ingredients such as cosurfactants and dissolved salts. The optimization of these systems presents a challenge to the formulator because of the astronomical number of possible compositions with different performance outcomes.

Conventional formulation practice requires literally years of laboratory experimentation to characterize and optimize products that depend on complex coacervate formation. Robotic combinatorial techniques that accelerate the characterization and optimization of complex coacervate formulations have been explored at the Institute for Formulation Science. There has been success in constructing compositional phase diagrams that "fingerprint" the compositional range of complex coacervate formation as a function of polymer and surfactant molecular characteristics and the presence of other ingredients. These diagrams quickly guide the formulator to compositions of interest, and dramatically reduce the time and effort required for the screening of new ingredients, the formulation of new products and optimization of existing products. This chapter briefly describes the application of combinatorial techniques to the detailed study of complex coacervation from the system: guar hydroxypropyltrimonium chloride (and) sodium lauryl ether sulfate (and) water (*aqua*) (GHCSL).[a]

Goddard's original research into the nature of the interaction of cationic polymers with anionic surfactants formed the technological platform for modern conditioning shampoos.[1] For systems comprised of a cationic hydroxyethylcellulose and anionic surfactants, Goddard showed that below the surfactant critical micelle concentration (CMC), an insoluble coacervate phase was formed and this phase was resolubilized at a surfactant concentration that was above the CMC. This mechanism formed the basis of the now familiar dilution-deposition concept for conditioning shampoos that relied on formulation of the solubilized coacervate in the shampoo and deposition of phase-separated coacervate as the system was diluted below the CMC upon rinsing.

However, behind this apparently simple mechanism there lies a complexity that continues to engage formulators to this day. Thus, patents continue to be issued in this area although more than 30 years have passed since the original discovery. The nature of the coacervate in these systems critically depends on factors such as polymer molecular weight, charge density, charge density distribution, and details of surfactant structure, cosurfactant ratio and the presence of electrolyte.

The coacervate properties must depend upon the conformation of the cationic polyelectrolyte and the hydration of that polyelectrolyte. The conformation of the polyelectrolyte depends, in turn, upon the

---

[a]INCI: name Guar hydroxypropyltrimonium chloride (and) sodium laureth sulfate and water (aqua)

ionic strength of the system as well as the exact nature of the ion-exchange process that causes surfactant to bind to the cationic sites.

The overall hydration will be affected by the availability of water binding groups such as hydroxyl groups on the polymer. Interaction of the cationic polymer with anionic surfactant micelles would be expected to change the micellar structure. It is well known that an increase in ionic strength will cause structural transitions from spherical to rod-like micelles, worm-like micelles or even lamellar phase. All of these micellar structures have distinct rheological properties and kinetics. Prediction and optimization of these systems is complicated by the complexities of the interactions. Alternatively, empirical formulation for ultimate understanding and optimization of the systems would require the study of a large number of possible polymers, charge densities, structures, molecular weights, surfactant types and ratios, ionic strength and electrolyte type. Such a study would require an army of formulators or a very long time to complete.

This challenge has been addressed by the Institute for Formulation Science with its development of robotic combinatorial methods for the study of these types of formulation problems requiring the generation of large data sets. At the present time researchers at the institute are engaged in developing their understanding of complex coacervates systems by the rapid generation and investigation of thousands of formulations in short time periods. The properties of these formulations are plotted as composition diagrams to guide the formulator.

The Combinatorial Investigation of Complex Coacervation

At the current time the preferred method for the preparation of complex mixtures at the institute is to utilize a robotic liquid handler[b] and to prepare mixtures in 96-well plates in which each well contains a sealable glass vial of appropriate size for the system being studied. The robotic equipment is limited to handling low-viscosity liquids. Therefore, researchers at the institute have developed multiple manual pipetting techniques to handle high-viscosity liquids.

[b]A product of Beckman-Coulter, Inc., Fullerton, Calif. USA

New pipette tips were used for each solution in order to avoid cross-contamination of the samples. When high throughput screening is conducted, it is necessary to include standard compositions to ensure the accuracy of the results; because instruments do drift with time, components such as pumps can fail. It is important to correct these deviations to avoid flawed data. With this in mind, at least two standard compositions in each 96–well plate were included and the measured values of these compositions were plotted. Any significant deviation was investigated immediately and, if necessary, corrective measures were taken.

The compositions were mixed by vortexing the 96-well plate. In order to ensure that the samples adequately were mixed, two dyed samples were included in each 96-well plate. Measurement of λ_{max} of the dye solution was a monitor for adequate mixing (see **Figure 1**).

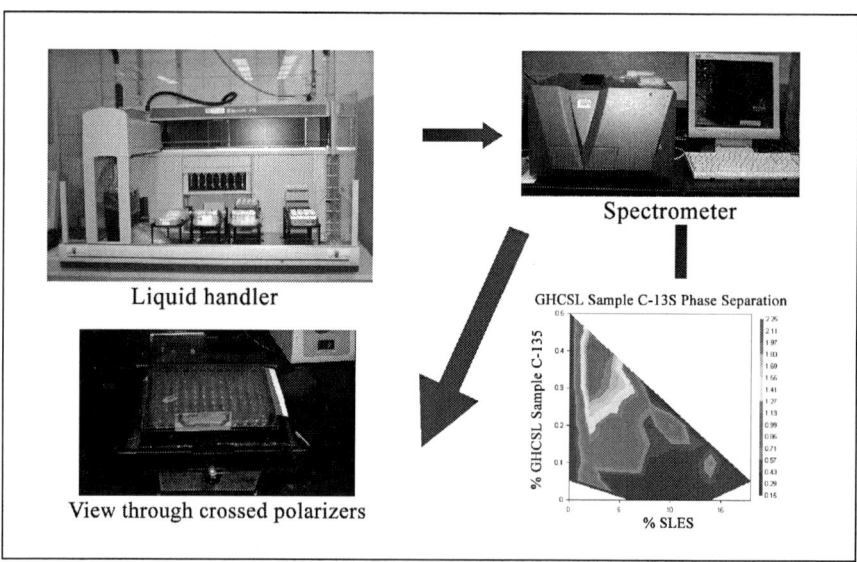

Figure 1: A combinatorial approach to the formulation of liquid products

High Throughput Analytical Techniques

Measurement using light or other common electromagnetic radiation is quick and nondestructive. Therefore, whenever possible, a spectrometer[c] capable of reading 96 samples as a single batch was

---

[c]The Safire UV/VIS is a product of Tecan Systems, Inc., San Jose, Calif. USA.

utilized. This instrument provided the capability to measure entire spectra, to measure wavelength shifts and to measure concentrations of desired species in a few minutes using Beers' Law.

The samples were viewed through crossed polarizers to detect birefringent phases such as liquid crystals. Microviscosities were measured by observing depolarization of biphenyls. The amount of coacervate in a sample was assessed by measurement of the absorbance in the visible region.

The data was collected in an interactive database and then visualized as color-coded composition maps. These composition maps showed the volume of complex coacervate formed as a function of polymer structure and composition, surfactant composition and electrolyte concentration. In original work to date, these maps have been shown to be distinctive for each polymer investigated. The precise mechanisms of coacervate formation and the driving forces involved were deduced from the characteristic patterns in the maps.

An important and usually time-consuming aspect of each of the studies is the validation of the high throughput experimentation methods with standard laboratory procedures and confidence that the methods will scale-up reliably.

Results

Cationic polymers, such as guar hydroxypropyltrimonium chloride, provide hair conditioning from shampoos. Guar hydroxypropyltrimonium chloride compounds, with varying molecular weights and charge densities, were combined with the anionic surfactant sodium lauryl ether (3EO) sulfate to form complex coacervates. Generating more than 350 compositions for each polymer/surfactant combination, researchers used high-throughput screening formulation methods to identify the structure and amount of coacervate formed. These results were represented using contour phase diagrams in order to map specific areas to study in detail. The detailed structures of the lyotropic association colloids that were selected from **Figures 2, 3** and **4**, were identified using polarized light microscopy.

One might expect that coacervate amount and composition range would increase with increase in polymer charge density. This indeed was observed as displayed in **Figure 2**, which shows increased amounts of coacervate as the polymer cationic charge density is increased from 0.14 to 0.17 moles per equivalent anhydroglucose unit.

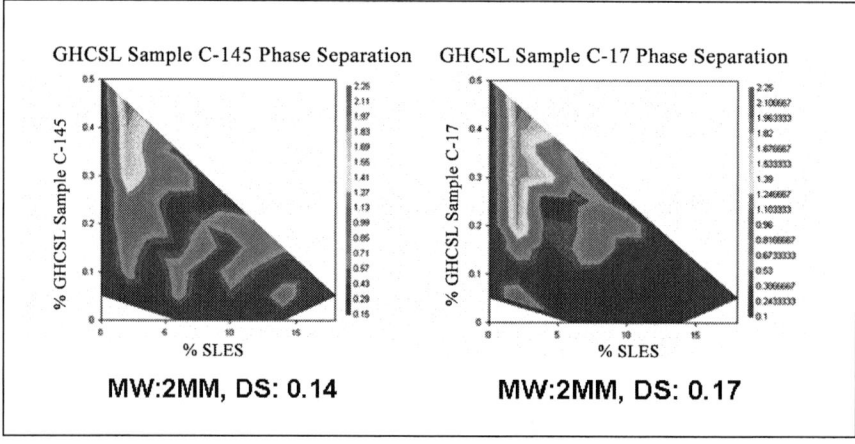

Figure 2: Composition diagrams for GHCSL. The diagrams are color-coded in accordance with the visual spectrum with blue representing the absence of coacervate and red indicating the maximum concentration of phase-separated coacervate. Each diagram was constructed from observations on at least 368 separate compositions and each composition was duplicated to check accuracy. The molecular weight was identical for both cationic guars but the degree of cationic substitution is 0.14 in diagram (a) and 0.17 in diagram (b).

The influence of polymer molecular weight on coacervate formation can be seen from **Figure 3**. Each of the three cationic guar samples possessed the same degree of cationic substitution (0.14), but they ranged in molecular weight from 1 million daltons (d) to 2 million d. It clearly is observed that the amount of coacervate formed increased in amount and concentration range as the polymer molecular weight was increased, despite the constancy of polymer charge density. There is a minimum polymer concentration that must be exceeded for coacervate formation to be observed. The lowest molecular weight polymer displays two islands of coacervate formation. It is suspected that this indicates two distinct mechanisms; one relying primarily on ion-exchange between the polymer and the anionic surfactant, and the other being driven by a change in surfactant micelle size and shape.

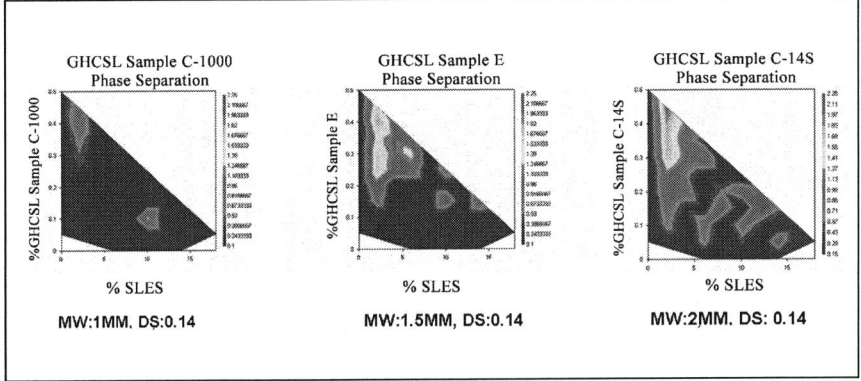

Figure 3: Composition diagrams showing regions of coacervate formation for GHCSL for cationic guars having the same change density but different molecular weights.

It is reasonable to assume that the interaction between oppositely charged polymer and surfactant should result in a collapse of the electrical double layers of both species. If this is the case, the response of the surfactant micelle should be to increase in size and to adopt a shape having lower surface curvature. Ultimately, the micelles might be expected to grow into lyotropic liquid crystals. Anisotropic lyotropic liquid crystals are optically birefringent; that is they rotate the plane of plane-polarized light. If lyotropic liquid crystals are present, they should be detectable by observing the compositions through crossed polarizers. This experiment was conducted for the systems shown in **Figure 3**. The result of the birefringence measurements are shown in **Figure 4**.

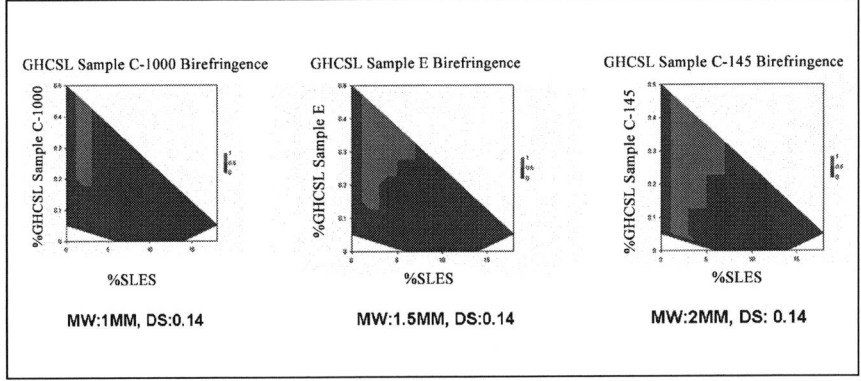

Figure 4: Composition diagrams showing regions of birefringent compositions for GHCSL for cationic guars having the same change density but different molecular weights. Birefringent compositions are shown in lighter gray.

It is notable that the compositional regions of birefringence correspond closely to the coacervate compositions reported in **Figure 3**. It was concluded, therefore, that the micellar structure of these coacervates is lyotropic liquid crystalline in nature.

Summary

Today's competitive environment demands that formulators produce tangible results at a greatly accelerated pace. Composition maps can be constructed rapidly to clearly show the effect of polymer molecular weight and charge density on the composition range of coacervation. Studies of birefringence indicate that the coacervates contain lyotropic liquid crystals. The composition maps provide valuable direction to formulators and can accelerate the development of new products and novel intellectual property.

Published March 2006 Cosmetics and Toiletries magazine

References

1. ED Goddard and KP Ananthapadmanabhan, eds, *Interactions of Surfactants with Polymers and Proteins*, CRC Press: Florida, Chapter 4 (1993)

CHAPTER 9

Advances in Polymers for Hair Styling

Robert Y. Lochhead and Lisa R. Huisinga
The School of Polymers & High Performance Materials, The University of Southern Mississippi, Hattiesburg, Mississippi USA

KEY WORDS: *Polymers, fixative, hair spray, styling, straightening, conditioning*

ABSTRACT: *Block and graft copolymers, including some produced by living free-radical polymerization, are among the new hair fixative polymers surveyed in this chapter. Other new polymers offer advantages in hair styling gels, hair straightening and hair conditioning.*

Hair spray consists of more than polymer. All components must be considered and these comprise fixative polymer, solvent, propellant, adjuvant and the valve system of the aerosol. Hair styling also has numerous components. In this chapter we'll discuss the hair styling components that depend on polymers. They include hair fixatives, styling gels, straighteners and conditioners. (For a brush up on the classes of polymer architecture discussed in this chapter, see **Figure 1**.)

Hair Fixatives

The desired attributes of hair fixatives include hair style hold improvement, ease of application on wet hair, ease of combing, no sticky feel, quick drying, not powdery or flaky during grooming, assurance of hair body and bounce, increased hair volume, no clumping of the hair, formation of a non-hygroscopic binding film that is removable by shampoo, good hair gloss, and no excessive stiffness.

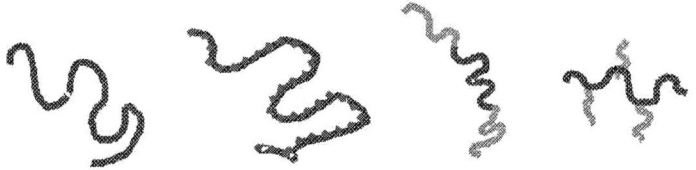

| Homopolymers consist of long molecular chains in which each link is an identical monomer. | Random copolymers consist of long molecular chains in which there are two different monomers and these are arranged randomly along the chain. | In Block copolymers the monomers are homopolymer blocks joined together. The figure depicts an ABA block copolymer. | In Graft or 'comb' copolymers branches consisting of one type of monomer are "hung" from a main chain consisting of another type of monomer. |

Figure 1. Contact angle greater than 90° causes the fibers to be pushed apart

Hair style hold improvement must be achieved with a minimal amount of fixative polymer applied easily from an aerosol spray, a pump spray, a gel or a mousse. For ease of application on wet hair, the solvent must be compatible with water and the polymer must not phase-separate as water permeates the system. The fixative system must also be safe; especially upon ocular exposure or inhalation.[1] For ease of combing, the cohesive strength of the polymer film must be less than the tensile strength and shear strength of the hair; and the adhesive bond of the film to the hair must be weaker than the shear strength of the hair. For conventional systems, sticky feel is avoided if the polymer in the dried film is immobile during the time of "touch" and has insufficient time to interact with the stratum corneum of the fingertips. Quick drying can be achieved either by judicious choice of solvent and propellant or by causing the system to gel. The mechanical property aesthetics of hair body and bounce, increased hair volume non-clumping and lack of extreme stiffness depend upon the hair matrix being lightly crosslinked rather than being coated by the applied polymer film. The film must be non-hygroscopic; otherwise it will be plasticized by absorbed water vapor under humid conditions. Such uncontrolled plasticization leads to loss of hold.

Random copolymers: During the last two decades the U.S. aerosol hair spray industry has been driven to develop low volatile organic compound (VOC) systems to comply with the Clean Air Act. In most cases this has meant the development of "aqueous" systems in which a significant portion of the solvent is replaced by water. This has posed two main challenges. First, the kinetics and thermodynamics of fiber wetting is less favorable for "aqueous" systems than the original solvent-based systems (see sidebar). This results in a reduction of capillarity and a concomitant loss of holding power due to the inter-fiber effects discussed above. The second challenge arises form the fact that the water rapidly penetrates into the hair cortex, plasticizing the hair and causing "droop" of the style.

Random copolymers have a solubility parameter that is intermediate between homopolymers made from the same monomers. Twenty years ago, conventional hair spray resins were designed to be soluble in a propellant mixture of ethanol solvent and propane/isobutane. As water was added to the polymer solution, the solvent mixture's solubility parameter could move out of range of that of the polymer and if this happened the polymer would phase separate. The configurational entropy of mixing increases as the polymer molecular weight decreases and this is manifested by solubility of the lower molecular-weight polymer in a wider range of solvents than a higher molecular-weight polymer. Therefore the polymer suppliers initially responded to the need for "aqueous-compatible" polymer by merely lowering the molecular weights of their polymer products. However, the lowering of molecular weight also resulted in poorer film properties and the consequent loss of holding properties imposed limitations on the extent to which this approach could be adopted.

Block and graft copolymers: Compared to random copolymers, block and graft copolymers can show dual solubility zones, with each zone corresponding to the solubility parameter of the respective homopolymers. Homopolymer mixtures do not, in general, form compatible blends because the large molecules have low entropies of mixing, and in the absence of large enthalpies of mixing, the free energies of mixing favor segregation of the polymer mixture into two phases – one rich in one of the homopolymers and the other phase that is rich in the other homopolymer.

Each of the component "molecular blocks" of block and graft copolymers also display such segregative phase separation. However, in this case because the molecular blocks are constituent parts of the same molecule, the segregation is limited to microdomain or nanodomain dimensions. This limited segregation leads to polymer alloys in which glassy microdomains confer mechanical rigidity and rubbery microdomains confer rubbery and shock-absorbing properties. These materials are thermoplastic elastomers and they often display enhanced mechanical properties. Thermoplastic elastomers comprise block copolymers containing rigid glassy blocks and soft rubbery blocks incorporated within each molecule and precise control of molecular weight of the blocks produces separation into exact micro- and nano-structures that can be "tuned" to display exact mechanical properties. Moreover, if the block copolymer is amphipathic (that is it comprises at least one hydrophilic polymeric segment and at least one hydrophobic polymer segment) it may form films that exhibit the desired resistance to humidity but susceptibility to shampoo.

Wetting of the Hair

Wetting of the hair by an applied polymer solution is extremely important because capillary forces are necessary to pull adjacent fibers together in order to form inter-fiber seam-welds and to cause migration of the solution to inter-fiber cross-points where the solution will be captured owing to a balance of Laplace pressure between the curvature at the hair-liquid interface and opposite curvature at the air-liquid interface. This phenomenon is commonly observed as the adhesion between the bristles when a paint-brush is loaded with paint. Dewetting of the hair can cause the fibers to be driven apart (**Figure 2**) and this would inhibit migration of the fixative solution to crosspoints of the hair matrix and prevent the formation of seam welds between fibers.

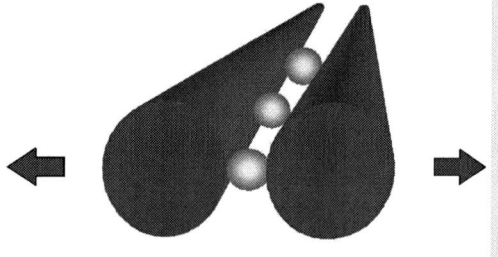

Figure 2. Contact angle greater than 90° causes the fibers to be pushed apart

In this context, it is interesting that Dubief et al[2] have reported that the inclusion of a non-thickening amphiphilic block copolymer in a fixative formulation with a conventional hair fixative polymer enhances the cosmetic and styling properties of the conventional polymer fixatives. The improvements are manifested by an increase in conditioning or styling power without increasing the total polymer concentration in the formula, or the same conditioning and styling benefits at reduced polymer concentration. The non-thickening polymer in this case is defined as a copolymer which when dispersed or dissolved in water leads to dynamic viscosities that are less than 0.1 Pa.s measured at a shear rate of 200 sec^{-1}. Examples of such amphiphilic block copolymer/ fixative polymer blends are demonstrated in **Table 1**.

Table 1
Examples of amphilic block copolymer/fixative polymer blends from Dubief[2]

Fixative Polymer	Amphiphilic Block Copolymer
Vinylpyrrolidone/vinylcaprolactam copolymer (Luvitec VPC 55K65W, BASF)	Poly(styrene-b-2-hydroxyethyl methacrylate) having block molecular weights: PS = 1500; PHEMA = 44,000
Vinylpyrrolidone/dimethylaminoethylmethacrylate copolymer (Copolymer 845, ISP)	Poly(styrene-b-acrylic acid) having block molecular weights: PS = 1500; PAA = 44,000
Polyurethane (Luviset PUR,BASF)	Poly(methylmethacrylate-b-acrylic acid) having block molecular weights: PMMA = 1200; PAA = 38,000
PPG-1/IPDI/DMPA copolymer (Avalure UR 450, Noveon)	—
Acrylic copolymer (Avalure AC115, Noveon)	—

The influence of the block copolymer on the morphology of the bulk material and/or on the adhesion of the fixatives to the hair surface could be speculated to follow the following scheme:

- Block copolymers tend to exhibit morphology of separated microdomains, each of which is rich in one of the blocks.
- Separation of discontinuous glassy domains in rubbery matrix would confer the properties of an elastomer

- Separation of rubbery domains in a glassy matrix would confer impact resistance.
- Separation of ionic microdomains within a nonpolar matrix would confer increases in toughness and tensile modulus.
- Ionic microdomains might be expected to confer susceptibility to shampoo that would lead to ease of removability from the hair after use.
- Alternatively, preferred adsorption of the block copolymer at the hair/fixative interface could lead to improved adhesion and consequently higher fixing of the hair.

The polydimethylsiloxone (dimethicone) chain is extremely flexible and hydrophobic and, as a consequence, this material is an excellent lubricant that confers conditioning benefits such as softness, disentangling and feel to hair. Thus, Dupuis[3] has claimed a terpolymer consisting of t-butyl acrylate, acrylic acid and a silicone macromer that is taught to provide softness, disentangling and feel benefits with simultaneous excellent styling and fixing properties.

Hair fixatives with improved flexibility are needed in Asia and in the United States. They should have good hold, natural feel, good combability, and they should be tack-free. BASF has sought to address this need by synthesizing a polyurethane/silicone polymer that provides smoothness and sleekness to the hair while being easy to wash out.[4] It is interesting that independent claim 1 of this patent lists polysiloxane as optional.

A polymer of *t*-butyl acrylate/methacrylic acid/N-butylacrylamide is taught to give easily washed-off hair hold with "soft touch".[5] The attributes in this case were tested by a curl-retention test and a panel-test for wash-off, hair feel and setting effect.

Improved shine, reduced flaking and better compatibility with modern solvent/propellant blends are taught for a product prepared from the polymerization of the following:[6]

- A C_2-C_{22} alkyl (e.g. *t*-butyl) (meth)acrylate
- A vinyllactam such as N-vinylpyrollidone
- A cationic acrylate or acrylamide monomer
- A silicone copolyol.

In another approach directed towards these combined attributes, BASF has introduced polyureas[7] prepared from a polyethoxylated diamine[a], an amine-containing or hydroxyl-containing polysiloxane[b] and a di-isocyanate.

Block copolymers from free radical polymerization: Block copolymers are well known. For example, styrene-butadiene, styrene-isoprene, styrene-ethylene, and styrene-propylene block copolymers have been available under the trademark Kraton for more than a quarter of a century. However, these are made by anionic living polymerization. This technique requires the absence of protons or abstractable hydrogen atoms and these constraints severely limit the choice of monomers and reaction media. Moreover, the costs of manufacture are relatively high due to the high reactant purity required for anionic polymerization.

These limitations are being overcome by the advent of living "free-radical" polymerization which offers the prospect of economically producing a wide range of block copolymer compositions in a broad array of reactant media. There are two main techniques for the polymerization of block copolymer elastomers by free radical living polymerization:

- The technique of free-radical polymerization by reaction with a nitroxide consists in blocking the growing free-radical species in the form of a bond of $C-ONR_1R_2$ type.[8-12]
- The RAFT (reversible addition-fragmentation chain transfer) polymerization technique consists in blocking the growing free-radical species in the form of a bond of C--S type.[13-14] Dithio compounds such as thiobenzoates, dithiocarbamates or xanthan disulfides are used to do this.

Mougin[15] has used free-radical living polymerization to prepare hair fixative polymers comprising (a) at least one rigid block having a glass transition temperature (Tg) of greater than or equal to 20°C, consisting of units derived from one or more ethylenic monomers, and (b) at least one flexible block having a glass transition temperature (Tg) of less than 20°C, consisting of units derived from one or more ethylenic monomers. These block copolymers produce a film having

---

[a]An example is Poly ESP 520 from Rachig.
[b]Examples include MAN and MAR brands from Degussa-Huls or the FINISH brands from Wacker.

an instantaneous recovery of between 5% and 100%. Such mechanical properties are characteristic of elastomers and the physical properties of these block copolymers should be distinctly different from the hard, glassy, brittle properties of conventional hair spray resins. Block copolymers having flexible blocks consisting exclusively of ethylene, propylene, butylene, butadiene and/or isoprene units are excluded in the patent claim.

Restylable fixatives: In a drive to satisfy a market that is moving towards water-soluble, low-VOC fixatives, National Starch has introduced nonionic derivatized starches,[16] poly-N-vinylacetamide,[17] amphoteric urethanes,[18] and dehydroxanthan gum.[19] Dehydroxanthan gum provides both thickening and hair fixative properties with high holding even in humid conditions. An added advantage is that it can be restyled by merely spritzing with water and combing or brushing.

Restyling has become an important attribute and several approaches have been adopted to bring restylable fixatives to market. These approaches include:

- Products similar to hot melt adhesives that allow remodeling of the hair style under the influence of a hair dryer.[20-22] These are based upon a National Starch product[c] that is reported to consist of 10 weight percent acrylic acid and 90 weight percent n-octadecyl methacrylate, and to have a crystalline melting point of 46°C.
- Semi-solids products that are prepared by including a polyalkylene glycol in which the hair-fixative resins is soluble.[23] This provides "reformable welds" that are liquid or semisolid at ambient temperature.

Hair Styling Gels

Hair styling gels are largely aqueous compositions and they are easily formulated to comply with the VOC requirements of the Clean Air Act but most preferred hair fixative polymers are incompatible with carbomer gels and this has restricted the formulations in this category to the early "workhorse" fixative polymers PVP and PVP/VA. These

---

[c]Structure 0 from National Starch

fixatives are marginally effective in hair styling, especially in conditions of high humidity. Moreover, PVP and PVP/VA copolymers impart an undesirable tacky or sticky feel to the hair. It has been reported that the tack can be reduced by the use of a reactive non-silicone polymer that produces tack on the hair that does not transfer to the hands.[24]

Some new polymers have been developed to be compatible with the traditional carbomer thickeners of this category. For example, National Starch introduced poly-N-vinylacetamide[25] to this market segment and researchers at Nalco have prepared fixative polymers that contain up to 10 weight percent of 2-acrylamido-2-methyl-1-propane sulfonic acid or its salts in combination with anionic or nonionic monomers.[26] These polymer fixatives provide a better balance between conflicting requirements of good curl retention at high humidity augmented by rapid and complete removal from the hair when rinsed with water. The additional polymers of this invention are also compatible with anionic thickening systems.

A possible extension of this class of polymers has been introduced by Clariant in the form of fluorine-modified comb polymers based on acryloyldimethyltaurine acid.[27] These polymers can be optimally crosslinked to improved their efficiency as associative thickeners. Perfluorocarbon chains do not easily associate or mix with hydrocarbon chains and the use of these thickeners could offer more formulation versatility.

Ease of dispersibility is water is an important criterion that is desired by gel manufacturers who wish fast process times or who are sensitive to the capital cost of mixing equipment. To meet this need, some polymer manufacturers have supplied inverse emulsion polymers or dispersions of thickening polymers in oil. However, the hydrocarbon oil vehicles have not always been desirable in personal care products. In this context, it is interesting that Ciba researchers have addressed the challenge by developing inverse emulsion polymeric thickeners as dispersions in silicone fluids.[28] As with other inverse emulsion polymers these are supplied with high HLB "activating" surfactant to enable the polymer to be dispersed and to thicken quickly when the phase is inverted when flooding with large amounts of water.

A new family of polymers has been introduced to simultaneously deliver thickening and film-forming capabilities. These polyacrylate-14 polymers[d] from Noveon are reported to provide thickening and hair fixing from aqueous and/or hydro-alcoholic systems.[29] The polymers, called rheology modifying hair setting (RMHS) polymers, contain:

- An acidic vinyl monomer (for example methacrylic acid)
- A nonionic monomer (for example ethyl acrylate)
- An associative monomer (for example a long chain alkyl ethoxylated methacrylate)
- Optionally a semi-hydrophobic monomer (for example an alkyl polyethoxylated methacrylate) and a cross linker (for example trimethylolpropanetriacrylate).

Hair Straightening

There are two main processes for relaxing or straightening hair:

- Hair treatment with a reducing agent to cleave of the disulphide cystine bridges (S--S) within the hair structure, mechanical "stretching" followed by an oxidizing treatment to reset the disulphide cystine bridges in a new, desired straightened hair conformation.
- Treatment of stretched hair with a strong alkaline agent.

Repeated relaxation treatments can result in rough hair that tends to become tangled.

The fundamental hair structure is damaged by the process of alkaline relaxing. Cationic and amphoteric polymers such as Polyquaternium-6, Polyquaternium-7 and Polyquaternium-39 are added to hair relaxer formulations to mitigate degradation of the hair structure.

The extent of damage can be assessed by measuring the porosity of the hair and the porosity of the keratin fibers can be measured by fixing 2-nitro-para-phenylenediamine at 0.25% in an ethanol/buffer mixture (10/90 volume ratio) at pH 10 at 37°C for 2 minutes.[30] Samain et al[30] reveal that the inclusion of high molecular-weight (>106 g/mole)

---

[d]Fixate Plus polymers from Noveon

polymers in the relaxing formula results in significant reduction in the hair structural damage caused by alkaline relaxation. The polymers are synthesized by precipitation polymerization in salt solution. The salt solution is of sufficient in strength to cause the growing polymer to precipitate upon reaching a critical molecular weight. The polymers are delivered to the substrate as a particulate dispersion in a concentrated salt solution. The claimed polyelectrolytes can be anionic, nonionic or cationic. The anionic polymers can be made from acrylic acid, methacrylic acid, acrylamido-2-methylpropanesulphonic acid, and itaconic acid. The nonionic monomers can be polymerized from the monomers acrylamide, methacrylamide, N-vinylformamide, N-vinylacetonamide, hydroxypropyl acrylate, and hydroxypropyl methacrylate. The cationic polymer can be, for example, copolymers of acrylamide and diallyldimethyl ammonium chloride, acryloyloxytrimethylammonium chloride, or acryloyloxyethyldimethylbenzylammonium chloride. Interestingly, these polymers are not effective for oxidation-reduction restyling.

Hair Conditioning

Conventional conditioner formulations are based upon either ceto-stearyl trimethylammonium chloride plus ceto-stearyl alcohol or distearyldimethylammonium chloride. These have been the workhorses of conditioners for decades and they do provide excellent detangling, wet- and dry-combing, and good anti-static properties, but they can leave the hair feeing lank and greasy. Polymeric conditioners can improve wet combability and ameliorate electrostatic charging of the hair (manifested by flyaway). For example, polyquaternium-10 can be applied as a conditioner to confer such benefits. Polyquaternium-7, a copolymer of acrylamide and diallyldimethylammonium chloride, and the homopolymer of polydiallyldimethylammonium chloride (polyquaternium-6) are found in conditioner formulations.

Recently, a patent was granted to Alzo International for polyurethane conditioners with enhanced conditioning properties.[31] These are made by reacting trialkanolamine (preferably triethanolamine) with a hydroxy fatty acid (ricinoleic acid, lactic acid or salicylic acid) to make a mono-, di- or triester, then reacting with a di-isocyanate to produce a polyurethane with tertiary amine functionality, then quaternizing the tertiary amines. The benefits claimed are better adhesion to hair and skin than conventional cationic conditioners. This leads to lower usage levels that in turn result in cost savings. The polyurethane conditioners confer excellent surfactancy, sheen, wet combing, dry combing, antistatic and conditioning properties.

Leave-on silicone conditioners specifically targeted to non-shampoo applications have been revealed by Unilever.[32] These contain emulsified vinyl-terminated silicones applied in combination with a conventional cationic conditioner. A preferred product type is a mousse. The significance of this claimed invention rests on the basis that these silicone block copolymers can achieve excellent conditioning at relatively high viscosities (100 KPa.s^{-1}). Aqueous foaming shampoo compositions containing emulsified vinyl silicone polymers are described in a copending application.[33]

Effective clear conditioners have been one of the long-standing challenges of cosmetic formulators. Conventional conditioners, comprising cationic surfactant and long chain alkanols form a gel matrix that confers conditioning benefits from rinse-off products but they give a long-lasting slippery feel during rinsing and this is perceived by some consumers as unclean hair feel. There is a need for clear conditioning compositions with suitable "conditioning" rheology conferred from something other than a gel matrix (defined as having a Brookfield RT viscosity of 5,000 to 20,000 cps at 2 sec^{-1}) and rinse-off to leave a clean feel while depositing sufficient material to confer benefits such as softness and reduced tangling of wet hair, and good wet-combing. Crystal clarity in the formulation is also desired as a visual cue to the consumer. Such conditioners should not weigh down the hair and should offer the opportunity to volumize fine hair. A recent patent application[34] claims that these benefits can be achieved from aqueous-based conditions comprising a cationic crosslinked thickening polymer and nonionic, cationic surfactants or mixtures of these. It is notable that these claimed conditioners contain no water-insoluble high-melting-point oils or waxes. The cationic crosslinked polymers, such as polyquaternium-32[e], are copolymers of dimethylaminomethacrylate and acrylamide

---

[e]Examples include Salcare SC95 and SC96 from Ciba or Synthalen CR, CU and CV from 3V Sigma.

crosslinked with methylene-*bis*-acrylamide. A homopolymer of quaternized dimethylaminoethylmethacrylate crosslinked with methylene-*bis*-acrylamide is especially preferred.

Similarly, scientists at BASF have recently been awarded a patent for a process of conditioning hair by the application of a crosslinked cationic thickening polymer.[35] The polymer comprises N-vinylimidazoline or a derivative, an N-vinyllactam such as N-vinylpyrollidone, and a short chain alkyl (meth)acrylate.

The application of cross-linked cationic polymers could herald a new innovative era for hair conditioners.

Conclusions

From the many polymer concepts discussed in this chapter, one can draw the following conclusions:

- Advances in polymer synthesis technology are leading to the ability to precisely control molecular architecture. This promises to yield low-VOC hair fixatives with improved film-forming mechanical properties and ease of removal by shampoo.
- The trend in hair gels is towards new copolymers that display dual functionality as gels and fixatives with the capability of being restyled by merely spritzing with water and combing or brushing.
- New cationic polyelectrolytes are the enabling technology for hair conditioning products that are crystal clear.

Published May 2005 Cosmetics and Toiletries magazine

References

1. C Zviak, *The Science of Hair Care*, New York: Marcel Dekker (1986)
2. US Pat Application 2004/00338246, Hair treatment compositions containing at least one non-thickening of amphiphilic diblock copolymer and at least one film-forming polymer which is beneficial for the hair, C Dubief, F Giroud and I Rolla (Feb 19, 2004)
3. US Pat 6,592,854, C Dupuis, assigned to L'Oréal (Jul 15, 2003)
4. US Pat 6,579,517, SN Kim, A Samir and V Schehlman, assigned to BASF (Jun 17, 2003)
5. US Pat 6,482,393, V Schehlmann, K Sperling-Vietmeier, A Sanner and R Blankenburg, assigned to BASF (Nov 19, 2002)
6. US Pat 6,737,049, SN Kim, A Sanner and V Schehlmann, assigned to BASF (May 18, 2004)
7. US Pat 6,800,276, SN Kim, A Sanner, P Hossel, assigned to BASF (Oct 5, 2004)
8. Intl Pat Application WO 9718247 A1, Improved processes based on atom (or group) transfer radical polymerization and novel (co)polymers having useful structures and properties, K Matyjaszewski, S Coca, S Gaynor, D Greszta, T Patten, J Wang and J Xia (1997)

9. K Matyjasezwski et al, *J American Chem Soc* 117 5614 (1995)
10. S Kobatake, HJ Harwood, RP Quirk, Synthesis of nitroxy-functionalized polybutadiene by anionic polymerization using a nitroxy-functionalized terminator, *Macromolecules* 30 4238-4242 (1997)
11. Intl Pat Application WO 9903894 A1, Polymerizable compositions containing alkoxyamine initiators derived from nitroso- or nitrone compounds, P Nesvadba, A Kramer, A Steinmann and W Stauffer (1999)
12. E Malmstroem, C Hawker and J Craig, Macromolecular engineering via living free radical polymerizations, *Macromol Chem Phys* 199 923-935 (1998)
13. WO-A-98/58974, E Malmstroem, C Hawker and J Craig (1998)
14. Y K Chong, Tam PT Le, G Moad, E Rizzardo and SH Thang, A more versatile route to block copolymers and other polymers of complex architecture by living radical polymerization: the RAFT process, *Macromolecules* 32 2071-2074 (1999)
15. US Pat 6,805,872, N Mougin, assigned to L'Oréal, (Oct 19, 2004)
16. US Pat 6,562,325, Use of stabilized starches in low VOC, polyacrylic acid-containing hair cosmetic compositions, M Vitale, M Tolchinsky, G Martino, D Solarek and L Cottrell, assigned to National Starch (May 13, 2003)
17. US Pat 6,599,999, Hair care compositions containing polymeric N-vinyl acetamide and methods of treating hair, R Chandran, J-P Leblanc and H Hanazawa (Jul 29, 2003)
18. US Pat 6,737,069, Cosmetic compositions containing amphoteric polyurethanes, S Asaoka, K Koyama, T Tsuzuki and T Hashimoto (May 18, 2004)
19. H Cao, K Maurer and M Vitale, Dehydroxanthan gum, *Happi* (May 2004) p 82
20. US Pat Application 2003/0143180, Hairstyling composition which makes possible remodeling of the hairstyle and process for remodeling the hairstyle using such a composition, H Samain (Jul 31, 2003)
21. US Pat 6,667,378, Reshapable hair styling composition comprising heterogeneous (meth) acrylic copolymer particles, I Rollat, H Samain and O Morel (Dec 23, 2003)
22. US Pat 6,645,478, Reshapable hair styling composition comprising (meth)acrylic copolymers of four or more monomers, I Rollat, H Samain and O Morel (Nov 11, 2003)
23. US Pat 6,585,965, Hair care compositions comprising polyalkylene glycol styling agents, J Caballada, D Kuhlman and M Schneider (Jul 1, 2003)
24. US Pat Application 2003/0157136, Cosmetic composition forming a tackifying coating comprising a polymer with a non-silicone skeleton and reactive functional groups, H Samain, I Rolla-Corvol, F Giroud, N Mougin and A Livorel (Dec 26, 2002)
25. US Pat 6,599,999, Hair care compositions containing polymeric N-vinyl acetamide and methods of treating hair, R Chandran, J-P Lebranc and H Hanazawa (Jul 29, 2003)
26. US Pat 6,569,413, Hair fixative composition containing an anionic polymer, YZ Hessefort, DE Betts and WM Carlson, assigned to Ondeo Nalco Company (May 27, 2003)
27. US Pat 6,833,419, R Morschhauser, C Kayser and M Loffler, assigned to Clariant (Dec 21, 2004)
28. US Pat 6,833,406, M Green, HR Dungworth, DE Gavin and DB Ridley, assigned to Ciba (Dec 21, 2004)
29. US Pat Application 2003/0202953, Hair setting compositions, polymers and methods, K Tamaraselvy and KL Ramey (Oct 30, 2003)
30. US Pat Application 20040265256, H Samain and A Livoreil (Dec 30, 2004)
31. US Pat 6,800,716, A Zofchak and J Obeji, assigned to Alzo International (Sayreville, NJ) (Oct 5, 2004)
32. US Pat Application 20050002871, K Ivanova and SK Pratley, filed by Unilever (Jan 6, 2005)
33. Patent Application GB 0102657.4 (filed Feb 2, 2001)
34. US Pat Application 20050002892, GF Khan, SM Guskey and RL Wells (Jan 6, 2005)
35. US Pat 6,682,725, R Dieing, P Hossel, S Kothrade, A Sanner, K Zeitz, H-J Raubenheimer and V Schehlmann, assigned to BASF (Jan 27, 2004)

CHAPTER 10

Advances in Polymers for Hair Coloring

Robert Y. Lochhead
The University of Southern Mississippi, Hattiesburg, Mississippi USA

KEY WORDS: *polymer, hair care, hair dyes, color retention, lightening, associative thickeners, non-associative thickeners, HASE thickeners, HEUR thickeners*

ABSTRACT: *This chapter surveys patents and technical literature, principally from the past 10 years, to report advances in polymers used for dyeing hair, color retention, and hair lightening. Associative thickeners (anionic, cationic, amphoteric, nonionic, HASE, HEUR), non-associative thickeners, and silicones are discussed.*

Polymers play several roles in the coloring of hair. They act as thickeners for oxidation dyes. In this role polymers include a range of associative thickeners (anionic, cationic, amphoteric, nonionic, and hydrophobically modified alkali swellable) as well as hydrophobically modified ethoxylated urethanes. Alkylmethicones and aminosilicones play a role in color retention. Non-associative thickeners help in achieving hair lightening.

This chapter surveys patents and technical literature, principally from the past 10 years, to report advances in polymers for hair coloring.

Thickeners for Hair Dyes

Oxidation dyes are made up of dye precursors (such as **ortho**- and **para**-phenylenediamine, or **ortho**- and **para**-amino phenols). The dye precursors are colorless compounds that can penetrate the hair fiber and in the presence of oxidizing agent, they condense to become colored compounds. The color can be modified by including "couplers" such as meta-phenylenediamine.

The oxidation dye compositions are usually thickened to localize the dye action on the hair and to prevent the dye composition from flowing down the face and into the eyes. Originally, thickeners such as carbomers,[1] hydroxyethylcellulose, or low HLB surfactants were used. The structure of carbomers consists of microgels of cross-linked poly(acrylic acid), whereas hydroxyethylcellulose thickens by entanglement of the relatively rigid-backboned cellulose macromolecules. It has been reported that oxidation dye compositions thickened with these traditional thickeners result in a dull shade on the hair and as a result, high concentrations of dyes are required to obtain intense colors.[2]

The challenges that must be overcome with two-part dye systems are: prevention of separation during storage; enhancing the slow diffusion of dye precursor onto the hair fibers; and ensuring efficient rinseability of the colorant after application.[3] Casperson listed the following conditions of thickened oxidation dye compositions:[4]

- The formulations must be stable to insure a reasonable shelf life.
- The compositions formed by mixing the lotion and developer must have rheological properties to allow the applied composition to readily distribute the dye throughout the hair mass and avoid dripping or running from the hair during the color development period.
- The dye mixture, as applied to the hair, should allow rapid diffusion of the dye precursors from the dye mixture into the hair fiber.
- The thickened mixture should be readily rinseable from the hair with water.
- The mixture should contain conditioning agents that leave the hair easy to detangle while wet and should feel smooth and be readily managed when dry.
- The lotion and developer should preferably, but not necessarily, have comparable viscosities in order to facilitate mixing.
- The dyeing effect should be rapid, with a dyeing time preferably under 30 minutes.

Oxidation dyeing in the presence of a thickener is a complex process in which it is reasonable to assume that adsorption of the thickener and the structure of the thickener can alter the rate and mechanism of diffusion of dye precursor and condensate into the hair. Therefore, it is interesting to consider the structure of the thickeners with their reported performance in oxidation dyeing. In many modern oxidation dyes, associative thickeners are employed. A range of associative thickeners is now available.[5-7] Examples of 4 different types are shown next.

Anionic associative polymers: Steareth-10 allyl ether/acrylates copolymer is the INCI nomenclature for terpolymers of methacrylic acid ethyl acrylate and steareth-10 allyl ether (for example Salcare SC80 or SC90 from Ciba Specialty Chemicals).

Acrylates/Steareth-20 methacrylate copolymer is the INCI nomenclature for methacrylic acid/ethyl acrylate/stearyl methacrylate oxyalkylenated terpolymer (for example, Aculyn 22 from Rohm & Haas).

Acrylates/C10-C30 alkyl acrylate crosspolymer are cross-linked copolymers of acrylic acid and C10-C30 alkyl (meth)acrylates (for example, Pemulen polymeric emulsifiers and selected Carbopol resins from Noveon; Coatex polymers from Seppic).

Maleic anhydride/C30-C38 alpha olefin/alkyl maleate terpolymers (for example Performa V from New Phase Technologies) are another example.

Polyacrylate-3 is a copolymer of methacrylic acid, methyl methacrylate, methylstyreneisopropyl isocyanate and PEG-40 behenate monomers. (Examples include the anionic associative polyurethanes, Viscophobe DB 1000 from Dow Chemical.)

Cationic associative polymers: These include associative polyurethanes, such as polyureas or polythioureas, prepared by reaction of selected amines, diisocyanates and hydrophobic compounds that are capable of coupling to form telechelic end groups on the polymer.

Polyquaternium-24 is the quaternized ammonium salt of hydroxyethylcellulose reacted with a lauryl dimethyl ammonium substituted epoxies. (An example is the Quatrisoft family of polymers from the Amerchol division of Dow Chemical Company.)

PG hydroxyethylcellulose coco-dimonium chloride, PG hydroxyethylcellulose lauryldimonium chloride, and PG hydroxyethylcellulose stearyldimonium chloride are quaternary ammonium salts of hydroxyethylcellulose. (An example is the Crodacel family of polymers from the Croda Company.)

Amphoteric associative polymer: One example is acrylic acid/(meth)acrylamidopropyl-trimethylammonium chloride/stearyl methacrylate terpolymers.

Nonionic associative polymers: Cetyl hydroxyethylcellulose is the cetyl ether of hydroxyethylcellulose (for example, Natrosol Plus CS modified hydroxyethylcellulose from Aqualon).

Hydroxyethyl ethylcellulose is the ethylene glycol ether of ethylcellulose (for example, Bermocoll EHM 100 from Berol Nobel).

Alkyl hydroxypropyl guars are the alkyl ethers of hydroxy propyl guar. [Examples include Esaflor HM 22 (C22 alkyl chain) from Lamberti, and RE210-18 (C14 alkyl chain) and RE205-1 (C20 alkyl chain) from Rhone-Poulenc.]

VP/Hexadecene copolymer and VP/Eicosene copolymer are copolymers of N-vinyl pyrrolidine with hexadecane and eicosene, respectively. [For example, Antaron V216 and Ganex V216 (vinylpyrrolidone/hexadecene copolymer), and Antaron V220 or Ganex V220 (vinylpyrrolidone/eicosene copolymer) from I.S.P.]

PEG-150/stearyl alcohol/SMDI copolymer is a copolymer of PEG-150 saturated methylene diphenyldiisocyanate and stearyl alcohol monomers. (Examples include the HEUR thickeners Aculyn 46 and Aculyn 48 from Rohm & Haas.)

PPG-14 palmeth-60 hexyl dicarbamate is the carbamic acid diester of the polypropylene, polyoxyethylene ether of the fatty alcohols derived form **Elaeis guineensis** (palm) kernel oil. (An example is the HEUR thickener Elfacos T212 from Akzo Nobel.)

Polyether-1 is a copolymer of PEG-180, Dodoxynol-5, PEG-25 tristyrylphenol, and tetramethoxy-methylglycouril monomers. The aminoplast skeleton of these thickeners offers enhanced stability. (Examples of polyether-1 include Pure Thix 1442, Pure Thix 1450 and Pure Thix HH from Sud-Chemie.)

Hydrophobically modified alkali swellable associative polymers: Pohl et al have reported that acrylates/steareth-20 methacrylate copolymer (Acrysol ICS-1 from Rohm and Haas) was capable of thickening hydrogen peroxide solution and this made it possible to prepare a 2-part system in which the acrylates/steareth-20 methacrylate copolymer, hydrogen peroxide and dye precursors in one part were thickened by adding a second part consisting of a base such as ammonium hydroxide.[8]

However, anionic acrylate thickeners tend to form complexes with the quaternary ammonium surfactant conditioners in the composition. Also, formulations thickened with simple aqueous polyacrylate are difficult to rinse from the hair and it is difficult to formulate to a consistent viscosity with Acrysol ICS-1.[4]

Casperson et al reported that the use of the acrylates/steareth-20 methacrylate copolymers Aculyn 22 and Aculyn 33 overcame these problems. Acrylates/steareth-20 methacrylate copolymer is a hydrophobically-modified alkali-swellable (HASE) thickener. In this case there are two mechanistic components that work jointly to produce the observed thickening.

- The first component is polyion swelling, which occurs when the polymer is neutralized with base and becomes a polyelectrolyte; the resulting polyion swells as a result of mutual ionic repulsion of the carboxylate ions that are covalently attached to the polymer chain.
- In the second mechanistic component, swollen thickener molecules are hydrophobically associated to form an overall network structure. The hydrophobic associations between the macromolecules are easily disrupted by shear and are reformed in a new conformation when the shear force is ceased.

The hydrophobic associations confer useful properties. For example, the efficiency of a molecular "network" is obtained without the elastic recoil that would normally be connected with crosslinked elastomers. However, steric hindrance of the polymer chains results in a significant proportion of the hydrophobic groups being isolated and unassociated in the aqueous environment.

This leads to the interesting observation that addition of surfactant causes first an increase in measured viscosity followed by a viscosity decrease when the surfactant concentration exceeds the critical micelle concentration. Such behavior is observed because co-micellization between the "isolated" polymer hydrophobes causes an increase in the number of "crosslink" sites. However, when sufficient micelles are present, the stoichiometry of co-micellization favors at most only one polymer hydrophobe per micelle and mutual repulsion between the micelles causes disruption of the network.

The effect of surfactant on the viscosity of HASE thickener solutions with a schematic molecular explanation is shown in **Figure 1**. Hydrophobic interactions between the macromolecules can be disrupted by associating surfactant micelles.

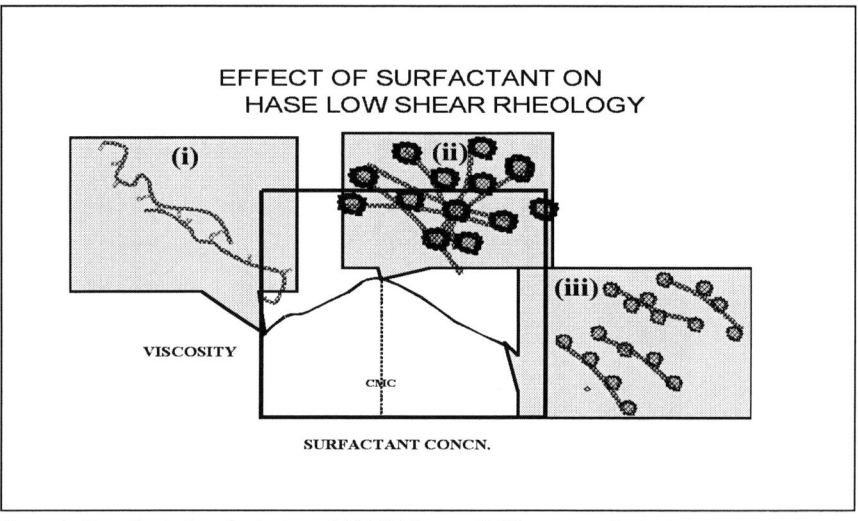

Figure 1. The effect of surfactant on HASE thickener. (i) When no surfactants are present some of the polymer hydrophobes are isolated and do not participate in network formation. (ii) In the vicinity of the cmc, the co-micelles enhance the associative network. (iii) Above the cmc the co-micelles mutually repel and the associative network is disrupted.

Consider the case of hydrophobically modified copolymers of acrylamidopropane sulphonic acid or salt and methacrylate esters of ethoxylated or propoxylated fatty alcohols. When these ingredients are incorporated with hydrogen peroxide in a developer formula used with an oxidation dye precursor compound, they have been claimed to achieve improved stability against separation that leads to an enhancement of hair coloration.[3] The polymer in this case is ammonium acryloyldimethyltaurates/beheneth-25 methacrylate crosspolymer (Aristoflex HMB from Clariant Corporation).

Hydrophobically modified ethoxylated urethanes: Enhanced color intensity from thickened oxidation dyes is achieved if the thickener is an amphiphilic polyether urethane.[2] These thickeners are commonly called hydrophobically modified ethoxylated urethanes, often shortened to the acronym HEUR.[10-12] In this particular case, the HEUR that is revealed is PPG-14 palmeth-60 hexyl dicarbamate (Elfacos T-212 and T-210 from Akzo Nobel).

The HEUR thickeners are ABA triblock copolymers in which the A blocks are hydrophobic and the B blocks are hydrophilic poly (alkoxylate).

HEURs are also available as graft/block copolymers with comb architecture. In the micelle, these molecules are bent into "hair-pin" confirmation with the hydrophobic ends in the micelle core and the hydrophilic "middle" interacting with water in the micelle corona (**Figure 2**).

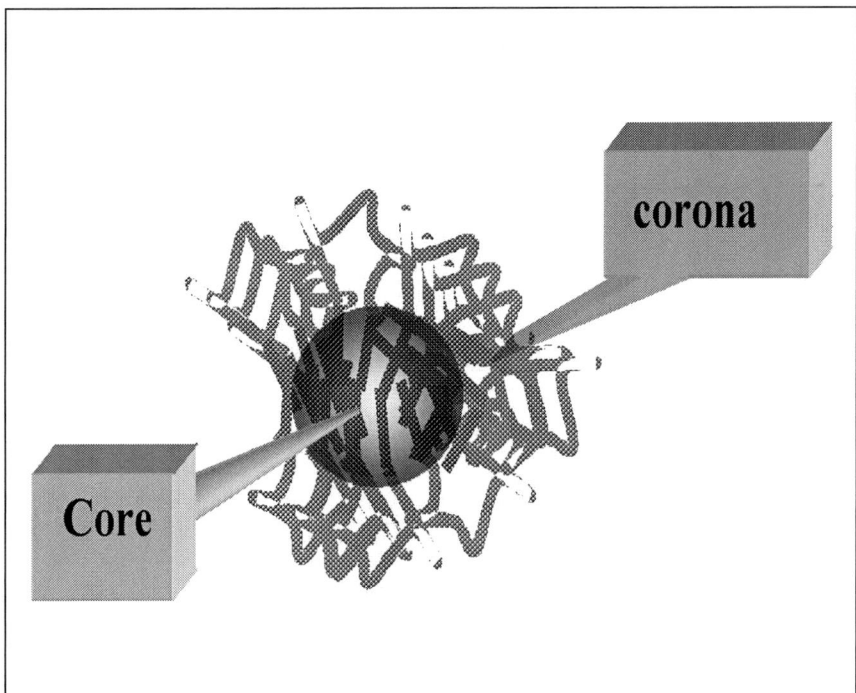

Figure 2. The HEUR molecules form multimolecular micelles with hydrophobic cores and poly(alkoxylate) coronas that are hydrophilic.

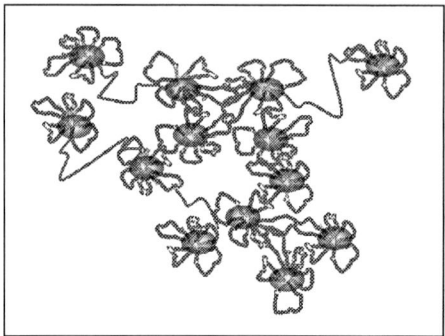

Figure 3. The HEUR molecules form micelles that are connected into networks by molecules that stretch between micelles.

A network is formed by some HEUR molecules that stretch between and link the micelles (**Figure 3**).[13] Comb-type HEURS show low aqueous solution viscosity, but they do offer better network formation and co-micelle association.[14-16]

Systems thickened by HEURS display pronounced shear thinning when the shear stress exceeds a critical value that corresponds to the stress that is necessary to extract the linking molecules from the micelles (**Figure 4**).[17] This model is supported by the fact that these systems can display a single relaxation time that corresponds to the process of the hydrophobic group being extracted from the micelle.[18]

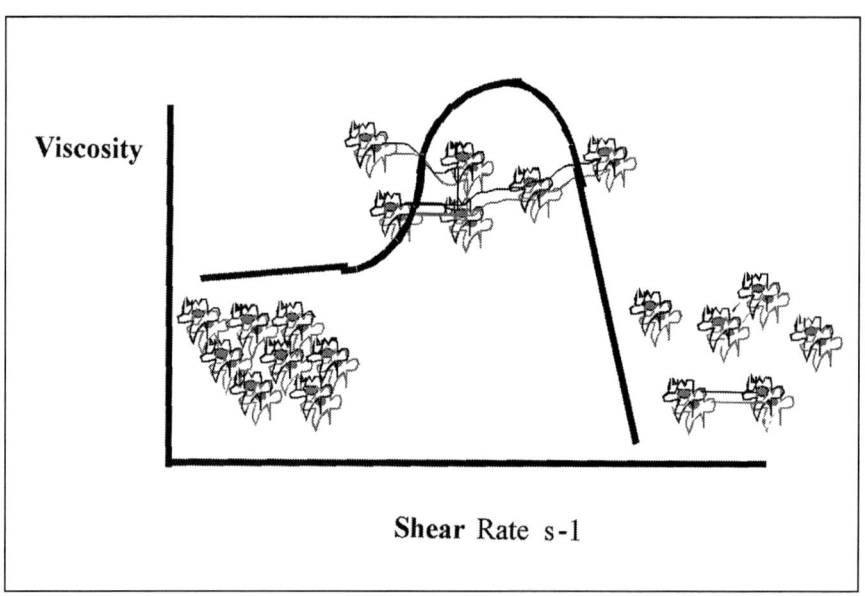

Figure 4. Shear thinning occurs when the shear rate exceeds the value that is necessary to "pull out" the linking molecules between the micelles.

The addition of even low concentrations of conventional surfactants to HEUR-thickened systems results in a dramatic loss of viscosity due to competition for residence of the micelle core between the surfactants and the HEUR linking molecules (**Figure 5**).[13]

Aminoplast thickeners function by similar rheological mechanisms as HEUR thickeners. Aminoplast reagents are the aldehyde reaction products of melamines, ureas, benzoguanamines, and glycolurils (**Figure 6**).[19]

The aminoplast thickeners are taught to cause bleaching[20]

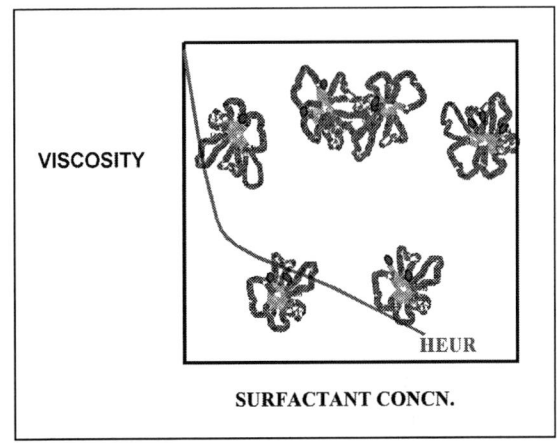

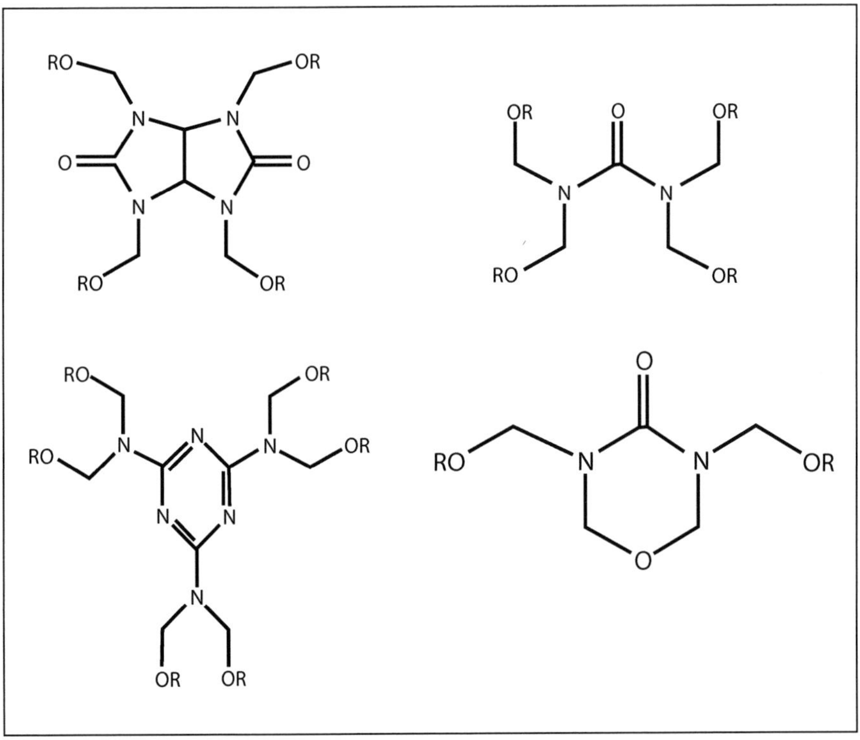

Figure 5. Surfactants cause a dramatic loss of viscosity in HEUR-thickened systems. This is due to loss of network as a result of displacement of "linking" molecules by comicellization with surfactant.

Figure 6. Aminoplast thickeners

and dyeing[21] formulations to remain localized at the position of application on the hair so that they do not run over the face. They are claimed to leave the hair less coarse than the currently used thickeners. The polymers described in this work include PEG-180/octoxynol-40/TMMG copolymer, PEG-180/laureth-50/TMMG copolymer, and polyether-1 (Pure Thix L, M, and HH, respectively, from Sud-Chemie).

Color Retention

Once the hair has been dyed with either a direct dye or an oxidative dye, the color must be maintained. Color retention can be enhanced by the addition of silicones during the hair coloring process.

Longer-lasting hair color retention and volumizing has been claimed by the addition of alkylmethicones either before, during or after the hair has been dyed.[22] Suitable alkylmethicones are hexylmethicone (Silcare 41 M10 from Clariant or DC2-1731 from Dow Coming), octylmethicone (Silsost 034 from Crompton & Knowles or DC2-1732 from Dow Corning), caprilylmethicone (Silcare 41 M15 from Clariant) and stearoxytrimethylsilane (Silcare 1 M71 from Clariant). In this study, the color retention was evaluated by half head tests in which the color was measured at root, middle and tip of hair by a chromometer.[23]

Pretreatment of hair with an aminosilicone is claimed to confer better color retention from direct dyes and oxidative dyes.[24] Preferred aminosilicones are Belsil ADM 652 and Fluid WR 1300 and microemulsions such as Finish CT 964 or SLM 28020 from Wacker Silicones. These compositions confer water contact-angles greater than 90° on the hair surface measured by the Wilhelmy plate method using the hair fiber as the plate.

Adsorption of silicones to hair has been claimed to be too weak to provide lasting protection. On the other hand, covalent binding of silicones to hair causes damage to and weakening of the fiber. However, the covalent attachment of trimethylpyridinium "molecular hooks" to the silicone chain is claimed to produce a silicone that adsorbs to the hair and is durable, while maintaining intact hair structure.[25-26]

Hair Lightening

Hair can be lightened with bleaching agents such as hydroquinone or kojic acid but hydroquinone is known to be cytotoxic to melanocytes and kojic acid derivatives are expensive.

It has been revealed that hair lightening can be achieved by application of compositions containing a fluorescent dye and a cationic polymer and it appears that these compositions give improved fixing of the dye on the hair surface. The cationic polymer must have a charge density of at least 1 meq/g.[27] The fluorescent dye absorbs light in spectral wavelengths between 360 and 760 nanometers and converts it into light of longer wavelength that is emitted in the visible region. This is distinguished from optical brighteners, which absorb only ultraviolet light (200 to 400 nanometers).

It has also been claimed that hair lightening can be achieved by application of compositions containing a fluorescent dye and a non-associative thickener. Suitable non-associative thickeners can be found among crosslinked acrylic acid homopolymers, nonionic guar gums, and dimethylaminoethyl methacrylate homopolymers and copolymers quaternized with methyl chloride.

Crosslinked acrylic acid homopolymers:

- Carbopol 980, 981, 954, 2984, and 5984 from Noveon
- Synthalen M and Synthalen K from 3 VSA
- Crosslinked 2-acrylamido-2-methyl-propanesulphonic acid homopolymers and their partially or totally neutralized acrylamide crosslinked copolymers
- Ammonium acrylate homopolymers or copolymers of ammonium acrylate and of acrylamide

Nonionic guar gums:

- Vidogum GH form Unipectine
- Jaguar C, Jaguar HP and Jaguar DC series from Meyhall
- Galactasol 4H4FD2 from Aqualon
- Biopolysaccharide gums of microbial origin, such as scleroglucan gum or xanthan gum
- Gums derived from plant exudates, such as gum arabic, ghatti gum, karaya gum and gum tragacanth

- Hydroxypropyl or carboxymethyl celluloses
- Pectins
- Alginates

Dimethylaminoethyl methacrylate homopolymers and copolymers quaternized with methyl chloride:

- Microsap PAS 5193, Bozepol C Nouveau or PAS 5193 and PAS 5194 from Hoechst
- Salcare 95, 96 and SC92 from Ciba

Conclusion

Hair coloring is the second-largest market in hair care and we can expect to see significant advances in this segment during the upcoming years. Polymers are important ingredients in hair-coloring products.

In the initial stages, thickeners ease application on the hair, mediate the diffusion of the dye precursor and prevent the highly alkaline compositions from dripping into the eyes. The precise mechanism of associative thickeners in this respect still requires investigation to gain a fundamental understanding of their role and their function in optimizing performance.

Polymers are also used to maintain color in the hair and to alleviate hair damage caused by the coloring process. There is a need to thoroughly understand the mechanisms involved in color protection and minimization of hair damage. Advances in spin echo pulsed gradient NMR and fluorescence microscopy may allow us to follow the diffusion of molecular components through the formulation and into hair. Advances in atomic force microscopy should allow us to view the effects at the molecular level on the hair surface.

Published July 2005 Cosmetics and Toiletries magazine

References

1. US Pat 4,130,501, Stable viscous hydrogen peroxide solutions containing a surfactant and a method of preparing the same, CW Lutz and LE Cohen, assigned to FMC (Dec 19, 1978)
2. US Pat 6,010,541, Oxidation dye composition for keratin fibers comprising a nonionic amphiphilic polymer, R De la Mettrie and F Boudy, assigned to L'Oréal (Jan 4, 2000)
3. US Pat App 2004/0255399, Method and compositions for coloring hair with taurate copolymers, J Yang, filed by Unilever (Dec 23, 2004)

4. US Pat 5,376,146, Two-part aqueous composition for coloring hair, which forms a gel on mixing of the two parts, S Casperson, S Pohl and M Wong, assigned to Bristol-Myers Squibb (Dec 27, 1994)
5. US Pat App 2005/0000037, Dye composition comprising 2-chloro-6-methyl-3-aminophenol as coupler, para-aminophenol and 3-methyl-4-aminophenol as oxidation bases and at least one associative thickening polymer, M-P Audousset (Jan 6, 2005)
6. US Pat App 2005/0000038, Dye composition comprising 2-chloro-6-methyl-3-aminophenol, at least two oxidation bases chosen from para-phenylenediamine derivatives and at least one associative thickening polymer, M-P Audousset (Jan 6, 2005)
7. US Pat App 2005/0000039, Composition comprising at least one coupler chosen from 2-chloro-6-methyl-3-aminophenol and addition salts thereof, at least one oxidation base, and at least one associative polymer comprising at least one C8-C30 fatty chain, M-P Audousset (Jan 6, 2005)
8. US Pat RE 33,786, S Pohl and M Hnatchenko, assigned to Clairol (Jan 7, 1992)
9. LM Landoll and AC Sau, Synthesis and solution properties of hydrophobically modified (hydroxyethyl) cellulose, *ACS Adv Chem Ser* 223 343-364 (1989)
10. US Pats 4,079,028, 4,155,892, 4,426,485, 4,496,708 5,281,654, 4,499,233 and 5,023,309, describing HEURS with hydrophobes in bunches
11. US Pat 4,327,008, describing branched and terminal HEURS (Apr 27, 1982)
12. EU Pat Application 0498,442 A1, describing silicone HEURS
13. H Hoffmann and G Wanka, The aggregation behavior of poly(oxyethylene)-poly(oxypropylene)-poly(oxyethylene) block copolymers in aqueous solution, *Colloid Polym Sci* 268 101-117 (1990)
14. B Xu et al, *Langmuir* 13 6896 (1997)
15. B Xu et al, *Langmuir* 13 6903 (1997)
16. US Pat 5,496,908, B Xu et al
17. R Yekta and M Winnik, Fluorescence studies of associating polymers in water: Determination of the chain end aggregation number and a model for the association process, *Macromolecules* 28 956-966 (1995)
18. T Annable and R Buscall, The rheology of solutions of associating polymers: comparison of experimental behavior with transient network theory, *J Rheol* 37 695-726 (1993)
19. US Pat 5,914,373, Water soluble aminoplast-ether copolymers, CW Glancy and AL Steinmetz, assigned to United Catalysts, Inc (Jun 22, 1999)
20. US Pat 6,800,096, Composition, process and kit for bleaching keratin fibers comprising at least one thickening polymer with an aminoplast-ether skeleton, F Legrand and D Allard, assigned to L'Oréal SA (Oct 5, 2004)
21. US Pat 6,800,098, Oxidation dye composition for keratinic fibres containing a thickening polymer with an ether plastic skeleton, D Allard and F Legrand, assigned to L'Oréal SA (Oct 5, 2004)
22. US Pat 6,805,856, Hair care compositions which reduce color loss in hair and methods of using the compositions, M Wong and E Memisha, assigned to L'Oréal (Oct 19, 2004)
23. MD Berthiaume et al, Effects of silicon pretreatment on oxidative hair damage, *J Soc Cos Chem* 46 231-245 (Sep/Oct 1995)
24. US Pat 6,824,764, Use of particular aminosilicones as a pretreatment of processes for coloring keratin fibers with direct dyes or with oxidation dyes, P Devin-Baudoin and A Sabbagh, assigned to L'Oréal (Nov 30, 2004)
25. US Pat 6,841,164, Silicone compositions for personal care products and method for making, MD Butts, SA Nye, CM Byrne, AR Katritzky and JW Merkert, assigned to General Electric Company (Jan 11, 2005)
26. US Pat 6,844,002, Silicone compositions for personal care products and method for making, MD Butts, SA Nye, CM Byrne, AR Katritzky and JW Merkert, assigned to General Electric Company (Jan 18, 2005)
27. US Pat Appl 2004/0258641, Cosmetic composition for dyeing human keratin materials, comprising at least one fluorescent dye and at least one cationic polymer, and a dyeing process therefore, G Plos and H Samain (Dec 23, 2004)

CHAPTER 11

Innovations in Hair Styling Technology

Randy Schueller and Perry Romanowski
Alberto-Culver, Melrose Park, Illinois USA

KEY WORDS: *VOCs, aerosol hair spray, pomades, hair dressing, packaging, solvents, polymers*

ABSTRACT: *The regulatory climate for cosmetic products is becoming more difficult for formulators. Here, the authors describe how new rules have inspired cosmetic chemists to use a variety of strategies and partner with raw material suppliers and packaging houses in order to provide consumers with what they want.*

This chapter reviews how changes in technology and regulatory pressures have "inspired" innovation. In order to understand how and why chemists are innovating to accommodate regulations presently, we need to start by looking at where it all began.

A History of Styling Technology

For almost as long as there have been cosmetic chemists, there have existed regulatory agencies to control their work. The incursion of regulatory requirements has forced changes in hair styling products more than in any other type of hair product.

Since their introduction in the 1940s, hair sprays led the popularization of modern styling products. The first sprays were pump type systems, but public demand for a better product prompted the development of the aerosol hair spray. The aerosol spray was based on Goodhue and Sullivan's patent of low-pressure propellants (fluorocarbon 12) and Abplanalp's patented valve design.

The first aerosol hair spray was introduced in 1949 in Chicago by the Global Liqinet Corporation, and created a multi-million dollar business. These early formulas used shellac as the fixative polymer but shellac exhibited several major drawbacks – such as being difficult to wash out of hair – that led to the development of synthetic polymers with properties that could be better controlled.

For the next 20 years business boomed but by the late 1960s environmental and safety concerns began to threaten the industry. While styling formulations gave good fixative properties, many contained environmentally sensitive solvents and propellants. Chlorofluorocarbons (CFCs) were the first to gain notoriety because they depleted the ozone layer, prompting fears that an unhealthy amount of UV radiation could reach the Earth's surface.

In 1979, regulatory agencies banned CFC propellants from aerosol formulations in most industrialized nations. (Despite what anyone may tell you, CFCs are no longer used in hair care aerosols today.) Shortly thereafter, the popular co-solvent methylene chloride came under scrutiny after it was discovered to be a potential carcinogen.

HISTORY OF CONSUMER PRODUCT VOC REGULATIONS IN THE USA

- 1978: CFC Ban
- 1983: South Coast AQMD (Los Angeles)
- 1988: California Clean Air Act
- 1989-1992: California Rules
- 1990: Federal Clean Air Act Revisions
- 1990-1995: Other State Rules
- 1996: EPA National Rule
- 1997-1999: More California Rules
- 2000: Reactivity-Based Aerosol Paint Rule in California Rule in California
- 2000-2004 Northeastern State Rules 2004
- 2003: New California Rule
- 2005-2010: More California Rules

Fortunately, the cosmetic chemists of the day found innovative solutions to these regulatory realities. Ethyl alcohol and alcohol/water systems became increasingly popular substitutes as solvents and dimethyl ether/hydrocarbon mixtures replaced CFCs as the primary propellant system. All was right in the world of cosmetic science – at least for a short while.

By the early 1980s this new breed of "eco-friendlier" formulations was coming under scrutiny because of concern for air pollution. These formulations relied heavily on ethanol and other hydrocarbons which belong to a class of chemicals known as volatile organic compounds (VOCs). Researchers found that when exposed to sunlight, VOCs were capable of combining with nitrogen oxides (NOx) to form ground level ozone, or smog. Ironically, the industry had swapped one material that destroyed ozone for another that created it. But this ozone stays near the Earth's surface and has negative health effects.

Concerns about smog led to VOC reductions in 1983, just after CFCs were banned. Originally, the South Coast Air District in California wanted to ban aerosols but industry activists succeeded in obtaining amendments to the law to preempt California Districts from doing just that. The result was the establishment of legal safeguards for development of regulations by the California Air Resources Board (CARB). These rules were developed through intense negotiations that occurred in the early 1990s. They ultimately limited the amount of VOCs that could be used in any cosmetic aerosol product.

Federal laws soon followed that supplemented an ever-growing number of state rules, but California remained the most stringent. California proposed still more rules during the late 1990s and the trend continued through the new millennium.

In 2000-2004 the Northeastern State Rules were first proposed and they were followed by still more California rules in 2003. As of 2005, California remains the state with the most stringent requirements. Texas, New York, Massachusetts, New Jersey, Delaware, Pennsylvania, Maryland and Virginia are somewhat less stringent than California, but more stringent than the National Rule. Arizona and Georgia have local rules that affect products other than aerosols. All states are subject to the EPA National Rule.

As of 2005 the rules state that hair mousse may contain no more than 6% VOCs, hair shine and hair holding sprays no more than 55%, and gels no more than 6%. And according to industry experts, we can expect to see even more rulings in California through 2010.

Strategies to Create Low VOC Formulas

What do all these rules mean to the formulator? Well, to begin with, we can no longer use ethyl alcohol as the major solvent in styling products. This limitation is a huge impediment because ethanol is really an ideal ingredient. It solubilizes holding polymers, has excellent spray properties, is easy to use, dries quickly, smells nice, and has no serious toxicological issues. Instead of ethanol, many manufacturers have resorted to adding water to their products. However, an increase in the water concentration can adversely affect the performance of a hair spray by accelerating the initial curl droop and/or increasing the dry time on the hair. Other styling products have similar issues related to drying time and application properties. Cosmetic formulators must rise to the challenge to do more with less, to create formulations that satisfy consumers despite rigorous regulatory constraints.

To achieve these goals, various strategic approaches have been suggested. Douglas Fratz, of the Consumer Specialty Products Association, listed several approaches for creating VOC-compliant products by using the following: exempt compounds, low vapor pressure compounds, water-based formulations, increased amounts of inorganic compounds and solids, innovative product exemptions, alternative compliance plans and product use instruction labeling.[2]

To achieve these goals, various strategic approaches have been suggested. At the 24th International Aerosol Congress in September, 2003, the Consumer Specialty Products Association's Douglas Fratz discussed creating VOC-compliant products and suggested the seven approaches described next.[2]

Use exempt compounds: This strategy involves formulating with compounds that the authorities consider exempt from VOC consideration. For example, hydroflourocarbons (HFCs) are exempt propellants and acetone is an exempt solvent. Certain types of silicones can be used in some products but they are very expensive.

Chemicals with negligible photochemical reactivity (e.g., compounds that have less ozone formation potential than ethane) are also exempt. There is also an exemption for materials with vapor pressures less than 0.1 mm Hg at 20°C. Similarly, fragrances are exempt. It is best to check with the Cosmetic, Toiletry and Fragrance Association (CTFA) or the Consumer Specialty Products Association (CSPA) to find a list of exempt compounds.

Use low vapor pressure compounds: Materials with low vapor pressure such as glycol ethers and propylene glycol can be used without affecting VOC content. This strategy is useful for products such as gels but less useful for hair sprays.

Use water-based formulations: By using water-based formulas the amount of VOCs is easily reduced. Unfortunately, adding water usually requires surfactants or emulsifiers to be added to the formula. These compounds will have various effects on the product performance, many of which are not desirable. Water itself also has negative impacts on the finished products such as increasing drying time and decreasing hold. To date, most hair spray manufacturers have used this formulation strategy even though it results in an arguably inferior product.

Use increased amounts of inorganic compounds and solids: Compressed gas propellants like carbon dioxide and nitrogen are not considered VOCs so they could be used as substitutes. However, their use is limited due to technological challenges. The major hurdle yet to be solved is the loss of pressure that products using compressed gas experience. A consumer using such a product will notice a weaker spray over time until eventually nothing gets dispensed. If product remains in the container but can not be removed, the consumer will be turned off and likely never purchase the product again.

This strategy is more effective for products like antiperspirants, where VOC levels can be decreased by adding non-volatile organic solids, such as surfactants and polymers.

Use innovative product exemptions: CARB allows an exemption for certain innovative formulations. To use this strategy, the chemist has to be able to provide "clear and convincing evidence' that, due to some characteristic of the product formulation, design, delivery systems or other factors, the use of the product will result in less VOC emissions…"[3] than a product with a comparable amount of VOCs. For example, a concentrated hair spray can be produced to have more active ingredients but be dispensed with less solvent.

Use alternative compliance plans: California allows the VOC emissions of some products to be averaged, or grouped together. This allows mixing products that can be over-reduced with others than cannot be reduced much at all. To use this strategy, cosmetic manufacturers have to submit an application to show the VOC content of the products in the plan, a sales verification method, and other emission tracking information.

Use product use instruction labeling: Another way to reduce VOC emissions is to educate consumers on an alternative method for using a product. This approach attempts to change consumer behavior to increase use efficiency and deter excessive VOC emissions. For example, instructing consumers to use less hair spray at a given time will make the product last longer and reduce emissions over a given time. While this method is not currently applied to hair care products, it could be in the future.

Styling Technology Today

All of the strategies have been attempted (with various degrees of success) to face the challenges of ever-increasing regulations of hair care products and more specifically, styling products. Let's take a closer look at some of the specific innovations that have been employed by formulators in today's styling products.

A quick review of some recent patents shows how formulators have compensated for VOC regulations in all types of styling categories including hair sprays, gels, and mousses. We'll begin with aerosol hair sprays because they are arguably the most complex, dynamic systems of all personal care products, and have also been subject to the most difficult regulations.

Aerosol hair spray: Aerosols face all the "standard" formulation problems imaginable such as phase separation, sedimentation, malodor generation, discoloration, pH drift, and so on. But additionally, they have a set of potential problems unique to their delivery system, including can corrosion, poor spray-ability, dry time, film formation, Department of Transportation pressure issues, can evacuation, dip-tube elongation, and so forth.

The two most successful methods for creating new VOC-compliant aerosol products are as follows.

- First, the formulator can try to modify the solvent/propellant mix to optimize its properties. This approach typically involves finding substitutes for ethanol as a solvent or replacing hydrocarbon propellants. In the latter case, a choice between using either HFC-152a propellant (a non-VOC classified material which allows for anhydrous systems) or dimethyl ether (DME) with hydrocarbon combinations (which allow water-compatible systems) is the norm.
- Second, the formulator may choose to alter the holding resins in the formula to improve the way the product functions. The technical literature indicates formulators have had some degree of success with both approaches. Optimizing the solvent/propellant mix is the most common solution to the VOC issue. While using HFC-152a propellant in an aerosol formulation is a straightforward replacement, it usually results in a product that is of significantly higher cost. DME formulations can be made less costly but have required innovative solutions to deal with the presence of water. Ethanol replacements have been harder to develop, but progress has been made. Consider the following three patents which deal with optimized solvent systems.
- U.S. Patent No. 6,752,983 discloses the replacement of ethanol and isopropanol by alkyl acetates, particularly methyl acetate and t-butyl acetate.4 These solvents can be problematic because they hydrolyze in the presence of water to form harmful acids. They may also have pungent chemical odors and may stain clothing. This patent discloses a way to mix alkyl acetates with lower levels of alcohols to over come these difficulties while lowering VOC content.
- U.S. Patent No. 6,464,960 involves the use of acetone as a solvent.5 Acetone is not widely used in hair sprays because it has an unacceptable odor, it evaporates too quickly, and it is a poor solvent for some polymers. This patent discloses the

use of a hair-setting polymer in a solvent/propellant system containing a 1- to 4-carbon alcohol, water, a cosolvent such as acetone, and a propellant mixture consisting of dimethyl ether and a fluorocarbon. According to the patent, this invention allows for water containing, reduced VOC hair spray that approximates the performance properties of conventional water-free hair sprays.
- In a similar vein, U.S. Patent No. 6,432,390 uses a concentrate blend of alcohol and methyl acetate along with dimethyl ether propellant.6 The composition consists of 50 to 90 weight percent concentrate and 10 to 50 weight percent propellant and it provides competitive styling properties with minimal VOC emissions. Recent examples of formulators changing styling polymer properties can also be found.
- U.S. Patent No. 6,638,992 discloses a styling product that involves the incorporation of latex chemistry in the formula.7 It uses a spray-dried hybrid-graft copolymer of a sulfopolyester and an acid-functional polymer segment. Purportedly, such compositions exhibit superior curl retention even at high humidity and they may be prepared over a wide range of VOC concentrations.
- U.S. Patent No. 6,562,325 relates to a non-aerosol hair spray based on polyacrylic acid and nonionically derivatized starches.8 The starches are hydrolyzed and modified by cationic substitution to give a clear solution with a stable viscosity. Furthermore, this formula provides a clear film which is not tacky, that has good stiffness and improved humidity resistance and is substantive to hair.

Gels and mousses: Hair sprays are not the only product category of interest. Other styling product categories such as gels and mousses have their own unique formulation challenges as well.

While not necessarily focused on low VOC content, U.S. Patent No. 6,663,855 does reveal a clever approach to formulating a mousse.[9] It uses graft copolymers which allow physical and chemical attributes like glass transition temperature and solubility to be varied independently. The result is a novel class of polymers that can be tailored to the particular application, particularly related to providing longer-lasting hold and/or improved feel.

Hairdressings and pomades: Finally, no discussion of styling products would be complete without a reference to hairdressings and pomades. U.S. Patent 6,649,154 discloses a method to make conventional hairdressings less sticky and oily-feeling.[10] This is accomplished by incorporating a polysaccharide such as beta-1,3-glucan. Formulas based on this type of polymer provide an excellent hairdressing effect and hair-setting power when applied with heat at reduced VOC levels.

U.S. Patent No. 6,579,517 reveals a way to make a dual component system using at least one cross-linked, water-soluble or water-dispersible polyurethane combined with at least one polymer having isocyanate-reactive groups.[11] This is a new way to achieve benefits of these polymers from a low VOC system.

The Role of Packaging

As you can see from even this brief review, VOC regulations have prompted a tremendous innovation effort for new hair styling formulations – but the story does not end there. Packaging companies have been busily innovating to help aid formulators in the development of lower VOC products.

Typically, changes in formulation technology help drive packaging development and the recent low VOC formulas are no different. Consider these recent attempts by packaging suppliers to develop new, more functional packaging and dispensers. For example, TricorBraun has a new line of special fine mist sprayers designed for lower VOC hair sprays and spray gels. Similarly, SeaquistPerfect Dispensing now offers actuators for new high viscosity styling products.

Companies have developed new anti-clog pumps that do not clog even with high resin content products. Some of these dispensers are also available in a 360° spray version that can be used upside down. Emsar offers a directional spray pump that provides precise application that is ideal for concentrated products such as root volumizers. Similarly, Saint-Gobain Calmar markets the Mark VI fine mist sprayer with a spray extender. It is a pressure build-up type of sprayer that delivers performance for 55% VOC formulations.

Finally, there is Airspray International, who has introduced the first foam pump on the market, the Finger Pump Foamer. It is a mechanical foamer and therefore does not require gas propellant to create thick foam. The dispenser is suitable for simple water-based (non-VOC) formulations such as mousses. Packaging companies have also aided formulators in dealing with low VOC issues by creating options for different kinds of styling products. While hair spray is still the biggest part of the styling category sub-segment, waxes and gels are rapidly growing in popularity. A recent trend in styling products is the use of putties and pastes which tend to have fewer VOC issues. This shift in product choice is attributed to the consumer's desire for a messy, matte look, but could also be a reaction to the lower performing, VOC-compliant products now being produced.

Pastes and putties are typically sold in tubes and jars and these containers dictate a certain formula texture and viscosity which chemists must take into consideration when formulating. The trend toward hair that is grungy, unkempt and wild has led to products which support that look. These include products that can create a tousled or stringy look like D:fi Beach Bum, Estée Lauder's Bumble and Bumble Surf Spray, Redken's In the Loop, and Sebastian's Bondage.

Packaging technology allows these products to match the look that the consumers want. For example, they give the packaging a matte look with special resins such as Velva-soft. Or they can use bi-injection molding to give the package a different, softer feel. In addition to making them VOC-compliant, formulators are also using newer types of styling polymers to help meet consumer expectations for these products.

Conclusion

The regulatory climate for cosmetic products is arguably becoming more and more difficult for formulators. Different states have different regulations that are constantly changing. This does not even take into consideration regulations proposed around the world. And these new rules have been particularly hard on cosmetic chemists who are responsible for developing styling products.

Fortunately, innovation is alive and well in the styling field of cosmetic chemistry. By using a variety of strategies and partnering with raw material suppliers and packaging houses, formulators have found ways to reduce VOCs released and still provide the consumers with what they want. Future regulations will likely make the formulating job even more difficult, but they will also spark true innovation – and that can't be all bad, right?

Published May 2005 Cosmetics and Toiletries magazine

References

1. P Romanowski and R Schueller, Aerosols for apprentices, *Cosm Toil* 111(5) 35-40 (1996)
2. D Fratz, USA VOC Regulations and Compliance Alternatives for Aerosol Products, presented at the 24th International Aerosol Congress, Consumer Specialty Products Association (September 2003) Available at: http://www.aerosols-info.org/nic02/t_cspa.pdf
3. California Air Resources Board (CARB) regulations 94511, Innovative Products, Div. 3, Ch. 1, Sub 8.5, Consumer Prod. Art. 2 (2004)
4. US Pat 6,752,983, Hair spray and consumer sprays with reduced volatile organic compounds (2004)
5. US Pat 6,464,960, Water containing aerosol hair spray with a reduced content of volatile organic compounds (2002)
6. US Pat 6,432,390, Low VOC methyl acetate hair sprays (2002)
7. US Pat 6,638,992, Hair care compositions (2003)
8. US Pat 6,562,325, Use of stabilized starches in low VOC, polyacrylic acid-containing hair cosmetic compositions (2003)
9. US Pat 6,663,855, Cosmetic and personal care compositions (2003)
10. US Pat 6,649,154, Hairdressing cosmetic preparation and hairdressing method using the same (2003)
11. US Pat 6,579,517, Cosmetic product (2003)

Publications:

- M Sangiovanni, Sprays under pressure: EPA announces consumer products rule, Spray Technology & Marketing, Vol 6, no 5. pp 8-16 (May 1996)
- M Johnsan, The analysis of aerosol hair sprays, Spray Technology & Marketing, Vol 4, no 2. pp 19-24 (Feb 1994)
- Scientific basis for VOC reactivity issues raised by Section 183(e) of the Clean Air Act Amendments of 1990, J Air & Waste Management Assn 46 (Oct 1996)
- E Walls and HK Krummel, Low VOC Hair sprays: Formulation challenges for a changing industry, Cosmet Toil 108(3) 111-117 (1993) n

CHAPTER 12

Protecting the Hair with Natural Keratin Biopolymers

Alisa Roddick-Lanzilotta and Rob Kelly
Keratec Ltd., Christchurch, New Zealand

Sonya Scott
Canesis Network Ltd., Christchurch, New Zealand

Grant Mitchell and Surinder Chahal
Croda Chemicals Europe, East Yorkshire, England

KEY WORDS: Antiaging, keratin, intermediate filament protein, combing force, tryptophan fluorescence, UV, pollution

ABSTRACT: *UV protection and sacrificial targets for aggressive pollutants are two hair-protection strategies employed by a new keratin biopolymer manufactured from wool.*

Consumers are becoming ever more conscious of the damaging effects of environmental insults such as pollution and sunlight. Such concerns have helped to establish key trends within skin care and now are fueling innovation within the hair care arena where antiaging and antipollution technology is becoming increasingly relevant.

Hair is a complex biological system that has been designed by nature to perform specific functions. The intricate structure of hair is being discussed more than ever in articles and scientific meetings involving cosmetic chemists.[1] Increasingly, attention is directed to the relationship between the structure and function of hair and how this impacts on ensuring the delivery of effective and innovative ingredients.

Hair consists principally of keratin protein and a small amount of lipid. The chemistry of hair can be modified by aging, by lengthening and by environmental insults such as pollution and sunlight. When the hair chemistry is modified, some of the natural properties of hair are compromised. The mechanism by which this damage occurs is understood now more than ever.[2] For example, UV radiation photo-oxidizes proteins. Protein photo-oxidation leads to cleavage of disulfide bonds, cross-linking of proteins, and breaking of thioester bonds, resulting in the release of bound surface lipids. These reactions lead to a deterioration of the hair properties, noticeable to consumers in the form of poor manageability, dryness and brittleness, loss of shine and, in extreme cases, decreased strength (fiber breakage).[3] Actives that can address these negative issues and prevent them from occurring clearly have antiaging efficacy and have the potential to maintain youthful hair.

This chapter discusses two strategies to counter the damaging effects of age and pollution on hair: UV protection and the implementation of sacrificial target components. Both strategies are employed in a biopolymer made from intact keratin proteins and keratin peptides from the wool of New Zealand sheep.

Keratin Biopolymer

A keratin biopolymer[a] has been designed to operate by sacrificial and chemical protection means:

- It protects the hair's natural protein by providing preferential binding sites and degradation sites for aggressive influences. The protected cystine groups present in the keratin biopolymer provide a site for reactivity. The biopolymer components acting on the surface of the fiber provide a shielding effect.
- It provides antioxidant activity against aggressive influences.

This keratin biopolymer is a purified form of keratin intermediate filament protein (IFP). This purified form is manufactured solely from wool of New Zealand origin. This material is predominantly intact protein, meaning it has not been degraded in any form; it

---

[a]Keratec IFP [INCI: Water (aqua) (and) keratin (and) Hydrolyzed keratin] is a product of Keratec Ltd. distributed exclusively by Croda Chemicals Europe.

retains both its original size (molecular weight ~55 kD) and amino acid composition. It also contains a smaller amount of peptide (average molecular weight 3–4 kD). IFP (**Figure 1** and More on IFP from New Zealand) was selected as the protein source because it is the protein that gives natural hair fibers their strength. **Table 1** shows the amino acid profile of this proprietary keratin biopolymer, which will be called *keratin IFP* in this chapter to distinguish this keratin biopolymer from other existing keratin blends, especially those containing synthetics.

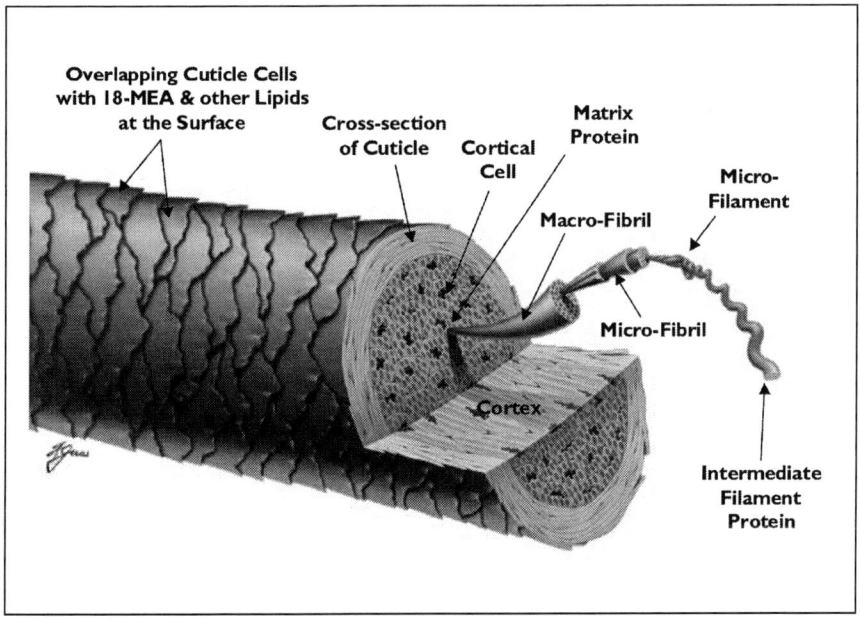

Figure 1. Hair structure

The intact keratin protein has excellent film-forming properties that allow it to be substantive to the hair from a range of hair care formulations. The lower molecular weight peptide component is capable of penetrating the cortex of the hair fiber. The dual action of surface coating and penetration of the peptide leads to antiaging efficacy (i.e., prevention of age-related damage) through a mechanism of sacrificial degradation of surface active proteins and antioxidant activity from the fractions within the cortex.

In summary, a liquid form of hair is being applied to the surface and interior of the fiber. This liquid form is somewhat more reactive than the hair itself. Hence any aggression that would normally react with the hair leading to deterioration of its properties will preferentially attack the applied keratin biopolymer, offering protection to the fiber.

Table 1
Amino acid profile of the keratin biopolymer

	Mole (%)
Aspartate	7.9
Glutamate	15.3
Serine	11.0
Glycine	8.2
Histidine	0.9
Arginine	7.7
Threonine	6.5
Alanine	7.5
Proline	5.5
Tyrosine	1.1
Valine	6.5
Methionine	0.2
Lanthionine	0.2
Isoleucine	3.6
Leucine	8.7
Phenylalanine	2.4
Lysine	2.1
Cystine	4.3

Environmental Pollution and Hair Damage

The impact of environmental pollutants on the hair is well-recognized and becoming increasingly important as pollution levels continue to be of concern. Work was undertaken to determine how hair properties are affected by pollutants commonly found in the environment. These pollutants include cigarette smoke, and gaseous sulfur dioxide ozone.

Combing force analysis and hair tryptophan content analysis were used to assess the condition of hair. Combing force analysis is an accepted method for measuring the hair surface health, and is related to the consumer perception of manageability.[3] Tryptophan is an amino acid that is sensitive to damage from reactants and UV radiation and is therefore a useful indicator of age-related damage in hair.[4] **Figure 2** shows the steady decrease in tryptophan content from root to tip in hair from a healthy volunteer. The regular decrease illustrates the effect of environmental exposure over time and validates the use of tryptophan analysis as a probe for hair damage.

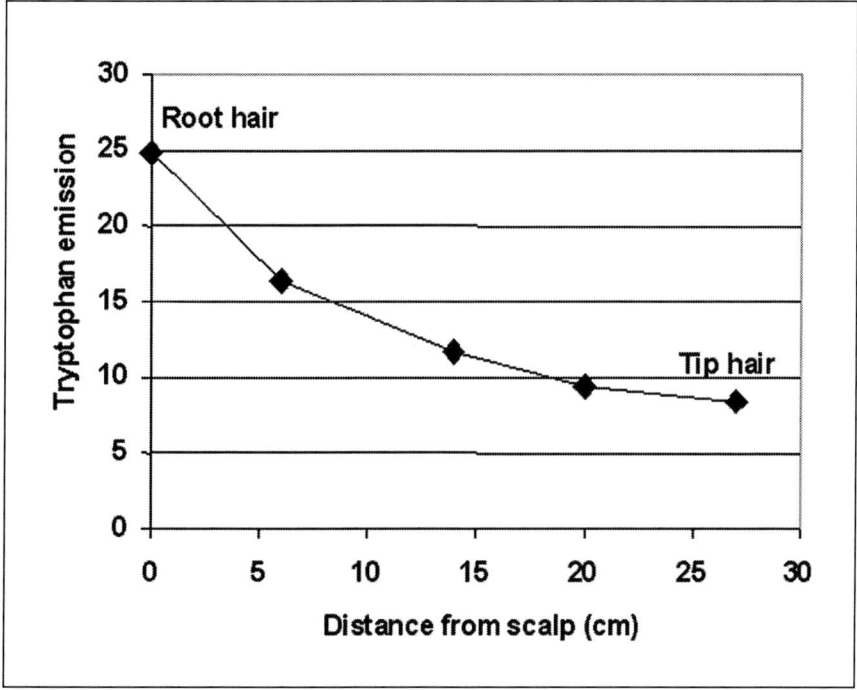

Figure 2. Tryptophan content on the hair surface measured at different distances from the scalp

Cigarette smoke: Cigarette smoke contains more than 4,000 components, including many that are known to be aggressive toward biological materials. Among the aggressors are formaldehyde, carbon monoxide, ammonia and reactive oxygen species (ROS).

Combing force analysis was used to investigate the effect of cigarette smoke exposure on untreated (virgin) hair, hair treated with a base conditioner and hair treated with 1% keratin biopolymer added to the conditioner base. A rinse-off protocol was used. Tresses were exposed to smoke from eight cigarettes with application of conditioner prior to initial exposure and reapplication after four cigarettes. The results following smoke exposure (**Figure 3**) indicate that compared to the force required to comb the untreated hair, only 38% as much combing force was required in the keratin IFP-treated hair (and 68% for the conditioner base without keratin IFP).

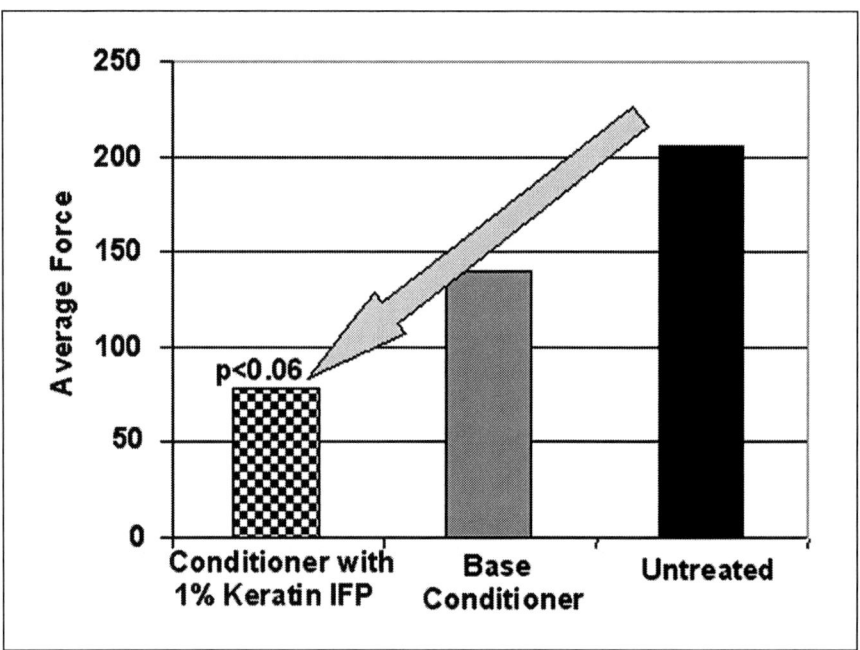

Figure 3. Effect of smoke exposure on average force to comb hair tresses

Sulfur dioxide gas: Sulfur dioxide (SO_2) gas is produced by burning coal, high-sulfur oil and diesel fuel, and together with particulates makes up the main pollutant load in many cities. It is a reducing gas and thus can potentially cleave disulfide bonds that hold the hair together.

Experiments were carried out to investigate the effect of SO_2 on hair fiber properties. Tresses were exposed to 40 ppm of gaseous SO_2, which decayed to 0 ppm over 12 h. **Figure 4** shows combing force and tryptophan analysis of sulfur-exposed hair that was untreated or pre-treated with either a conditioner base or the conditioner containing 1% keratin biopolymer. Application of the keratin conditioner decreased the combing force to 80% of the force required to comb the control untreated sample. No improvement was observed when the conditioner base was used. The keratin conditioner treatment also provided complete protection of the tryptophan in the cuticle, whereas in the absence of treatment the SO_2 gas decreased the tryptophan content of the hair to approximately 80% of its original value.

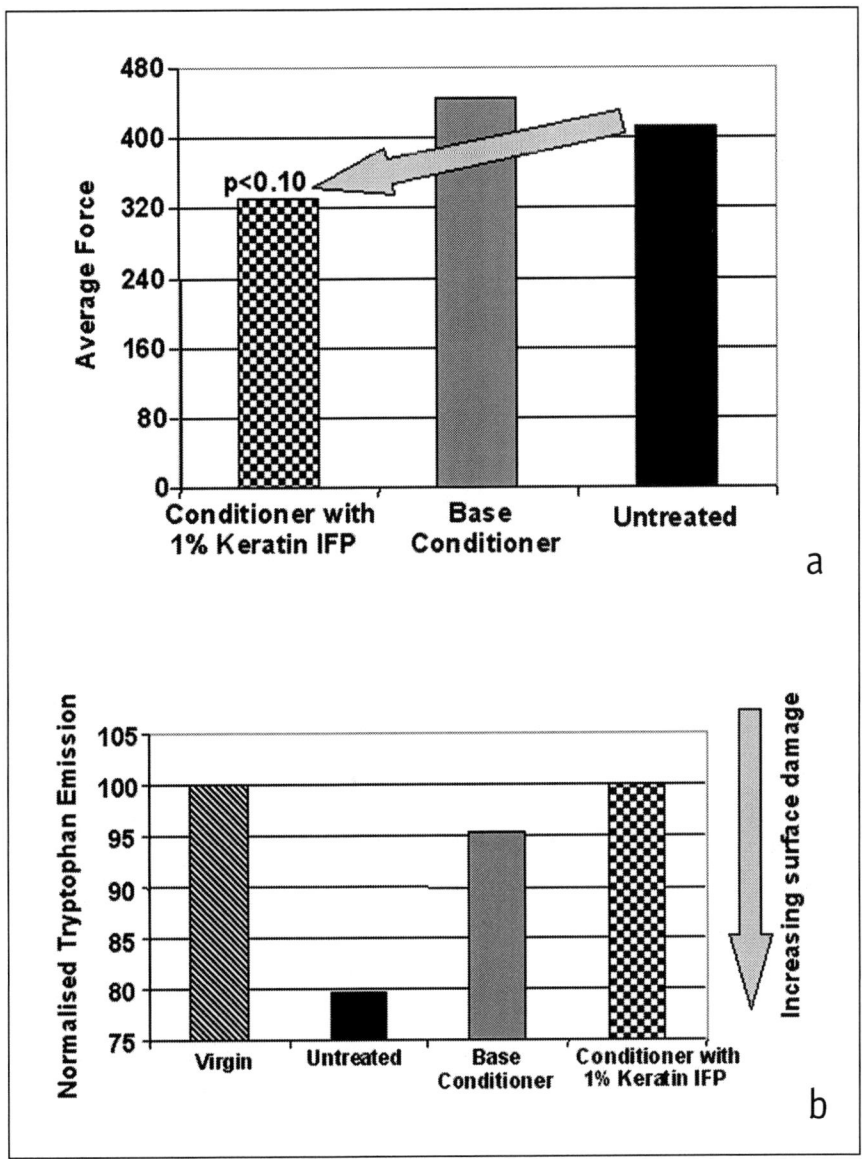

Figure 4. Effect of sulfur dioxide exposure on hair: a) 40 ppm for 12 h on average force to comb hair tresses, and b) 4 ppm for 60 h on relative tryptophan content of hair tresses

Ozone: The pollutant ozone is formed by the reaction of nitrogen oxides, hydrocarbons and sunlight, and is a component of photochemical smog. This extremely powerful oxidant reacts with proteins, attacking amino acids such as cystine and tryptophan. Even very small amounts of ozone can cause significant damage to the hair, particularly when it is wet. This is illustrated in **Figure 5a**, which shows a scanning electron micrograph of a wet hair fiber exposed to 0.1 ppm of ozone for 30 sec. In this instance a bubbling effect was observed and holes were generated in the outer cuticle layer, exposing the cortex of the fiber and likely causing cuticle loss during routine grooming practices.

Combing force and tryptophan analysis studies were used to assess the effect of ozone on untreated hair, and hair to which a conditioner base or 1% keratin IFP conditioner had been applied using a rinse-off protocol. Wet hair tresses were exposed to 20 ppm ozone for 2 min.

The results of the combing force study are displayed in **Figure 5b**. Addition of the keratin IFP had the effect of decreasing the combing force (i.e., increasing manageability) of ozone-exposed hair to 59% of the untreated control.

Interestingly, treatment with the conditioner base alone had a detrimental effect, markedly increasing the required combing force (to 169% of the control). It is believed that this increase arises from reaction between the substantive conditioning agents and the ozone. The reaction exacerbates the damage to the fiber surface. This was supported by SEM investigations (not shown).

Ozone is known to react quickly with organic matter that contains double bonds, activated aromatic groups or amines, and it reacts more rapidly with ionized and dissociated organic compounds, such as quaternaries found in conditioning systems. These reactions in turn lead to bi-products such as peroxide and carboxyl compounds. It is thought that in the presence of keratin IFP, ozone reacts preferentially with the active, protecting the hair fiber from damage associated with these reactions. Further work is being undertaken to investigate whether this effect is typical of many conditioning systems.

Tryptophan fluorescence studies also were carried out on the ozone-exposed fibers and the results are shown in **Figure 5c**. It was found that exposing untreated control hair to ozone reduced the emission intensity due to tryptophan. Treatment with the conditioner base also resulted in tryptophan loss, but no loss was observed in hair treated with the conditioner containing keratin biopolymer.

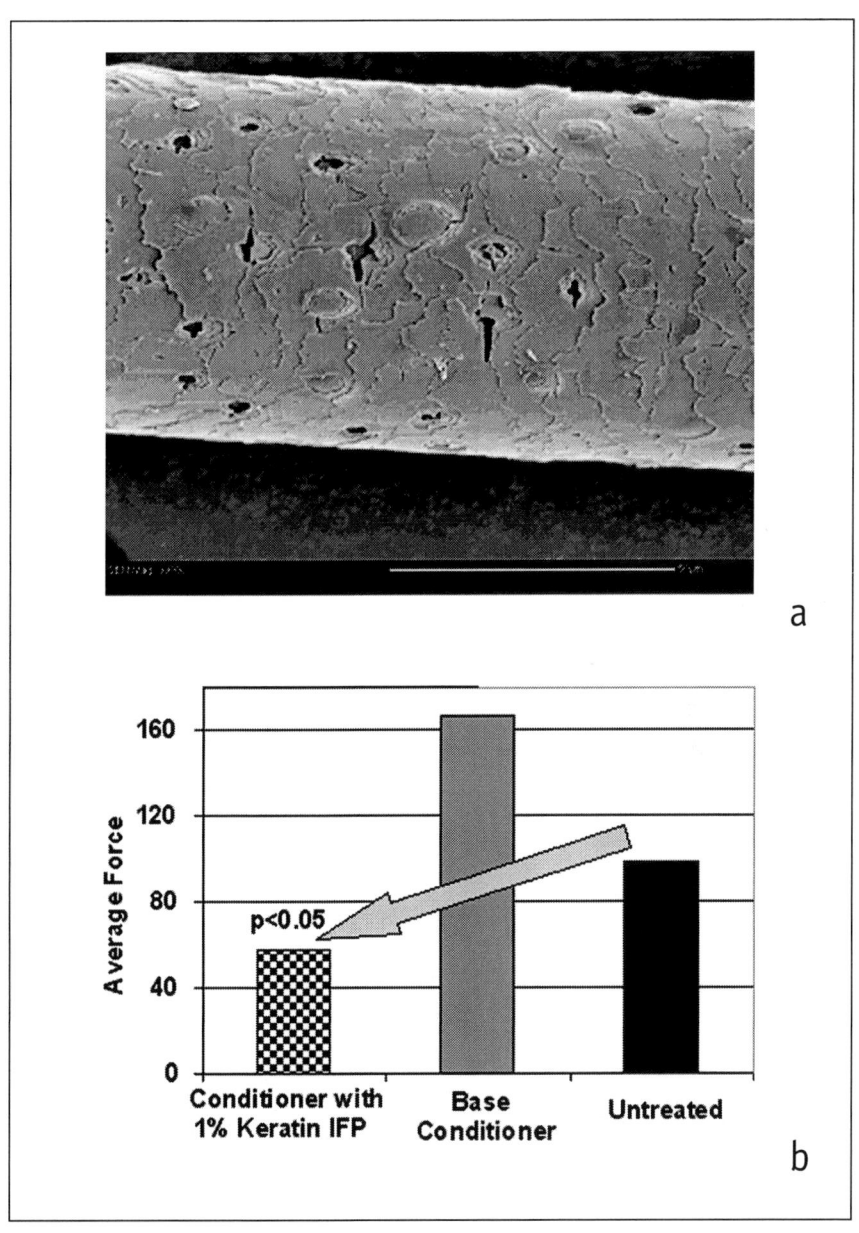

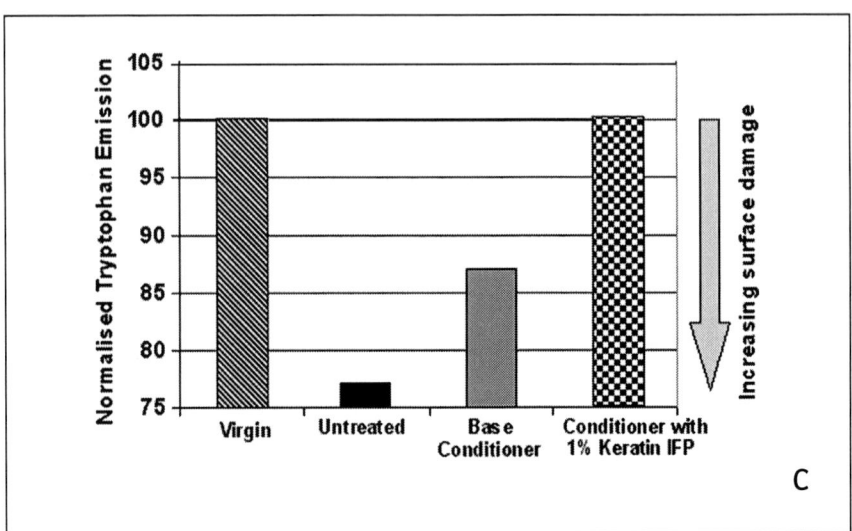

Figure 5. Effect of ozone exposure on hair:
a) Scanning electron micrograph of untreated wet hair exposed to 0.1 ppm of ozone for 30 sec
b) 20 ppm for 2 min on average force to comb hair tresses
c) 20 ppm for 2 min on relative tryptophan content of hair tresses

UV Radiation and Hair Damage

Ultraviolet radiation, particularly UVB, is another major source of hair damage from the environment. The effect of UVB on hair and the protective properties of keratin biopolymers were examined using tryptophan analysis and single fiber tensile strength measurements. Tryptophan is particularly sensitive to UVB radiation, being readily destroyed, and thus is an extremely sensitive probe for photo-oxidative damage of hair. Fiber tensile strength is a recognized method for assessing the structural integrity of the fiber cortex, giving a useful indication of overall health.

An experiment was performed to mimic the progressive hair damage from exposure to sunlight and grooming practices. The baseline tryptophan content was measured using a fluorescence spectrophotometer. The hair then was irradiated with UVB for the equivalent of 96 h of sunshine, and washed with surfactant shampoo. This cycle of irradiation and wash was repeated several times. The resulting decay in tryptophan content is shown in **Figure 6a**.

This experiment then was repeated, with the modification that this time the hair was treated with a 5% solution of keratin IFP using a rinse-off protocol before UVB irradiation in each cycle. The results of the tryptophan assessment are displayed in **Figure 6b**. It was observed that treatment with the keratin IFP protected the tryptophan of the hair, leaving it in an undamaged state.

A further fluorescence experiment was performed using a rinse-off protocol to investigate the delivery of the keratin IFP from a conditioner formulation. The results are displayed in **Figure 6c**. The tryptophan levels of the untreated hair and conditioner base-treated hair decreased to approximately 60%–70% of the initial value, whereas treatment with the base conditioner formulation containing the keratin biopolymer at a level of 1% maintained the surface fluorescence levels of the hair fiber.

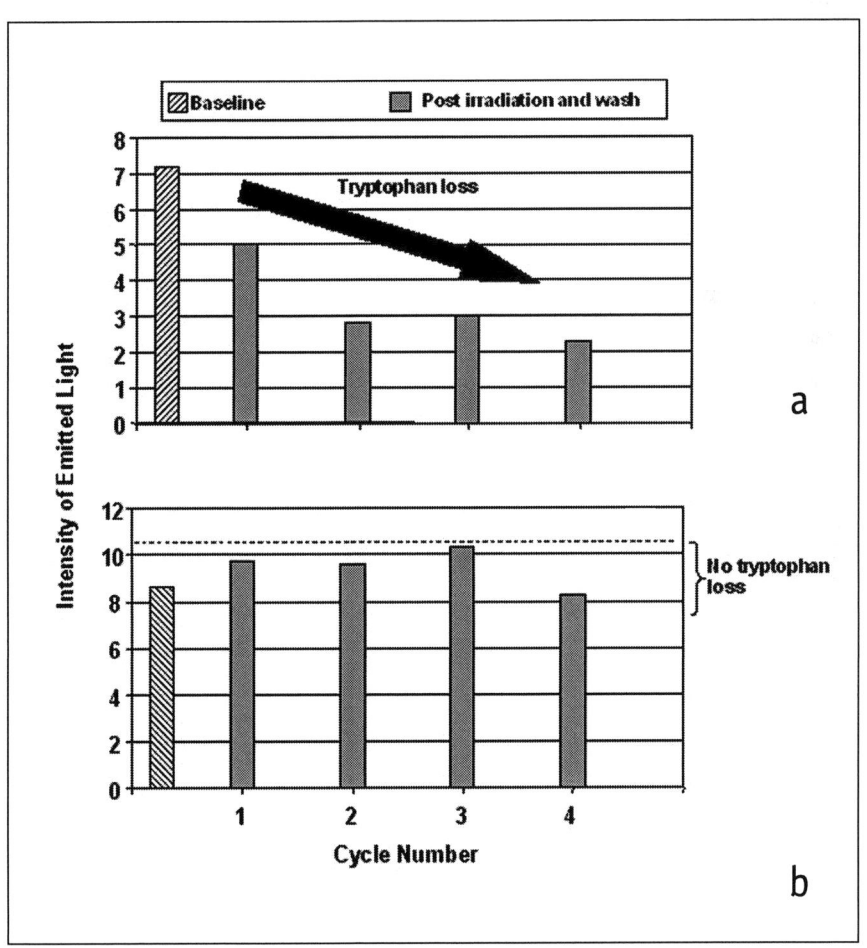

Finally to assess the effect of UV radiation on the bulk mechanical properties of hair, tensile measurement was applied to UVB-exposed hair with and without treatment with the keratin biopolymer at a level of 5% in a conditioner. The resulting data are displayed in **Figure 6d**. The effect of UVB light exposure on

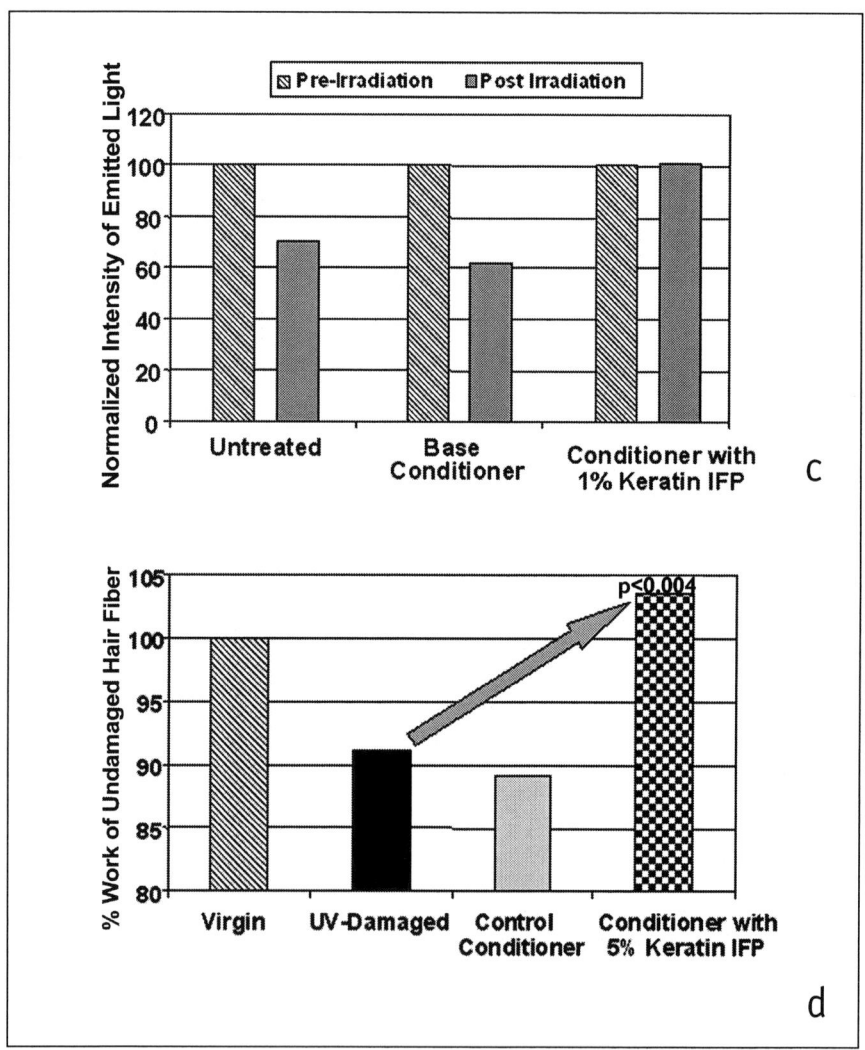

Figure 6. Effect of UVB exposure on hair:
a) Equivalent of 96 h sunshine on tryptophan content of surfactant-washed untreated hair tresses
b) Equivalent of 96 h sunshine on tryptophan content of surfactant-washed hair tresses pre-treated with 5% solution of keratin IFP
c) Equivalent to 96 h sunshine on tryptophan content of hair tresses
d) Equivalent to 125 h sunshine on work required to achieve a 20% extension of wet hair fibers

virgin untreated hair was to decrease the work required to extend the fiber by 20%; in other words, the fiber was damaged and thus weakened. Application of the conditioner base did not protect the underlying hair fibers from UV damage as evidenced by a reduction in the amount of work required for fiber extension. However, applying conditioner base formulation containing 5% of the keratin biopolymer resulted in tensile properties that were very similar to the tensile properties of the fiber before exposure, indicating that the biopolymer was successfully preventing aging damage to the fiber, and maintaining the fiber in its original condition.

Conclusions

Age-related damage to hair occurs as a result of exposure to the external environment. The detrimental effect of commonly encountered pollutants (cigarette smoke, ozone and sulfur dioxide) and sunlight has been demonstrated using a combination of analysis techniques and consumer-relevant measurements. Damage to the proteins and lipids of the hair cuticle and cortex can be prevented through the sacrificial effect of a unique keratin biopolymer ingredient that essentially undergoes the same degradation processes in preference to the hair fiber.

Published May 2006 Cosmetics and Toiletries magazine

References

1. R Schueller and P Romanowski, Inside the hair—An advanced biology model, *Cosmet Toil* 120(11) 53–58 (2005)
2. V F Monteiro, AS Pinheiro, ER Leite, JAM Agnella, MA Pereira-Da Silva and E Longo, UV radiation: Aggressive agent to the hair—AFM, a new methodology of evaluation, *J Cosmet Sci* 54 271–281 (2003)
3. P Maillan, Measurement of UV protection in the hair, *Business Brieifing: Global Cosmetics Manufacturing* 1–5 (2004)
4. C M Pande and J Jachowicz, Hair photodamage—Measurement and prevention, *J Soc Cosmet Chem* 44 109–122 (1993)

CHAPTER 13

Advances in Polymers for Hair Conditioning Shampoos

Robert Y. Lochhead and Lisa R. Huisinga
The School of Polymers & High Performance Materials, The University of Southern Mississippi Hattiesburg, Mississippi USA

KEY WORDS: *polymers, hair conditioning, shampoos*

ABSTRACT: *The dilution-deposition mechanism is the core of the modern conditioning shampoo. It is described here, along with polymer inventions that enhance benefits and improve the clarity of conditioning shampoos, and enable conditioning from shampoos that do not contain a cationic polymer.*

Cationic polymers, specifically polyquaternium-10 and guar hydroxypropyltrimonium chloride, have been included in shampoos to confer wet-conditioning benefits and style to the hair after drying. Interest in these systems has recently been revived due to advances in our knowledge of the nanoscience of self-assembling systems and polymer-surfactant coacervates. The trend has been driven commercially by the desire to enhance deposition of "actives" and benefit agents from cleansing compositions during the rinsing.

Conditioning Shampoos

The origin of conditioning shampoos can be traced to the Balsam Shampoos of the 1960s followed by the introduction of polyquaternium-10 and the groundbreaking work and scientific insight of Des Goddard[1] in the 1970s and 1980s in which he introduced the concept of polymer-surfactant complex coacervates that phase-separated and deposited on the hair during rinsing. During the 1980s and into the 1990s, complex coacervates were employed as vehicles for the deposition of silicone on hair as conditioning shampoos evolved.[2] This trend continues today and the two original polyelectrolytes – polyquaternium-10 and guar hydroxypropyltrimonium chloride – continue to be the dominant "polymer actives" in conditioning shampoos.

Polyions in aqueous solution are surrounded by small-molecule counterions (**Figure 1**). If the counterions are very soluble in water they will be driven by chemical potential to diffuse to regions of lower counterion concentration and away from the polyion and towards the free water. However, because the polyion and the counterions carry charges of opposite sign, the counterion diffusion

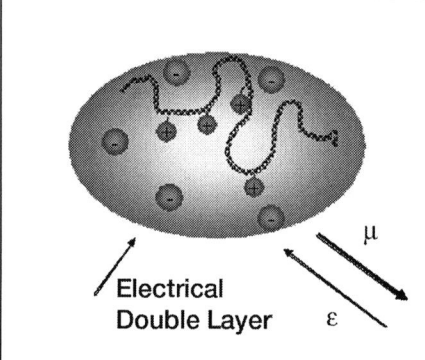

- Chemical Potential μ drives counterions into solution, increasing entropy

- Electrochemical Potential ε attracts counterions towards PE

- Equilibrium between μ and ε creates an Electrical Double Layer, the region with the highest colume of counterions

Figure 1. Polyelectrolyte solubility in water is governed by Donnan Equilibrium

Wetting of the Hair

Wetting of the hair by the applied polymer solution is extremely important because capillary forces are necessary to pull adjacent fibers together to form inter-fiber seam-welds and to cause migration of the solution to inter-fiber cross-points where it will be captured due to a balance of Laplace Pressure between the curvature at the hair-liquid curvature and opposite curvature at the air-liquid interface. This phenomenon is commonly observed as the adhesion between the bristles when a paint-brush is loaded with paint. Dewetting of the hair can cause the fibers to be driven apart and this would inhibit migration of the fixative solution to crosspoints of the hair matrix and prevent the formation of seam welds between fibers.

away from the polyion chain is restrained by the electrochemical potential due to ion-ion attraction. The balance between counterion chemical potential and electrochemical potential determines the ultimate location of the counterions with respect to the polyion chain. This balance between chemical potential and electrochemical potential is called the "Donnan Equilibrium." If the counterions diffuse far away from the polyion chain, then the like charges that are covalently attached to the polyion will mutually repel and the polyion will swell.

Surfactant ions contain a large hydrophobic group and this makes them intrinsically less soluble in water than inorganic ions such as chloride or bromide. When surfactant ions interact with an oppositely charged polyion, they bind strongly and displace the water-soluble inorganic ions from the polyion; that is, they ion-exchange (**Figure 2a**). Once the surfactant ions bind, hydrophobic interaction between the hydrophobic surfactant tails causes the polymer-surfactant complex to collapse (**Figure 2b**). If the surfactant concentration is sufficiently high to form micelles or hemi-micelles along the polyion chain, then the charge on the polyion is reversed and the polymer-surfactant complex will re-expand and will be solubilized (**Figure 2g**).

Conditioning shampoos are formulated within the range of surfactant concentrations that correspond to this solubilized regime. If this solubilized complex (shampoo) is diluted to a concentration in the vicinity of the critical micelle concentration, then the complex coacervate phase-separates (**Figure 2f**). If the separated phase has the correct mechanical and electrical properties it will be deposited on the hair during rinsing. This so-called dilution-deposition mechanism lies at the heart of modern conditioning shampoos.

Conditioning shampoos are expected to confer the wet hair attributes of hair softness and ease of wet-combing, and the dry hair attributes of manageability, good cleansing efficacy, long-lasting moisturized feel, with no greasy feel. Recent research efforts have been directed towards:

- Optimizing polymer and surfactant structure and formulation variables to seek enhanced benefits
- Adding other components to enhance the conditioning benefits

- Improving the clarity of conditioning shampoos, and
- Seeking new methods of conferring conditioning from shampoos that do not contain a cationic polymer.

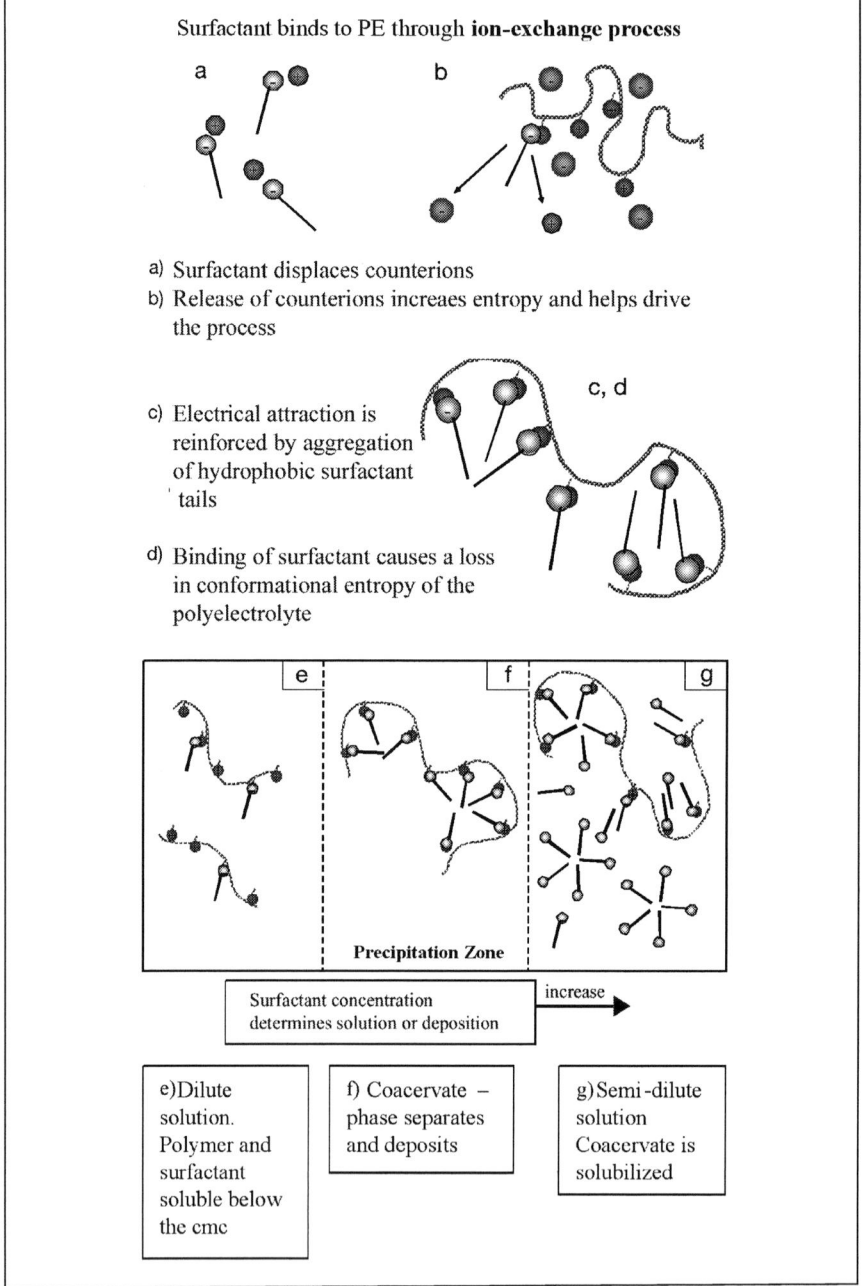

Figure 2. The dilution-deposition mechanism of modern conditioning shampoos

Optimizing Polymer and Surfactant Structure and Formulation Variables

A combination of anionic detersive surfactant with guar hydroxypropyltrimonium chloride in the molecular weight range 10,000 to 10 million and charge density from 1.25 to 7 meq/g is taught to form coacervates that confer excellent conditioning benefits.[3]

Precise optimization of a conditioning shampoo formulation is exemplified in a patent application by Peffly et al[4] who teach optimization of coacervate in a conditioning shampoo from a composition comprising:

- From about 0.01 to about 5 wt. % of a cationic cellulose polymer, wherein the cationic cellulose polymer has a molecular weight of at least 800,000; and
- From about 5 to about 50 wt. % of an anionic surfactant system having specified levels of ethoxylate and sulfate. The ethoxylate level is in the amount of 1.04 multiplied by the molecular weight of the cationic cellulose polymer divided by 1,000,000 plus from about 0.75 to about 3.25. The sulfate level is in the amount of 0.42 multiplied by the charge density of the cationic cellulose polymer plus from about 1.1 to about 3.6; and
- From about 0.01 to about 5 wt. % of a mono or divalent salt; and
- At least about 20 wt. % of an aqueous carrier.

Adding Other Components to Enhance Conditioning Benefits

By the use of microscopic identification, with and without dyes, Wells et al showed that the inclusion of polyalkylene oxide alkyl ether particles in a conditioning shampoo led to larger coacervate flocs (20-500 microns) that resulted in cohesive flocs that resisted shear and gave superior deposition efficiency on hair that conferred good wet conditioning.[5] Typical components of such a shampoo are shown in **Table 1**.

A conditioning shampoo containing a polyester oil formed from a condensate of a polyprotic acid and a polyprotic alcohol is taught to provide manageability for dry hair (possibly from reduced hair friction), no greasy feel, and a moisturized feel.[6] For example the polyester is a polycondensate of adipic acid and pentaerythritol polycondensate with a molecular weight in the range 800 to 10,000. This is exemplified by **Formula 1**.

Researchers at Johnson and Johnson teach that shampoos containing more than one cationic conditioning polymer and a quaternary silicone give more uniform deposition on hair than standard shampoos based on Polyquaternium-10 as the sole conditioning polymer.[7] According to claims in the invention, the conditioning polymer "cocktail" comprises poly(acrylamide-co-acrylamidopropyltrimonium) chloride[a], guar hydroxypropyltrimonium chloride, and silicone quaternium-13. The claims are based upon multiple testing and analysis, namely:

- A Multiple Attribute Consumer Assessment Study against "Pantene Pro-V" for normal hair and J&J's pH 5.5 regular shampoo. The attributes measured were cleaning, wet-comb, dry-comb, hair softness, lather amount and creaminess.
- Secondary Ion Mass spectrometry to detect silicon on the hair surface. This method revealed that "Pantene Pro-V concentrates silicone on cuticle edges" whereas the Patent Application shampoo "distributed silicone more evenly."
- X-Ray photoelectron Spectroscopy (XPS) to measure thickness of silicone polymer layer on hair from Si:C:O ratios. This method revealed that Pantene deposited a significant amount of silicone, and the Patent Application shampoo deposited only one or two molecular layers.
- Instron Ring Compression as a measure of combability.
- Elubiol and Salicylic Acid Skin Permeation studies to determine the efficiency of deposition.
- Complex coacervates can also be formed from mixtures of cationic and anionic polymers. This could be the underlying mechanism in shampoos that include a carbomer[b] with cationic polymer to enhance the deposition of silicone and to improve conditioning benefits.[8]

---

[a] An example is Salcare SC 60 from Ciba.
[b] Carbopol SF-1, Noveon

Table 1
Addin components to enhance the conditioning benefits of a shampoo

Function	Ingredient
Anionic cleansing detergents	Ammonium lauryl sulfate Sodium lauryl ether sulfate (2 or 3 EO)
Amphoteric surfactant	Cocamidopropyl betaine
Conditioning agent	Polyalkylene oxide alkyl ether (e.g. PPG-15 stearyl ether*) Particle size >l micron and <50 microns HLB <7
Water-soluble carrier	Ethanol
Cationic polymer	1-2 meq/g < charge density < 7 meq/g Molecular weight 100,000 to 3 million Polyquaternium-10 is preferred at concentration 0.1-1%. Ratio of cationic polymer to polyalkylene oxide alkyl ether is 1:2 to 1:10.
Silicone conditioning agent	Silicone fluid Silicone resin improves deposition and gloss (high refractive index)
Silicone conditioning agent	100,000 cSt < Viscosity < 1.5 million csks Small particle deposition (Number average particle diameters = 0.01-0.5 micron) Large particle deposition (Number average particle diameter from 12-181 micron) Particle sizes below 5 microns deposit more efficiently on hair.**

* Arlamol E, Uniqema

** Trapped within the coacervate upon dilution?

**Formula 1
Conditioning shampoo**

Function	Ingredient	Amount
Anionic detersive surfactant	Ammoniun lauteth-3-sulfate	10.00% w/w
Anionic detersive surfactant	Ammonium lauryl sulfate	2.00
Amphoteric surfactant	Cocamidopropyl betaine	2.00
Cosurfactant	Cetyl alcohol	0.60
Cosurfactant/foam builder	Cocamide MEA	0.80
Conditioner	Polyquaternium-10	0.50
Suspending agent	Ethylene glycol distearate	1.50
Conditioner	Dimethicone	2.00
Conditioning polyester	Pentaerythritol adipic acid	2.00
Fragrance	Polymeric ester perfume solution	0.70
Chelation	Sodium citrate	0.40
pH adjustment	Citric acid	0.40
	Water *(aqua)*	qs 100.00

Improving the Clarity of Conditioning Shampoos

Silicones are excellent for adsorbing at interfaces and spreading and wetting hair to provide smoothing and conditioning benefits but there are challenges in making stable suspensions of silicones in shampoos. Silicones also tend to reduce foaming and usually silicone shampoos are not visibly clear. Silicone copolyols were introduced to overcome these challenges. They have better solubility in shampoo compositions but their deposition onto hair is much lower. Therefore, conditioning performance is compromised.

Scientists at Kao Corporation have now invented a method to make clear conditioning shampoos that contain a hydrophobic silicone.[9] Adding a solubilizer reduced the silicone droplet size sufficiently to maintain a light transmission value of greater than 97%. The preferred solubilizer is trideceth-2 carboxamide MEA[c].

Peffly et al have reported clear conditioning shampoo formulations that include a silicone microemulsion in a conditioning shampoo containing guar hydroxypropyltrimonium chloride and an anionic detersive surfactant.[10,11]

---

[c]Aminol A15, Finetex

- The anionic surfactant has a specified level for ethoxylate and sulfate. The ethoxylate level is in the amount of about 1.97 multiplied by the molecular weight of the cationic guar polymer divided by 1,000,000 plus from about 0.15 to about 3.5 The sulfate level is in the amount of about 0.97 multiplied by the charge density.
- The cationic polymer is guarhydroxypropyltrimonium chloride having a molecular weight of at least 300,000 and a charge density of at least about 0.1 meq/g.
- The silicone microemulsion is selected from among several products[d] from Dow Corning.

Seeking New Methods of Conferring Conditioning from Shampoos

Organic conditioning oils such as polybutene[e] have been claimed to confer conditioning benefits from a shampoo.[12] Addition of polybutene is taught to increase the deposition of silicone conditioners, and provides improved conditioning benefits such as wet and dry feel and combing. It is interesting to try to figure out the mechanism by which these shampoos provide conditioning. Perhaps these oils are solubilized by the surfactant micelles in the shampoo and then released during rinsing when the system drops below the critical micelle concentration.

Conditioning can be achieved by including chain extended silicones in an anionic surfactant-based shampoo. Specific examples of useful silicones include a Dow Corning emulsion[f] containing divinyldimethicone/dimethicone copolymer with a viscosity about 1.30×10^8 to 1.5×10^8 cP.[13]

There is a need to increase hair volume and styling from conditioning shampoos, and an interesting method to meet this need is to include particles that can deposit on the hair to increase interfiber friction. Wells et al have revealed that cationic guar polymers can enhance the deposition of particles on hair.[14] In this

---

[d]Examples include DC2-5791, DC2-5791-sp, DC2-1470, DC2-1870, DC2-1845, DC2-1845HV and DC2-1550 from Dow Corning.
[e]L14 polybutene from Amoco Corp
[f]HMW2220 from Dow Corning

case the guar is specified to have a charge density less than 4.5 meq/g and a molecular weight in the range 100,000 to 3 million. Pigment particles can be included for color, friction-conferring particles for style (titanium dioxide, clay, pearlescent mica, silica), and platelet or spherical particles for slip and conditioning (hollow silica, hollow polymer). Shampoos containing ethoxylated alcohols have been found to enhance the deposition of large particle silicones (5 to 2000 microns) and in this case it is claimed that cationic polymer is not required.[15]

Hollow particles can be included in shampoo to increase hair volume in people with fine hair that tends to lie flat.[16,17] Factors that influence hair body and fullness include hair diameter, hair fiber-to-fiber interactions, natural configuration (kinky, straight, wavy), bending stiffness, hair density and hair length.

Deposited hollow particles that can increase fiber-fiber interaction comprise:

- Complexes of gas-encapsulated microspheres such as silica modified ethylene/methacrylate copolymer microsphere[g] and talc-modified ethylene/methacrylate copolymer microsphere[h] from Kobo
- Selected polyesters[i] from Akzo Nobel
- Selected inorganic hollow particles[j] from 3M.
- The deposition is claimed to be improved by including a cationic polymer of molecular weight 10,000 to 10 million and charge density 0.9 to 7.0 meq/g.

Cationic polysaccharide polymers having a molecular weight of from about 10,000 to about 10 million and a charge density from about 1.4 meq/gm to about 7.0 meq/gm have been claimed to enhance the deposition of antidandruff particulate ingredients on surfaces.[18]

---

[g]DSPCS-I2TM from Kobo
[h]SPCAT-I2TM from Kobo
[i]Examples include EXPANCELTM 091 DE and 551DE 50 from Akzo Nobel.
[j]Examples include 3M Scotchlite Glass Bubbles, 3M Zeeospheres ceramic microspheres, and 3M Z-Light Spheres ceramic microspheres.

Johnson & Johnson have also directed attention to new compositions for enhancement of actives deposition from shampoos.[19] The Johnson & Johnson shampoos comprise:

- A water-soluble silicone. More preferred silicones are silicone quaternium 13, cetyltriethylammonium dimethicone copolyol phthalate, stearalkonium dimethicone copolyol phthalate.
- A cationic conditioning agent. Most preferred conditioning agents include acrylamidopropyltrimonium chloride/acrylamide copolymer[k], guar hydroxypropyltrimonium chloride[l].
- A cleansing detergent
- Suspending agents are necessary to ensure homogeneous distribution of insoluble active ingredients. Among the preferred suspending agents are carbomer[m], hydroxyethylcellulose, and PVM MA decadiene crosspolymer[n]. Enhanced deposition of particulate actives, such as zinc pyrithione, was shown on cadaver skin treated in a Franz diffusion cell.

Conclusion

This chapter has traced advances in conditioning shampoos that have been announced in the last year or so. Significant progress has occurred driven by technological breakthroughs in our understanding of the nanoscience of coacervates and also the marketplace demand for stimuli-responsive compositions for enhanced deposition of benefit agents. We can expect this trend to accelerate due to five factors. First, the growing availability and awareness of advanced instrumental methods such as atomic force microscopy, nanoindentation, photo-acoustic spectroscopy, and small-angle neutron scattering. Second, the introduction of combinatorial methods for formulation that with allow investigation of the complete composition space in reasonably short times and this will allow the formulator to rapidly optimize systems of interest. Third, the international interest and focused national funding for nanoscience that will greatly enhance our

---

[k]Salcare SC 60 from Ciba
[l]Jaguar C-17 from Rhodia
[m]Carbopol resin from Noveon
[n]Stabilize 06 and QM from ISP

Antidandruff Discoveries at P&G

Procter & Gamble researchers have discovered that the coverage and bio-availability of the antidandruff agent is a better measure of antidandruff efficacy than the absolute deposited amount.20 Thus, the antidandruff active will be more bio-available if it is co-deposited on the surface of coacervate particles rather than if it is encapsulated inside the coacervates and if the coacervate is soft and spreadable rather than elastic on the hair surface.

These researchers also define a bioavailability coverage index that is measured by the following method. Samples of product, control, and placebo were applied to portions of pigskin, which were then lathered and rinsed. Agar contact plates inoculated with Malassezia furfur were exposed to the pigskin surface, and after an incubation period, the plates were analyzed using commercially available software to determine the area of the agar surface which had been colonized by M. furfur. An index was calculated comparing the area colonized in a control relative to the area colonized in each sample. The inhibition of M. furfur growth on the plates is indicative of the bioavailability of the antidandruff agent and coverage of the antidandruff agent, which together and independently are indicative of overall antidandruff efficacy.

Also, they defined first and second conditioning indexes that were measured respectively by wet-combing and expert panel "clean-feel" assessment. Based upon this, they claim improved antidandruff shampoos based upon

- An anionic surfactant that can be one of the following:
- Alkyl sulfates or alkyl ether sulfates
- Alkyl sulfonates alkyl / aryl sulfonates, beta-alkyloxyalkane sulfonates
- Sarcosinates or sarcosinate derivatives
- A non-volatile conditioning agent, such as silicones or organic conditioning oils
- An antidandruff agent. Zinc pyridinethiol-N-oxide is preferred.
- A cationic polymer. The preferred cationic polymers have a molecular weight in the range 350,000 to 500,000 and a charge density in the range 0.6 to 0.9 meq/g.

understanding of the structure/ property relationships of these complex fluids. Fourth, advances in polymer science, such as living free-radical polymerization and modern catalysis that will allow the syntheses of polymers with well-defined precise microstructures. Fifth, consolidation of the finished goods industry and the chemical suppliers will channel more and better technological resources to the production of advanced high performance products and will emphasize the importance of diligent protection of intellectual property. The end result will be a pronounced increase in the sophistication and diversity of products that will be offered to the consumer.

Published May 2005 Cosmetics and Toiletries magazine

References

1. ED Goddard, Polymer surfactant interaction, Parts I and II, chapters 4 and 5 in *Interactions of Surfactants with Polymers and Proteins*, ED Goddard and KP Ananthapadmanabhan, eds, Boca Raton, Florida: CRC Press (1993)
2. US Pats 5,104,646 and 5,106,609, R Bolich et al, assigned to Procter & Gamble (Apr 14, 1992)
3. US Pat Application 20030199403, RL Wells and ES Johnson, filed by Procter & Gamble (Oct 23, 2003)
4. US Pat Application 20040146475, MM Peffly, NW Geary and JA Staudigel, filed by Procter & Gamble (Jul 29, 2004)
5. US Pat application 20030143 74 AI, DR Royce and and R Wells, assigned to Procter & Gamble (Jul 31, 2003)
6. US Pat application 20030138392, DR Royce and R Wells, assigned to Procter & Gamble (Jul 24, 2003)
7. US Pat application 20030176303AI , SM Niemec, H Yeh, R Gallagher and KL Hoe, filed by Johnson & Johnson (Sep 18, 2003)
8. US Pat Application 20030108503, Cosmetic compositions containing a methacrylic acid copolymer, a silicone and a cationic polymer, and uses thereof, M Maubru and B Liebard (Jun 12, 2003)
9. US Pat 6,803,050, H Denzer, H Abe, M Pytlik, R Jansen and A Buhmann, assigned to Kao (Oct 12, 2004)
10. US Pat Application 20040234483, MM Peffly and DW Chang, assigned to Procter & Gamble (Nov 25, 2004)
11. US Pat Application 20040234484, MM Peffly and DW Chang, assigned to Procter & Gamble (Nov 25, 2004)
12. US Pat 6,221,817, Conditioning shampoo composition, SM Guskey, TW Coffindaffer, EM Schrader, RL Wells and JT Baravetto, assigned to Procter & Gamble (Apr 24, 2001)
13. US Pat Application 20030143177, Q Stella, assigned to Procter & Gamble (Jul 31, 2003)
14. US Pat application 20030199403AI, RL Wells and ES Johnson, assigned to Procter & Gamble (Oct 23, 2003)
15. US Pat 6,200,554, Conditioning shampoo compositions having improved silicone deposition, T Yeoh, TW Coffindaffer, H Uchiyama, JG Schroeder and Y Okuyama (Mar 13, 2001)

16. US Pat Application 20030086896, S Midha, BD Hofrichter and SR Thomson, assigned to Procter & Gamble (May 8, 2003)
17. US Pat Application 20030091521, S Midha and BD Hofrichter, assigned to Procter & Gamble (May 15, 2003)
18. US Pat Application 20030202952, RL Wells, ES Johnson and DA Royce, filed by Procter & Gamble (Oct 30, 2003)
19. US Pat Application 20030176303, SM Niemiec, H Yeh, R Gallagher and KL Ho, filed by Johnson & Johnson (Sep 18, 2003)
20. US Pat Application 20020102228, DS Dunlop, RA Boyd, SM Guskey, JR Schwartz and AR Marchetta, filed by Procter & Gamble (Aug 1, 2002)

CHAPTER 14

Polyquaternium-74: An Advanced Hair Conditioning Polymer

Eric Leroy
Rhodia Research, Aubervilliers, France

KEY WORDS: *polyquaternium-74, shampoo, hair conditioning, dimethicone emulsion, natural look, hair shine*

ABSTRACT: *Polyquaternium-74 is a synthetic high performance conditioning polymer whose flocculation and deposition characteristics enable it to match or outperform traditional conditioning polymers in detangling, overall hair conditioning, shine enhancement and build-up reduction when combined, as shown here, with a submicron dimethicone emulsion. Benefits are noted for 2-in-1 shampoo formulations.*

When using a hair conditioning product such as a shampoo, consumers expect their hair to be cleansed, repaired and nourished. But they also expect their hair to be soft and shiny, with volume and a light feel. In a word, consumers expect hair to look natural.

Shampoo formulations have evolved over the last decades, from simple cleansing and foaming bases with poor hair conditioning performance, to fairly sophisticated systems containing a variety of surfactants combined with one or more conditioning polymers and a silicone agent.

While the inclusion of silicones in shampoo has been common since the 1990s, many limitations have prevented a more widespread use of these effective systems. Current challenges are the ability to deposit conditioning actives effectively on different types of hair, such as damaged/oxidized and virgin zones, while enabling desired adjustments to the overall sensorial experience of hair management during and after shampoo. Among the conditioning and delivery polymers introduced recently in the cosmetic industry is polyquaternium-74, whose physico-chemical properties and hair surface modification abilities are described in this chapter.

Polyquaternium-74 Performance Mechanism

Conditioning polymers are usually of cationic nature and the most commonly used are derived from the chemical modification of polysaccharides such as guar and cellulose. It is well-known in the industry that this class of water-soluble polymers can deposit on the hair surface thanks to a mechanism variously called *flocculation* or *coacervation* that occurs while the shampoo is applied on a wet head.[1] Flocculation depends on the surfactant base, the pH and the ionic strength of the formulation. It has been reported that the nature of the polymer backbone has a significant effect on the polymer ability to flocculate. In that respect, cationic guars have always been the reference, outperforming synthetic and cellulose-based conditioning polymers.[2]

Polyquaternium-74 (PQ-74) is a novel synthetic polymer for hair conditioning. It was developed by Rhodia to be a highly flocculating polymer, one that deposits on hair as effectively as high molecular weight cationic guar. PQ-74 is an amphoteric copolymer of acrylic acid anionic monomer and its net charge density is a function of formulation pH.

Flocculation: The flocculation behavior of four conditioning polymers was evaluated by transmittance measurement with a UV spectrophotometer at 600 nm in a cell 10 mm by 10 mm, for different dilution ratios of shampoo compositions. The polymers tested were PQ-74, and the following conventional conditioning polymers: polyquaternium-10 (PQ-10), polyquaternium-7 (PQ-7) and guar hydroxypropyltrimonium chloride (cationic guar). This same group of polymers was used for all the tests reported in this chapter. Shampoos were formulated with 14% sodium laureth

Polyquaternium-74: An Advanced Hair Conditioning Polymer

sulfate (SLES-2EO), 2% cocamidopropyl betaine (CAPB) and 0.2% of conditioning polymers.

Figure 1 depicts the flocculation of PQ-74, which is similar to cationic guar. Images of PQ-74 shampoos at the dilution ratios 1, 2 and 3 in **Figure 2** illustrate how turbid the solutions are, which is linked to the quantity of polymer flocs.

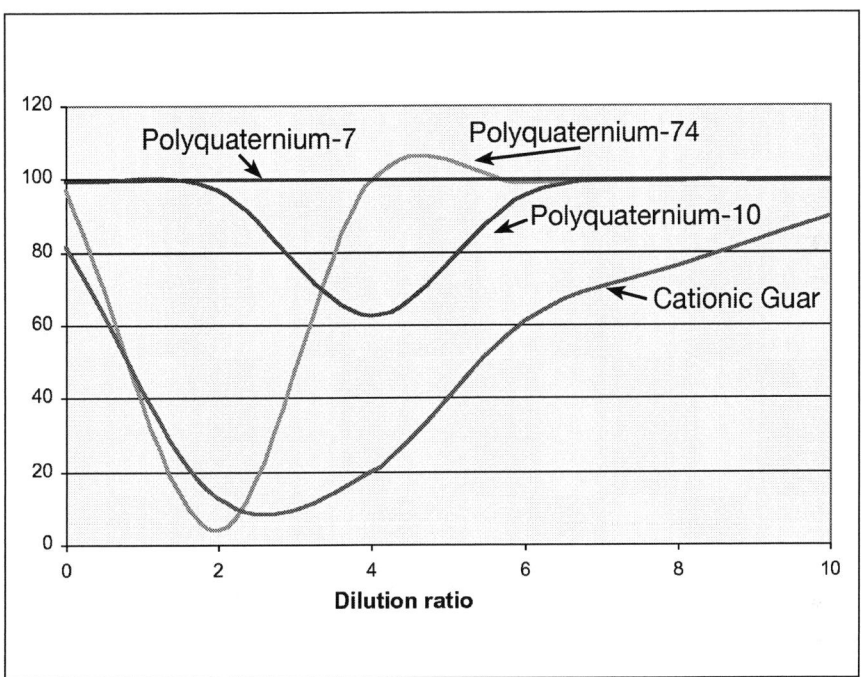

Figure1. Flocculations profiles of polyquaternium-74 and other conditioning polymers

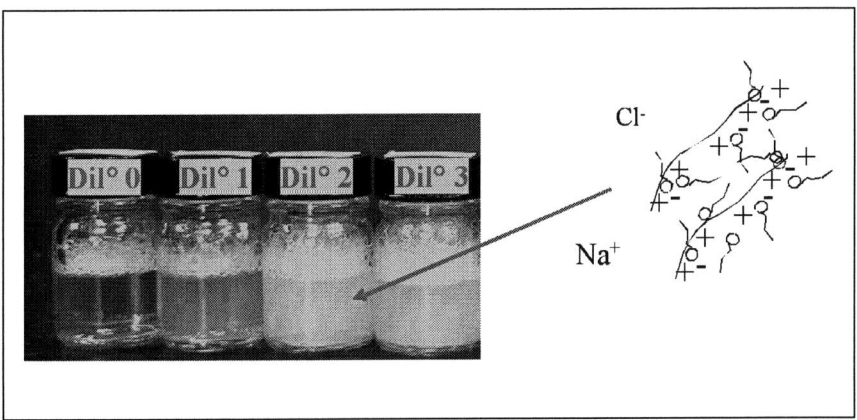

Figure 2. Polyquaternium-74 flocculation at dilution ratios 1, 2 and 3

On the other hand, it appears that PQ-7 does not flocculate in these conditions, and that PQ-10 has a different profile. The minimum of transmittance is obtained for a higher ratio of dilution and its value remains fairly high, which is a sign of only few hydrophobic flocs of PQ-10.

Deposition of PQ-74 on both virgin hair and damaged hair: *Damaged hair* is a generic term that encompasses various kinds of damages. The more frequent is oxidation when hair is dyed, but oxidation differs from damage due to UV or sun light, and also from damage caused by combing and brushing.

Oxidized hair is also called hydrophilic damaged hair. It is a hydrophilic surface of amphoteric nature with a high charge density. By contrast, virgin hair is hydrophobic, essentially of anionic nature with a low charge density.

Hydrophobic flocs deposit on the surface, but during the rinsing step these flocs are more easily washed out from the hydrophilic, amphoteric surface, than from the hydrophobic one. Moreover, the oxidized hair surface is very heterogeneous. It could be seen as a chess board, where black squares are hydrophobic areas and white squares hydrophilic ones. Indeed, these differences in the physical-chemistry of virgin and oxidized hair surfaces explain the poor deposition of conditioning ingredients on damaged zones.

There is direct correlation between the ability of conditioning polymers to form hydrophobic flocs during the shampoo process and their effective deposition on the hair surface. A simple method to evaluate the deposition of polymers bearing cationic charges is the Rubin dye test, also called the red dye test.

Upon shampooing, a conditioning polymer deposits on hair surface. The hair tress is then treated with a solution containing an anionic red dye. The dye reacts with cationic sites at the surface to produce a red-colored substrate whose color intensity is related to the amount of deposited cationic polymer. The red dye is then extracted at 60°C using a sodium chloride solution and titrated using UV spectrophotometric analysis.

For reasons already mentioned, depositing hydrophobic flocs on hydrophobic virgin hair is much simpler than the challenging task of depositing hydrophobic flocs on hydrophilic damaged or oxidized hair. In one red dye test conducted in house the ratio of PQ-74 deposition on virgin to damaged hair was close to 2:1. A ratio that low suggests that PQ-74 can be formulated for both virgin hair and damaged hair.

Deposition of silicone: Efficient conditioning polymers are those that flocculate during hair shampooing, i.e., before dilution in rinsing. Polymer that does not flocculate is not effective, as seen in **Figure 1**. Moreover, it also is possible to use polymers or formulate polymers in a way that flocs are preformed in the shampoo, prior to any dilution. This generally is done with a certain category of polymer chemistries that are not the most efficient with respect to deposition of silicone on hair.

The hydrophobic flocs that are formed vary in size with surfactant compositions and are generally a few tens of microns in size. These objects have come to be regarded as potential vehicles to deliver particulates dispersed in the shampoo base onto the hair surface, especially, silicone oil droplets and antidandruff agents such as zinc pyrithione.

An in-house test was conducted to determine the effect of droplet size on silicone deposition by PQ-74. Classic high viscosity dimethicone oil was emulsified with laureth-7 or laureth-8. Shampoos tested contained 1% of silicone and 0.2% of PQ-74 in a SLES/CAPB base. Dimethicone deposited on hair surface was extracted from the keratinous surface with tetrahydrofuran (THF) solvent and the silicone oil in THF was dosed using gel permeation chromatography (GPC). The results obtained with this method were quantitative. (By the way, this same technique was used to show that adding some common tertiary surfactants does not diminish dimethicone deposition by PQ-74 and may improve it. See **Table 1**.)

The most efficient combinations were created by associations of PQ-74 with submicron dimethicone emulsions. For an emulsion with droplets 3 μm in size, 245 ppm of dimethicone per gram of hair were deposited, which corresponds to a deposition yield of approximately 25%. For submicron emulsions, this yield increases to above 55%, and is constant over droplet sizes of 0.4 μm (500 ppm), 0.6 μm (550 ppm) and 1.0 μm (550 ppm). Therefore, a very interesting conditioning system is the association of a PQ-74 with a dimethicone emulsion of 0.6 μm. For the rest of this chapter, the term *PQ-74DIM* will be used to refer to this proprietary system[a] of PQ-74 and a submicron dimethicone emulsion.

Table 1
Influence of secondary and teriary surfactants on dimethicone deposition on virgin hair by PQ-74. The primary surfactant was SLES-2EO at 14%

Secondary surfactant	Tertiary surfactant	Dimethicone (ppm)
2% CAPB	-	550
1% CAPB	1% Coco glucoside	500
-	2% Coco glucoside	500
2% CAPB	2% Sodium laureth sulfosuccinate	560
2% CAPB	4% specialty blend (sodium cocoyl isethionate, sodium lauroamphoacetate, sodium methyl cocoyl taurate)	620

Once again using the GPC procedure already described, PQ-74DIM was benchmarked against cationic guar, PQ-10 and PQ-7 in association with the same submicron dimethicone emulsion. The measured values of dimethicone deposition onto virgin hair in ppm per gram of hair were 600, 600, 72 and 24, respectively. A simple correlation clearly appears when comparing these silicone deposition results with the polymer flocculation profiles in **Figure 1**. PQ-10 and PQ-7 poorly deposit dimethicone on virgin hair, while they weakly flocculate upon dilution. Similarly, PQ-74DIM deposits a high level of dimethicone, similar to cationic guar.

The major challenge of hair conditioning in rinse-off products is to maintain sufficient deposition of conditioning agents on hair after rinse cycles, and in that regard the selection of cationic polymer and silicone emulsion conditioning agents is crucial to the performance of the shampoo. PQ-74DIM has been shown to be an effective way to meet that challenge.

---

[a]Polycare Boost (INCI: Water (aqua) (and) Dimethicone (and) Polyquaternium-74 (and) Laureth-7) is a product of Rhodia Novecare, Cranbury, N.J., USA. Polycare is a registered trademark of Rhodia.

Hair Conditioning and Repairing

Detangling: Because PQ-74DIM deposits effectively on the hair surface, it was anticipated that this system would provide hair conditioning benefits such as wet hair combing and detangling. These benefits were evaluated using tensile testing equipment[b] that monitors the force developed to comb a hair tress from top to bottom.

Tresses of damaged/oxidized hair[c] were treated with shampoo containing 1.0% of a submicron dimethicone emulsion and 0.2% of PQ-74, cationic guar or PQ-10. For each treatment, six tresses were treated and combed 10 times. The percentage reduction of combing force versus untreated wet hair for PQ-74DIM, cationic guar, PQ-10 and the shampoo base was 25, 25, 6 and 1.5%.

These data indicate that PQ-74DIM had approximately the same level of reduction in wet combing force, i.e., ~25%, as the cationic guar with dimethicone. On the other hand, PQ-10 with dimethicone emulsion had a fairly low performance to improve the combing of oxidized hair tresses. This finding is not surprising and fully in agreement with the previous data on the ability of PQ-10 to deposit silicone on hair surface.

Overall hair conditioning of Caucasian hair: The overall hair conditioning properties that are brought by this system were evaluated in half-head salon tests carried out at the Schrader Institute in Germany on damaged hair, and compared to a PQ-74DIM-based shampoo. The shampoo composition was exactly the same as those tested in wet combing with the tensile equipment. The panel was composed of 10 women with damaged hair (oxidized, colored and dry hair). Most of the women had long hair. The hair dresser carried out two hair shampooings. The first was a pre-wash. The second came as the hair dresser judged the hair on various sensorial benefits while washing, combing and styling each panelist. As presented in **Figure 3**, four different hair conditioning attributes were assessed: wet hair detangling, wet hair feel, dry hair detangling and dry hair feel.

Figure 3 illustrates that PQ-74DIM outperformed PQ-10 with dimethicone for each of the four conditioning attributes evaluated.

---

[b]Diastron is a registered trademark of Dia-Stron Limited, Andover, Hampshire, UK.
[c]Supplied by International Hair Inc., Florence, S.C., USA.

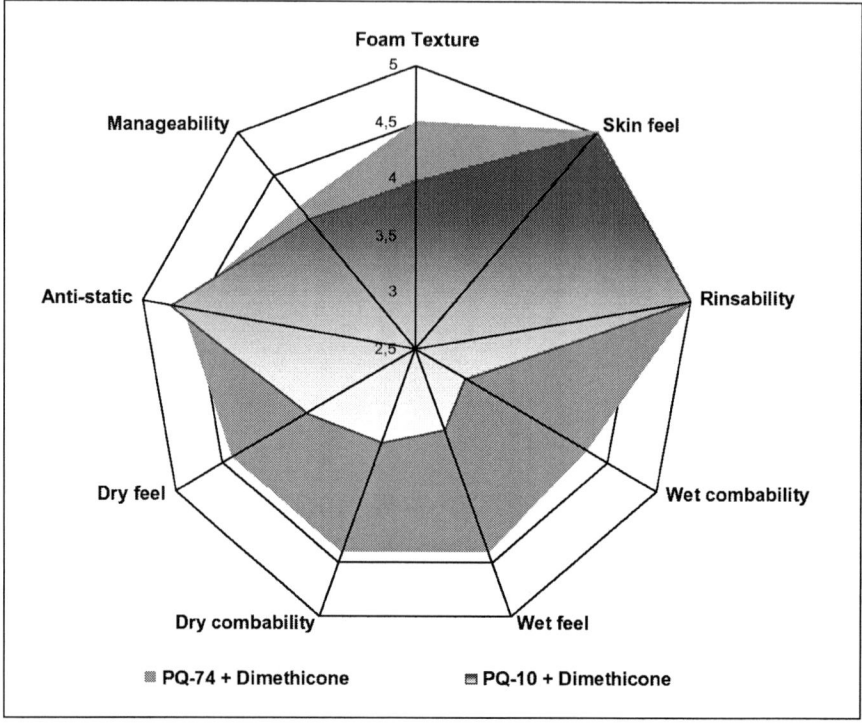

Figure 3. Half-head panel evaluation of a system of polyquaternium-74 and dimethicone versus a system of polyquaternium-10 an dimethicone in Germany

Damaged/oxidized hair is much more porous than virgin hair and can absorb large quantities of water while wet. In these conditions, damaged hair is far more fragile than in the dry stage. Thus, the ability to smoothly detangle this type of hair is critical to ensure the integrity of the fiber. The detangling performance of PQ-74DIM is linked to the ability of PQ-74 to flocculate and thus deposit on hair surface and deliver actives such as dimethicone submicron emulsion. That performance also is linked to the quality of the dimethicone emulsion. In the shampoo, silicone oil is dispersed in droplets, the quantity of which is a cubic function of the diameter of the droplets. For instance, an emulsion with droplets 0.6 μm in size such as the one associated in PQ-74DIM will have 100 times as many droplets as an emulsion with droplets 3 μm in size; i.e., one droplet 3 μm in diameter can be divided into 100 droplets 0.6 μm in diameter. Thus, the oil is deposited in a much more homogeneous way, which is key to quickly coating the hair fiber.

The advantages of PQ-74DIM over PQ-10 and dimethicone alone on wet and dry damaged hair were demonstrated by this in-use evaluation. This test was conducted in Germany on Caucasian hair. How would PQ-74DIM perform on Asian hair?

Overall hair conditioning of Asian hair: In Western countries, damaged hair is more and more common. Meanwhile, Asia is witnessing the increasing popularity of hair grooming. Essentially influenced by Japan and Korea and a trend more and more followed by young people, the coloring, dyeing and bleaching of hair has gained popularity in Asian countries since the end of the 1990s. Consequently, there is an increasing demand in Asia for products that provide a high degree of conditioning and protection to the hair fiber.

A panel test in China evaluated the performance of PQ-74DIM on the damaged/oxidized hair of 15 Asian women. The shampoo formulations tested were free of thickening polymers and were stabilized with a fine-tuned association of surfactants. Shampoo was applied in the same way as in the Caucasian hair study, and the same four hair conditioning attributes were assessed.

The results of half-head evaluations are depicted in **Figure 4** and show that PQ-74DIM outperforms the PQ-10 with dimethicone system on those four hair conditioning benefits. Differences in performance evaluated by the hair dresser were statistically significant and were in full agreement with the previous data generated on Caucasian hair.

This result confirms the versatility of this association, which is effective on virgin and damaged hair, for Asian and Caucasian hair types. Moreover, it demonstrated that the system is effective in different surfactant bases. In the Caucasian test, shampoos were formulated with a stabilizing polymer, whereas in the Asian test a cocamide MEA alkanolamide was incorporated to ensure formulation stability.

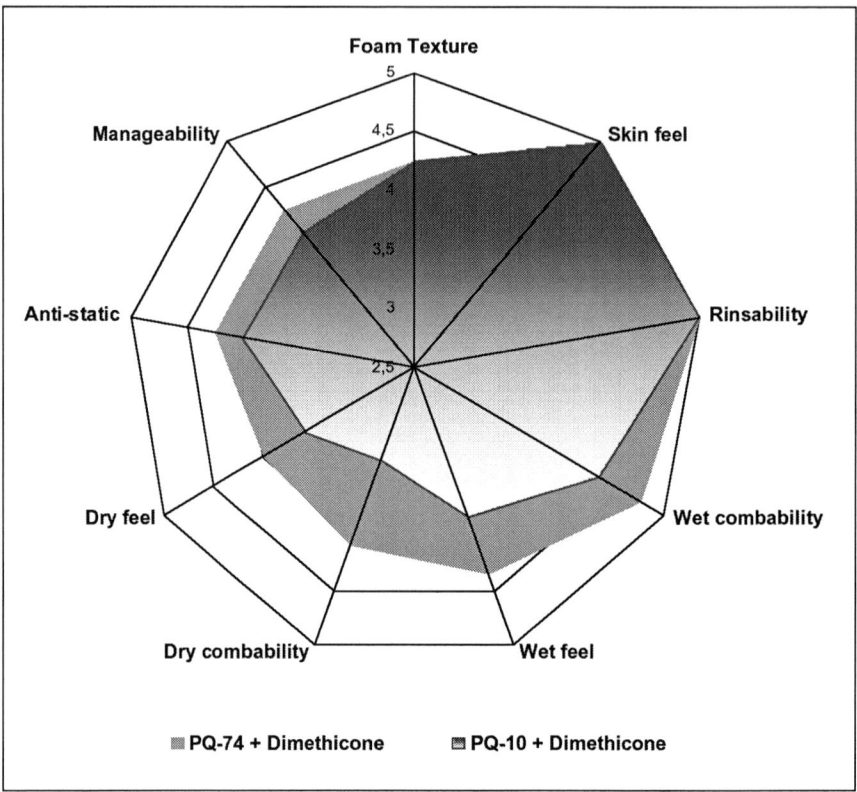

Figure 4. Half-head panel evaluation of a system of polyquaternium-74 and dimethicone versus a system of polyquaternium-10 and dimethicone in China

Enhancing Hair Shine and Natural Look

The most effective conditioning polymers such as high molecular weight cationic guar provide a strong after-feel to the wet hair. That after-feel can be perceived by consumers as an effective treatment and conditioning of the hair. However, in some cases consumers associate this strong feel to over-conditioned hair fibers and thus tend to over-rinse their hair. Hence, some consumers are looking for a conditioning system that provides a squeaky clean feel in the wet stage and also ensures the excellent hair detangling.

Build-up: The build-up of PQ-74, cationic guar and PQ-10 was evaluated from repeated shampoo applications on virgin hair. Hair tresses were treated 1, 3 and 10 times and polymer deposition was measured with the red dye test described previously. The amount of dye adsorbed by the hair surface is linked to the cationic charges on the polymer backbone and does not allow for a direct comparison of polymers. Thus, dye intensity measured by UV-spectrophotometry was normalized to 100% after the first shampoo application. The shampoo formulation was a simple surfactant base of 14% of SLES-2EO and 2% of CAPB at pH of 5.

Results displayed in **Figure 5** show that neither PQ-74 nor cationic guar builds up after multiple shampoo applications, but PQ-10 does build up. Therefore, PQ-74 is a sustainable choice for the formulator because it will not induce over-conditioning of the hair fiber and will be beneficial to the hair volume and styling. This absence of build-up was also confirmed in sensorial assessments by hair dressers at the Schrader Institute.

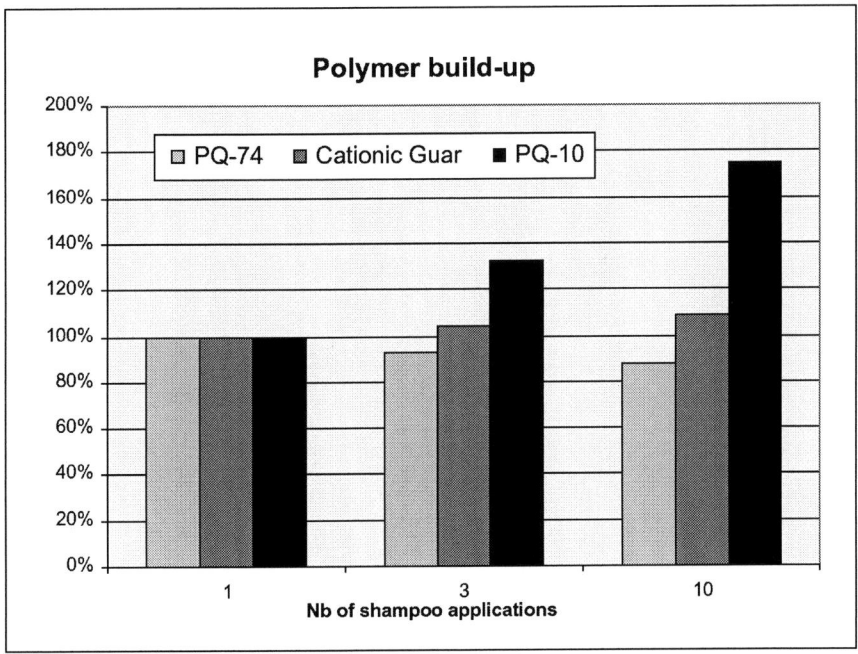

Figure 5. Buildup of polyquaternium-74 and other polymers

The build up of silicone on hair can be of concern for formulators developing 2-in-1 conditioning shampoos. Thus, repeated shampoo applications on virgin hair tresses were carried out with a formulation comprising 1.0% of a dimethicone emulsion of 0.6 μm and 0.2%

of one of these conditioning polymers: PQ-74, cationic guar or PQ-10. Two hair tresses were used per conditioning system and the deposition of the dimethicone was measured after extraction with THF by GPC. As shown in **Figure 6**, the system of cationic guar and dimethicone emulsion, widely used in 2-in-1 shampoos, produced a silicone deposition profile similar to that of PQ-74DIM after 1, 3, 5 and 10 repeated shampooings. Evaluation of the system based on PQ-10 provides little information because this polymer barely deposits the silicone oil.

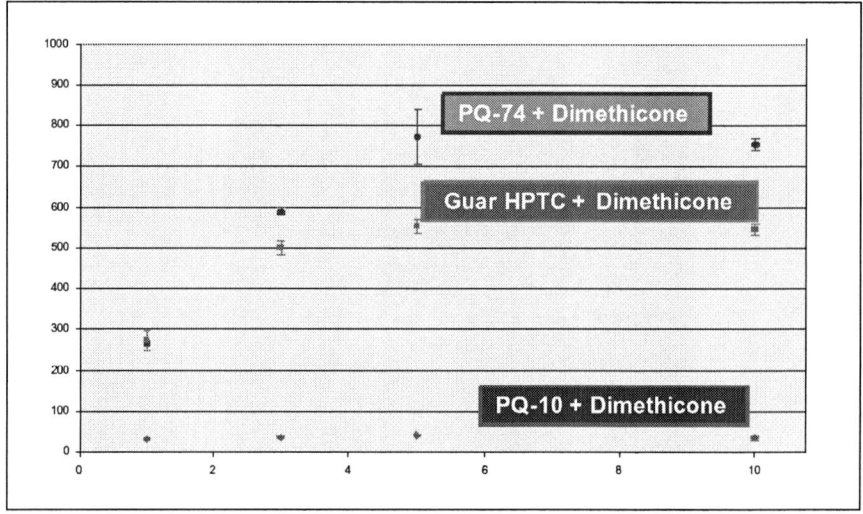

Figure 6. Buildup of dimethicone with selected conditioning polymers

Overall, it appears from the evaluations presented in **Figures 5 and 6** that PQ-74DIM does not build up on hair upon multiple applications (evaluated for up to 10 shampooings). The association of these conditioning actives is thus of great interest for the formulator because it provides benefits for hair detangling and repairing, light silky touch and squeaky clean feel during rinsing, and can be repeatedly used by the consumer without jeopardizing these performances.

Rinsability: The removal of dimethicone build-up by rinsing with a clarifying shampoo was tested on two hair tresses washed 10 times with a 2-in-1 conditioning shampoo containing PQ-74DIM at 2.5%, which corresponds to 0.2% PQ-74 and 1% dimethicome.

In the case presented here, the clarifying shampoo was a simple formulation of SLES-2EO. It appears (**Figure 7**) that after one application, 50% of the dimethicone was removed and 80% was removed after the third clarifying shampoo. Thus, dimethicone is only temporarily bound to hair surface and PQ-74 does not prevent its removal by a clarifying shampoo.

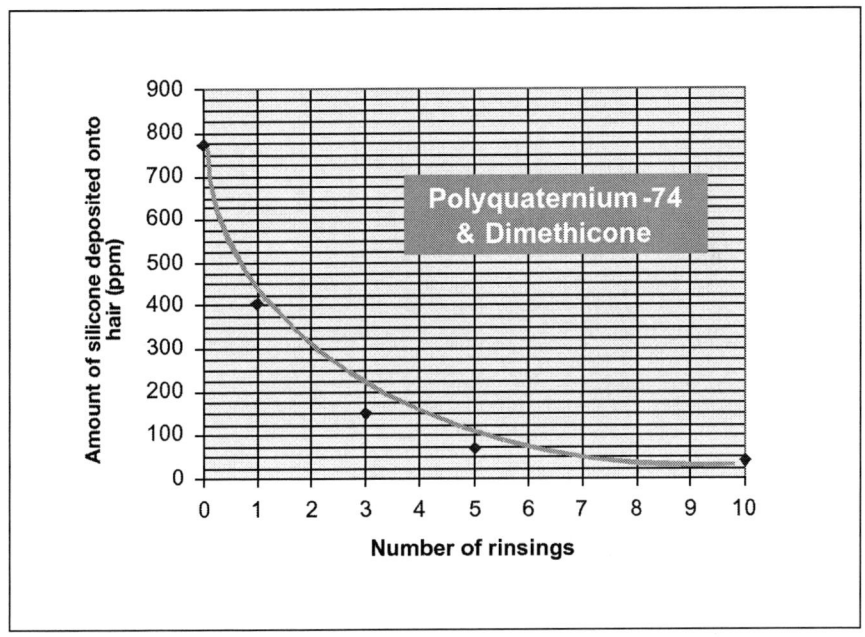

Figure 7. Dimethicone rinsability wiht a clarifying shampoo after 10 shampooings with a 2-in-1 shampoo containing PQ-74DIM

Shine: Hair oxidation from coloring, perming or waving treatments dramatically denatures the hair fiber. It changes from a hydrophobic, smooth surface to a hydrophilic, rough one. Repetition of these treatments results, especially at the tips, in severe hair damage. Consumers perceive this damage as unhealthy hair, without volume or shine, and with an overall hair style that does not look natural compared to the prior virgin state of hair.

Many attributes convey the signal of a healthy hair that looks natural. Volume and color are some of them, but more importantly, the luster or shine of the hair is the most significant property that recalls healthiness and the natural state of hair.

A 2-in-1 conditioning shampoo containing one of three polymers was evaluated for its effect on the shine of blond hair tresses. Three tresses were evaluated for each polymer. Shine was measured with a gloss meter after 10 consecutive shampooings. The shampoo was a surfactant base of SLES-2EO at 14% and cocamidopropyl betaine at 2% with one of three conditioning polymers: PQ-74DIM; a system of PQ-10 and PEG-12 dimethicone; or a system of PQ-10 and the submicron dimethicone emulsion. Results are shown in **Table 2**.

Table 2
Effect of selected conditioning polymers on relative percentage of shine enhancement compared to the surfactant base

Polymer	Ingredient
PQ-74DIM	43
PQ-10 (and) PQ-12 (and) dimethicone	23
PQ-10 (and) dimethicone	5

PQ-74DIM enabled a significant improvement in hair shine when formulated in the 2-in-1 conditioning shampoo. This result is first linked to the level of dimethicone deposited on hair surface, which explains why the PQ-10-based systems are under-performing. A second factor is PQ-74's unique chemical structure. High-depositing polymers of high molecular weight will not adsorb flat on a surface, and thus will tend to reduce the shiny appearance of hair. PQ-74 behaves differently. Because of its acrylic acid monomers, its cationic sites and the high flexibility of its backbone, it will adsorb flat and thus will not reduce the hair shine. Thus, PQ-74 is able to form a thin and homogeneous coating on the hair surface. That coating neither disrupts the light scattering nor reduces the intensity of the light reflected back.

Conclusion

The association of PQ-74 with a dimethicone emulsion in a single liquid product form is a means to efficiently restore the natural look of hair and maximize positive signals to consumers such as hair shine, smooth feel, hair volume and manageability.

In addition to these benefits, this novel system based on PQ-74 and dimethicone emulsion simplifies processes for the manufacturing of shampoos, does not require any sophisticated mixing tools and gives the formulator an access to a range of performances with only one conditioning ingredient. The formulator has now the possibility to meet demanding formulation projects aiming at improving hair wellness and consumer well-being.

Published March 2008 Cosmetics and Toiletries magazine

References

1. ED Goddard and RB Hannan, Cationic polymer / anionic surfactant interactions, J Colloid Interface Sci 55 73–78 (1976)
2. US Pat 5,085,857, Conditioning shampoo comprising a surfactant, a non-volatile silicone oil and guar hydroxypropyltrimonium chloride as a cationic conditioning polymer, ES Reid and AM Murray (Feb 4, 1992)
3. S Rogasik, N Martin, JM Ricca, W Wielinga and O Anthony, The challenge of damaged hair shampoos: Which links between benefits on damaged hair and measurable physical chemical parameters?, SOFW Journal 125(11) 32–39 (1999)

CHAPTER 15

Evaluating Polyimide-1, a Styling Resin for Gel and Mousse Formulations

Nancy Clements
International Specialty Products, Wayne, New Jersey USA

KEYWORDS: *Hair styling resin, gel, mousse, polyimide-1, testing and instrumentation*

ABSTRACT: *This chapter surveys a variety of tests used to evaluate polyimide-1, a new hair styling resin, by comparing its performance against that of PVP in gel and mousse formulations.*

Variations of hair gels and mousses comprise approximately half of the global styling product market and are the key growth area within the category. New technology is required to sustain this growth and to meet the challenge of providing longevity of style (style memory), volume creation, style definition, and a smooth/touchable hold while maintaining compatibility with polyacrylic acid rheology modifiers.

This chapter surveys a variety of tests ISP uses to evaluate new hair styling resins for gels and mousses. Tests for high humidity curl retention, film clarity, flexibility, durability, toughness, film surface friction and versatility/compatibility are used to compare the in-product performance of a new resin (polyamide-1) versus an established styling resin (polyvinylpyrrolidone).

Polyimide-1

Polyimide-1[a] was specifically designed by ISP to meet consumer needs for the gel and mousse market. It is a water-soluble, amphoteric polymer comprised of an isobutylene/dimethylaminopropylmaleimide polymer backbone derivatized with ethylene oxide/propylene oxide (EO/PO) oligomers and dimethylaminopropylamine (DMAPA) (**Figure 1**). ISP is the sole supplier of polyimide-1.

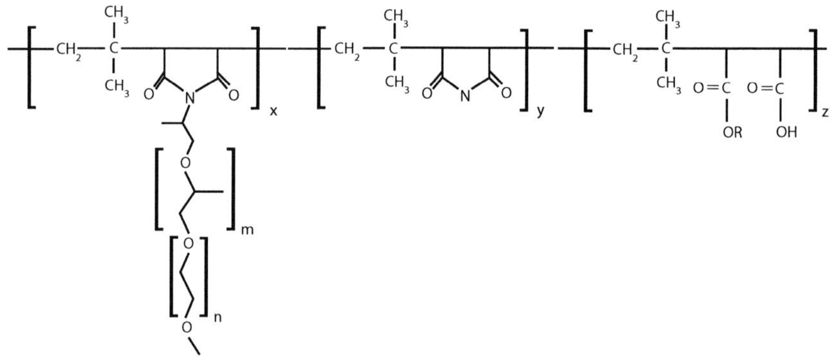

Figure 1. Structure of polyimide-1

EO/PO oligomers provide the unique, natural feel and water resistance properties of polyimide-1. These oligomers are typically used in other industries for their flexibility and natural humectant ability, i.e. the ability to take up water without impacting other properties. DMAPA is a self-associating, secondary amine that imparts good cohesive strength, toughness and overall good mechanical performance. The ratios of EO/PO and DMAPA in polyimide-1 were optimized to work synergistically with anionic rheology modifiers (especially polyacrylic acid-based rheology modifiers such as carbomer). Performance benefits of formulations with polyimide-1 and polyacrylic acid polymers can be tailored to provide customized functionality/esthetics and tactical differences based on the ratio of polyacrylic acid to polyimide-1.

[a] Aquaflex XL-30 (INCI: Polyimide-1) is a product of International Specialty Products.

Evaluating Polyimide-1, a Styling Resin for Gel and Mousse Formulations

To demonstrate the uniqueness and effectiveness of polyimide-1, various hair gel formulations containing polyimide-1 and carbomer and other typical styling products were prepared in ISP's laboratory to study performance properties. The following measurements were performed to determine the attributes and efficacy of polyimide-1/carbomer systems:

- High humidity curl retention
- Film clarity
- Flexibility, durability, and toughness
  - Dynamic Hair Spray Analysis (DHSA)
  - Cantilever 3-point bending
  - Stress/Strain testing
- Film surface properties: coefficient of friction
- Volume and consumer perception: salon studies
- Versatility/compatibility: formulation stability

Half-head salon evaluations were also conducted in ISP's applications laboratory to ascertain consumer perceptions and to corroborate our experimental results.

Water Resistance and High Humidity Curl Retention

Polyimide-1 is a water-based polymer that produces hydrophobic films that are easily removed from hair by shampooing; there is no resulting buildup of polymer on the hair. Polyvinylpyrrolidone (PVP) is an established styling resin used by a significant portion of the current hair gel market. PVP K-30 is a specific grade of PVP offered by multiple suppliers. We used PVP K-30 for all tests reported here, so for the remainder of this chapter we will use only the term "PVP" and it will refer to PVP K-30.

Figure 2 illustrates a hair swatch treated with a 2% polyimide-1 / 0.5% carbomer gel (4:1 blend ratio), dried as a flat ribbon spike, dipped in water for 5 seconds and then held horizontally to demonstrate resistance to water. The polyimide tress maintains its holding ability after the 5 second immersion while the PVP/carbomer tress fails.

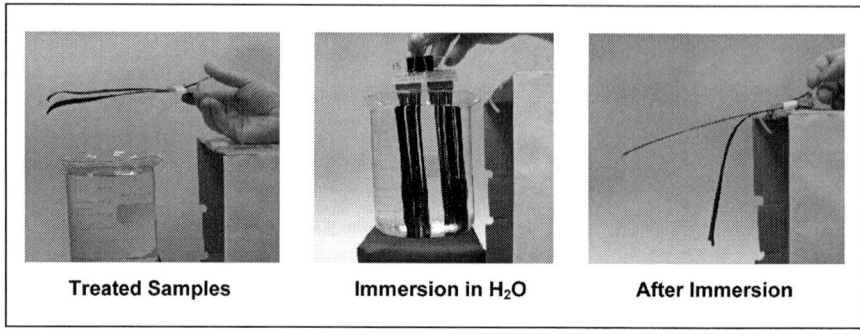

Figure 2. Water resistance and high humidity curl retention of hair swatches treated with 2% polyimide-1 / 0.5% carbomer gel (upper) or 2% PVP / 0.5% carbomer gel (lower) dipped in water for 5 seconds

Water resistance for a measurable time period is only one of the key benefits of polyimide -1. Its films are also resistant to high humidity. **Figure 3**, shows a comparison chart of high humidity curl retention of polyimide-1/carbomer systems versus the most popular hair gel system, PVP/carbomer. The test was conducted by applying 0.5 g styling gel per 2 g tress of 6.5" European dark brown hair and then rolling the tress in spiral curl. The graph depicts the significant humidity resistance of the polyimide-1 formulations, even at very low use levels of polymer, demonstrating the superior curl retention properties of this polymer.

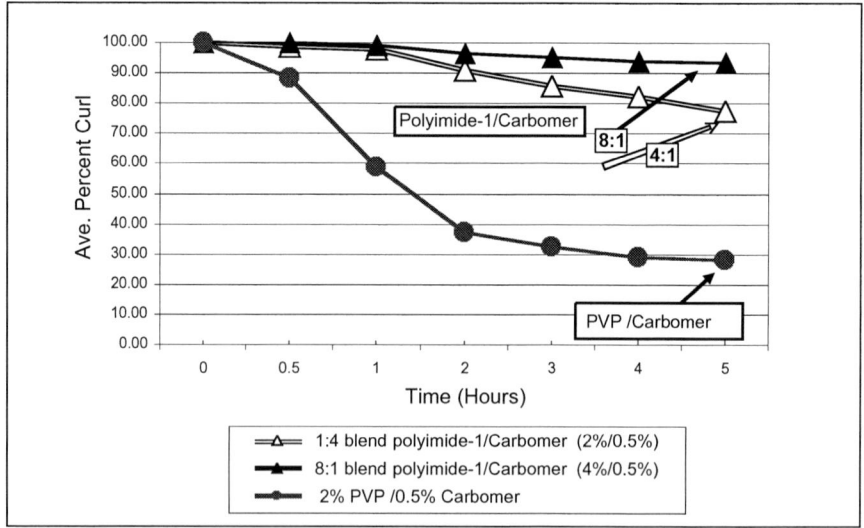

Figure 3. High humidity curl retention of polyimide-1/carbomer blends versus PVP/carbomer over 5 hours at 90% RH and 80°F

High humidity resistance is an essential factor for creating and maintaining a hairstyle, but there are other consumer perceivable features that are also important to a multifunctional resin, including stiffness, durability and conditioning benefits.

Gel Film Clarity

Dry film properties are a key attribute for evaluation of polymer performance on hair. Typical hair gel formulations containing polyimide-1 and carbomer were compared to the most widely used formulations on the market. Films were drawn on a glass plate using a Bird Applicator 0.003" and allowed to dry at 70°F and 50% relative humidity. As can be seen in **Figure 4**, the dry films of polyimide-1 are clear while PVP/carbomer films are hazy.

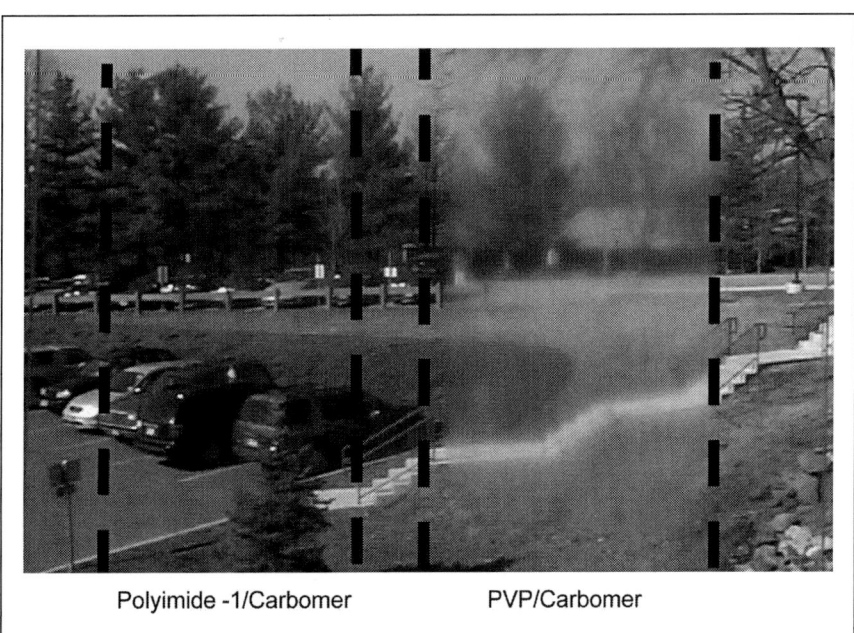

Figure 4. Clarity of dry films of polyimide-1/carbomer (left) and PVP/carbomer (right)

Formulation Clarity

Formulation clarity is an important factor for any hair gel system, especially those with polyacrylic acid or anionic rheology modifiers. Anionic rheology modifiers are acidic polymers that are insoluble in water until they have been neutralized. They need time or heat to hydrolyze fully before adding other ingredients or neutralizing. When hydrolyzed, they are in the acidic form and may form insoluble complexes with other ingredients. Therefore, the order of addition is crucial to formulate clear gels. This is especially true for polyimide-1 formulations because polyimide-1 has been designed to complex with carbomer to create synergistic performance benefits.

Polyimide-1 was tested with a variety of rheology modifiers including carbomer, acrylates C20-30 alkyl acrylate copolymer, PVM/MA decadiene crosspolymer, and acrylates/beheneth-25 methacrylate copolymer. Within this group of rheology modifiers, acrylates C20-30 alkyl acrylate copolymer furnished gels with the highest clarity when using typical component ratios. An acrylates C20-30 alkyl acrylate copolymer gel measured 25 NTU as opposed to 45 NTU with carbomer using the same component ratios. Viscosities are typically in the 20-30,000 cps range using 2% polyimide-1 and 0.5% of the rheology modifier.

Acrylates C20-30 alkyl acrylate copolymer was used to observe the effects of: changes to the neutralizer; concentration; and addition of ethanol. It was found that reduction of the polyimide-1 / acrylates C20-30 alkyl acrylate copolymer ratio from 4:1 to 2:1 not only reduced haze by 50%, but also resulted in a more flexible film.

Addition of ethanol to carbomer gels can prove to be a problem, even in the absence of polyimide-1, because it reduces both the ability of carbomer to be quickly dispersed in the solvent system and the extent of solvation. It was found that addition of ethanol after a gel is fully neutralized and mixed is superior to adding it prior to neutralization.

Use of increasingly more hydrophilic amines (particularly inorganic bases) resulted in gels having increased haze and decreased viscosity. Use of the more hydrophobic bases, such as triisopropanolamine, drastically improved hydroalcoholic gels in terms of both clarity and viscosity. A hydroalcoholic gel prepared with NaOH measured 37 NTU and 8800 cps while the same gel prepared with triisopropanolamine measured 23 NTU and 20000 cps.

A typical procedure for preparing a gel formulation of polyimide-1 is:

1. Prepare a diluted solution of the thickener;
2. Achieve 100% neutralization of the thickener solution to form the gel;
3. Add polyimide-1.

Flexibility, Toughness and Durability

By conducting studies with the Dynamic Hair Spray Analysis (DHSA) on omega loops of hair and the Cantilever 3-Point Bending method (**Figure 6**) on flat hair tresses, the stiffness, stiffness ratio, flexibility and durability under normal and high relative humidity of polyimide-1 have been quantified.

DHSA: When a treated omega loop of hair is depressed and bent 10 times at 50% RH using DHSA, the maximum force needed to depress the curl and the resiliency of the curl is obtained (**Figure 5**). The smooth curve at the top of the peaks and the overlapping multiple hysteresis loops indicate the flexibility of the polymer film on hair and durability of the hair set. The vertical Y axis shows the number of grams of force needed to depress the curl at the depth (in mm) shown on the X axis.

Using DHSA, the resiliency and durability of polyimide-1, carbomer, PVP/carbomer and polyimide-1/carbomer were compared on hair set into omega loops. F_1 is the maximum force attained during the first 4 mm depression. The stiffness ratio can be calculated from the force needed to depress the set hair to 1 mm (a region that is mostly elastic and reproducible after several depressions if 1 mm isn't exceeded) divided by the force needed to depress untreated hair 1 mm. Then resilience and durability measurements are calculated by the ratios of the maximum force at the first depression compared to the maximum force at the 10th depression (F_1/F_{10}), the slope of the 1st depression curve versus the 10th (E_1/E_{10}), and the depth of penetration into the hair loop in order to sense plasticity, 1st versus 10th (H_1/H_{10}). The data in **Figure 5** shows that polyimide-1 + carbomer provides significantly improved resiliency as compared to carbomer alone or PVP/carbomer systems.

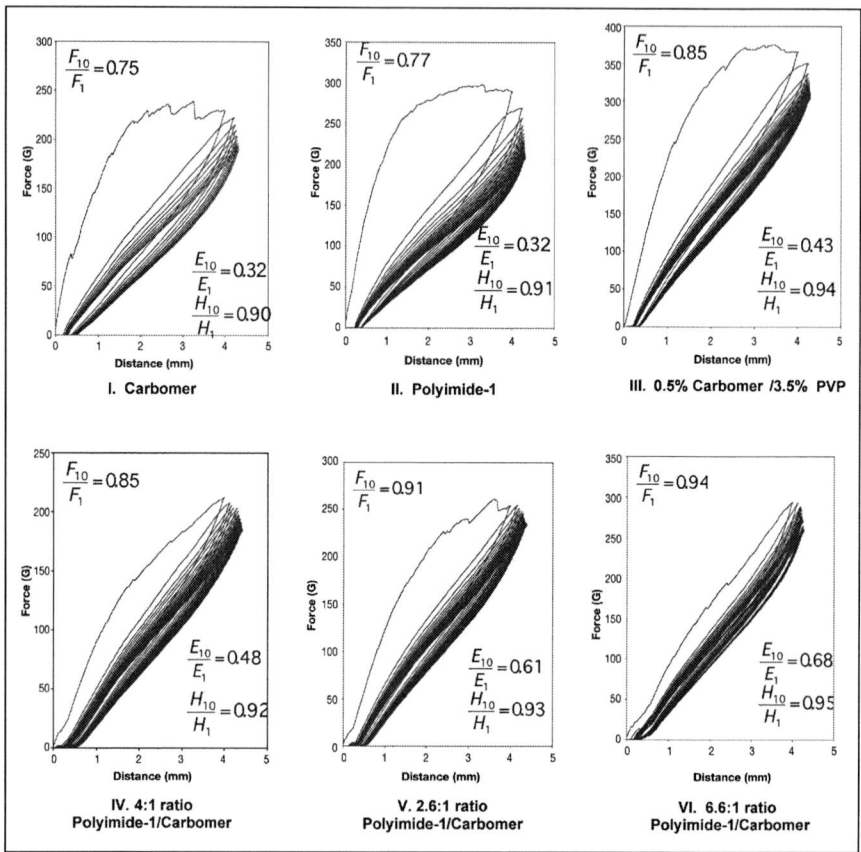

Figure 5. Flexibility of the polymer film on hair and durability of the hair set, from Dynamic Hair Spray Analysis on omega loops of hair treated with selected polymer combinations

Examination of the DSHA curves indicates the importance of the ratio of carbomer to polyimide-1. Chart I shows a carbomer film on hair. Notice the roughness of the first curve. This roughness indicates that the film is deforming to the point of fracture.

Chart II shows a polyimide-1 film. The first curve is smooth, indicating deformation without fracture of the film. Chart IV shows a 4:1 ratio of polyimide-1 to carbomer film. Notice the tightness of all 10 curves, indicative of a resilient film. Deformation occurs and the system returns to almost its initial state.

Chart V shows a profile of a 2.6:1 ratio of polyimide-1 to carbomer film. This profile indicates some film fracture; the 2.6:1 ratio blend begins to exhibit properties of a carbomer system.

Chart VI shows a profile of a 6.6:1 ratio blend. All 10 curves are extremely tight without much deformation. The 6.6:1 ratio blend exhibits both stiffness (no deformation) and elasticity (returns to the same position). As with gel clarity, our data indicates that this synergistic effect with carbomer is also seen with other polyacrylic rheology modifiers, acrylic-based resins and VP-based resins. The ratios of polymer to polyimide-1 are dependent on the composition of the polymer.

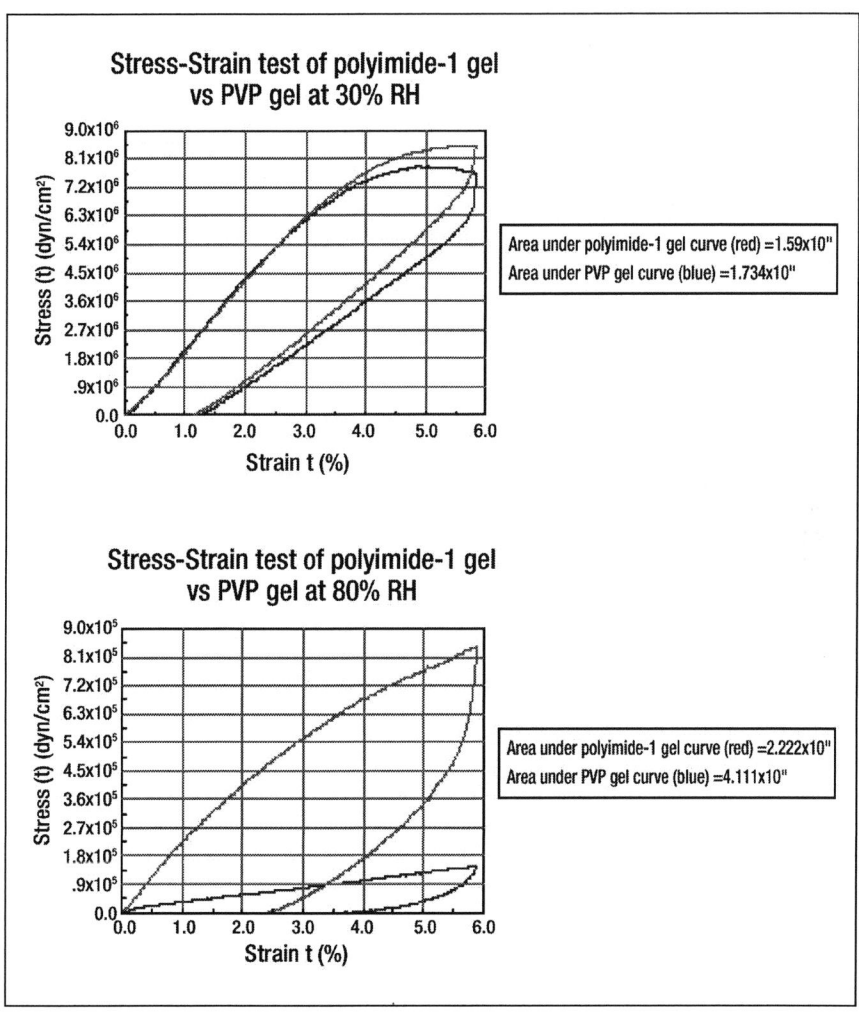

Figure 6. Stress-Strain test on a felt substrate treated with polyimide-1 / carbomer gel (red) versus a PVP/carbomer gel (blue) at moderate and high humidity

Cantilever 3-point bending: Three-point bending measurements were also preformed utilizing a texture analyzer equipped with a cantilever apparatus. 2 g tresses of 6.5" European dark brown hair were treated with 1 g of styling gel formulated with 4:1 ratio of polyimide-1 to carbomer (2.0% active to 0.5% active in water) and compared to gels formulated with a 1:1 ratio of 2% PVP to 2.0% carbomer. The tresses were allowed to dry straight. The probe pressed the hair sample until a 2.0 g force was detected and then a 3.00 mm deformation of the fiber assembly was performed. The probe returned to the control height and repeated the cycle for a total of 10 deformations.

We plotted the maximum force ratio of the first to the tenth deformation at 50% and 90% relative humidity (RH). The force ratio for the polyimide-1 gel at 90% was close to the value at 50% RH; the values were 0.835 and 0.695, respectively. For the PVP gel, the corresponding force ratios were 0.912 and 0.050. Thus, polyimide-1 retains its film integrity even upon exposure to high humidity, while the PVP fails.

Stress/Strain testing: DSHA and cantilever 3-point bending help to assess the toughness and durability of a polymer film on a consumer's hair when touched, but these tests do not take into account a consumer's motion and activity. ISP is investigating new methods to more fully quantify and understand polymer performance on consumer's hair in real life conditions. One such test evaluates the stress of a polymer film on a felt substrate as a function of percent of strain during a twisting motion.

While more work is required to fully validate this method, some conclusions can be drawn from the results. By examining the curves in **Figure 6**, it is easy to conclude that as humidity increases, 4:1 polyimide-1/carbomer gel film retains its strength, while a PVP/carbomer gel film fails.

Film Surface Properties: Coefficient of Friction

The coefficient of friction has been used to quantify a measurement for a consumer sense of touch. The coefficient of friction (COF) is determined by the ease with which two surfaces slide against each other and is calculated as the ratio of the force required to slide the surfaces to the force perpendicular to the surfaces. A lower COF indicates that a surface is smoother, i.e. there is less resistance to the sliding motion.

Polymers were tested instrumentally[b] as dry films on a glass substrate at 25°C and 50% relative humidity. The results shown in **Table 1** indicate that polyimide-1/carbomer systems are smoother than glass or satin and much smoother than the current gel systems on the market.

Table 1
Film surface properties of selected materials

Material	Average Coefficient of Friction
Teflon	0.341
Polyimide-1/Carbomer gel	0.502
Satin	0.739
Polyimide-1	0.828
PVP K-30/Carbomer gel	0.972
Glass	1.053
PVP K-30	1.101
Sandpaper	1.948

Salon Evaluation of Volume and Body

Better performance in the laboratory does provide information on how well a styling polymer will perform, but it is not a substitute for consumer-rated performance of a formulation on a consumer's hair. The results of a 10 person half-head blind-coded salon study comparing polyimide-1 in a styling gel formulation versus a commercial PVP styling gel are shown in **Figure 7**. Polyimide-1 rendered noticeable body versus PVP. Eight out of ten panelists were of the opinion that hair treated with polyimide-1 provided longer lasting style and more volume. Other attributes that consumers expect from styling products performed well.

---

[b]SP-2000 Slip/Peel Tester from IMASS Inc.

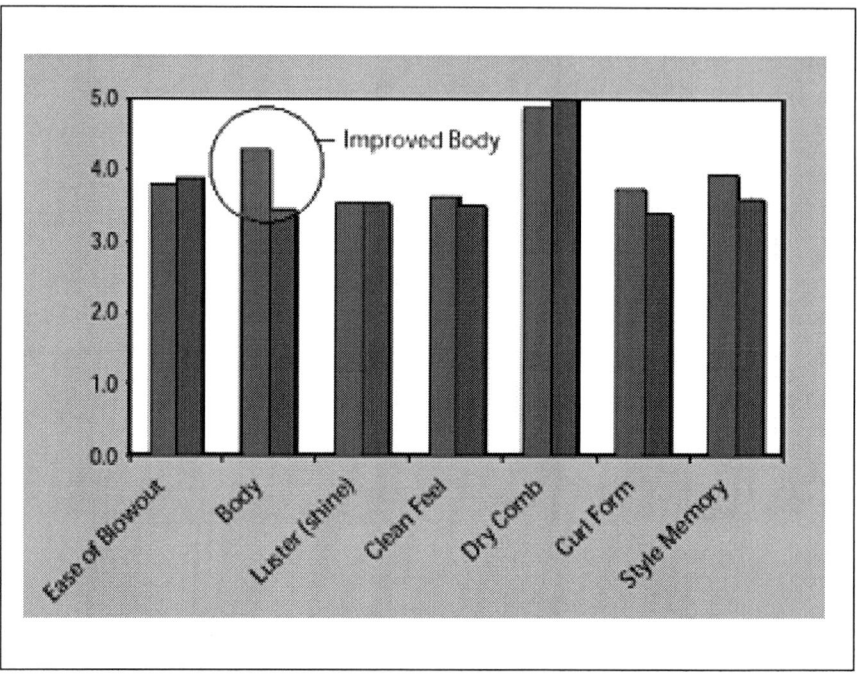

Figure 7. Consumer-rated blow drying performance of a polyimide-1 styling gel (red) versus a commercial PVP styling gel (blue) in a salon evaluation

Formulation Versatility and Compatibility

The last key factor for a polymer to be successful in the styling marketplace is formulation versatility and compatibility with other polymers and materials typically used in hair styling formulations. Two prototype formulations demonstrate the versatility of polyimide-1 in typical styling formulations.

Formula 1 shows a traditional styling gel that delivers a smooth feel to hair yet provides a long-lasting, durable style with body and volume. This product eases blow dryer styling and does not stick to a curling iron. The end result is manageable hair that can easily be restyled.

Formula 2 demonstrates polyimide-1 functionality in mousse applications. This high-powered root lifter leaves hair feeling textured, yet smooth, with excellent volume and manageability.

Formula 1
Classic styling gel

A. Water (aqua)	49.26
Carbomer	25.00
Propylene glycol (and) diazolidinyl urea (and)	
iodopropynyl butylcarbamate (Liquid Germall Plus, ISP)	0.50
Disodium EDTA (Versene NA, Dow)	0.05
B. Triethanolamine, 99%	0.26
C. Water (aqua)	18.00
Polyimide-1 (Aquaflex XL-30, ISP)	6.67
Triethanolamine, 99%	0.26
	100.00

Procedure: Mix A. Add B after A is uniform. Premix C separately. Add C to AB with sweep mixing to avoid aeration. Continue mixing until uniform.
Physical Properties: Appearance - viscous gel; pH - 6.8; Viscosity - 26,000 cps (DV II/T-C/10 rpm/1 min, 25° C).

Formula 2
6% VOC root-lifting spray foam

Water (aqua)	69.56
Polyimide-1 (Aquaflex XL-30, ISP)	13.34
PEG/PPG-25/25 dimethicone (Si-Tec DMC 6031, ISP)	0.15
Polysorbate 20 (Tween 20, Uniqema)	0.15
Cetrimonium chloride (Carsoquat CT-429, Lonza)	0.15
Caprylyl pyrrolidone (Surfadone LP-100, ISP)	0.10
Glyceryl polymethacrylate (and) propylene glycol (and)	
PVM/MA copolymer (Lubrajel Oil, ISP)	0.05
Propylene glycol (and) diazolidinyl urea (and) iodopropynl butylcarbamate	
(Liquid Germall Plus, ISP)	0.50
Hydrofluorocarbon 152a (Dymel 152a, DuPont)	10.00
Isobutane	6.00
	100.00

Procedure: Add ingredients in order listed, mixing well between each addition. Fill into lined aluminum cans and charge with propellant. Valve: Precision; Stem S90 013, Body 013 S90 Capillary DT, 040 Capillary Diptube; Actuator: Precision; Kosmos Ext/Nozzle 020 x 041 FT; 01-8894

Conclusions

The complex styling needs of today's marketplace demand styling products that provide style longevity, smooth feel and durability in high humidity conditions. Various test methodologies are needed to demonstrate a new styling product's performance. The tests surveyed here demonstrate that polyimide-1 meets consumer demands and outperforms current products on the gel and mousse market.

Published March 2005 Cosmetics and Toiletries magazine

CHAPTER 16

Polyurethane-14 AMP-Acrylates Copolymer: A Hair Fixative Technology with "Memory"

Gary Martino, Melissa Vitale and Penny Vanemon
National Starch Personal Care, Bridgewater, New Jersey USA

KEY WORDS: *Polymer, hair styling, fixative, flexibility, viscosity, tack, film toughness, bond strength, memory*

ABSTRACT: *Polyurethane and acrylates chemistry have produced a hair styling polymer that delivers hold, flexibility and "shape memory" in tests of viscosity, particle size, drying time, tack, film toughness and spot weld bond strength.*

With current market offerings for hair styling products, today's consumer must choose between two different types of styling products. One type of styling product offers a strong hold, allowing the creation of a dramatic difference in styled hair versus unstyled hair. The other type of styling product offers the natural or flexible look. However, both approaches have drawbacks.

This paper reviews a new hair styling technology[a], called DynamX, that builds upon both approaches to styling, offering both excellent hold and a natural, flexible look. In addition, this new technology adds the dimension of shape memory to hair styling. The combination of these three parameters – hold, flexibility and shape memory – define a new standard in hair fixative performance: truly durable hold.

[a]DynamX is a trademark of National Starch Personal Care, Bridgewater, New Jersey.

Drawbacks of Existing Technology

Styling polymers that offer "strong hold" are typically based on acrylate, acetate, methyl vinyl ether/maleic anhydride, PVP, or other traditional copolymer technology. Polymer technologies introduced over the past year have also focused on the strong stiff hold.

While offering excellent initial styling, strong hold products can feel stiff, raspy or crunchy to the touch. They do not provide natural movement to hair. Hair-to-hair bonds made with this type of product tend to be brittle, and vigorous movement will cause bonds to break. As a result, styles lose shape and require re-styling or touch-up to maintain a freshly styled look over the course of a day.

"Flexible" hold styling polymers are typically based on acrylate/silicone technology. The silicone copolymer chemistry provides weak holding power, meaning that consumers are limited in the styles that they can create. Hair-to-hair bonds created with this technology tend to be weak and easily break when forces have been applied to the hair. As a result, styles will lose their shape and require re-styling or touch-up to maintain a styled look over the course of a normal day.

Polyurethane-14 AMP-Acrylates Copolymer

The advance behind this new DynamX technology is a patented polymer composition based on polyurethane and acrylates chemistry. The INCI name for this new polymer is polyurethane-14 AMP-acrylates copolymer. We will call it Polymer PA in this chapter. The keys to the performance of this new technology are the characteristics of the film that is created when Polymer PA is applied to hair.

Polymer PA is characterized by optimized physical properties such as viscosity and interfacial energy that affect spray particle size and flowability on hair. It also offers new levels of functionality for the hair-polymer-hair bond that affect bond duration and integrity, polymer toughness and polymer adhesion.

The enabling technology is based on the polyurethane/acrylate system diagrammed in **Figure 1** as a generic structure. Polyurethanes contain blocks of soft segments (IPDI/PPG blocks are flexible) and hard segments (IPDI/rigid diol blocks are stiff). The soft segments absorb energy when the polymer is deformed, while the harder segments provide rigidity to the polymer. The polyurethane contributes properties such as bond strength, style memory, style flexibility and sprayability. The acrylate provides high humidity curl retention, shampoo removability and additional hair-polymer-hair bond strength.

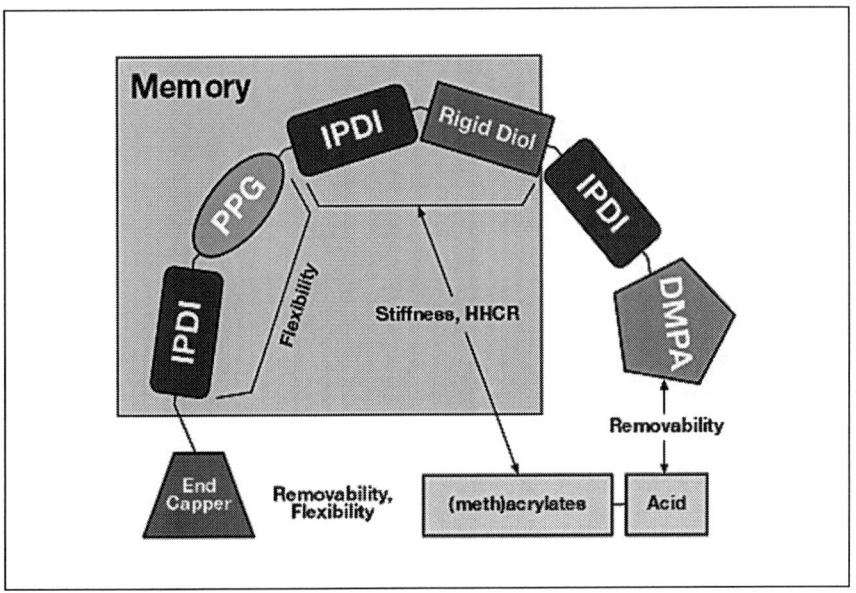

Figure 1. Generic structure of Polymer PA
IPDI = isophorone diisocyanate
PPG = polypropylene glycol
DMPA = dimethylol propionic acid
Rigid Diol = a proprietary ingredient
End Capper = amino-terminated polyether
HHCR = high humidity curl retention

The polymer is supplied as a 28% solution in ethanol (25%) /water (47%). The anionic polymers are pre-neutralized with aminomethylpropanol, facilitating production and reducing compounding costs, compared to dry polymers, which need to be dissolved.

The durable hold performance is especially strong when delivered from hairsprays (low and high VOC), but is applicable to all styling products (such as gels, spray gels, mousses, creams, lotion and pomades).

To describe how this new technology translates to a durable hold, we must describe the mechanism of style maintenance, as delivered from a hairspray. There are three main aspects that control the holding of hair:

- Hairspray formula properties;
- Polymer film properties;
- Hair-polymer-hair bonding.

We will discuss each of these aspects and compare the performance of Polymer PA against other commonly used hair styling polymers listed in **Table 1**. (No examples of "flexible" hold styling polymers were available for testing because the acrylate/silicone technology is proprietary.)

Table 1
Hair styling polymers studied in comparisons against Polymer PA

Polymer Abbreviation	INCI name	Trade name	Supplier
PA	Polyurethane-14 AMP-acrylates copolymer	DynamX*	National Starch
A	Isobutylene/ethylmaleimide/ hydroxyethylmaleimide copolymer	Aquaflex** FX-64	ISP
B	Polyurethane-1	Luviset*** PUR	BASF
C	Acrylates copolymer	Balance* 0/55	National Starch
D	Octylacrylamide/acrylates/ butylaminoethyl methacrylate copolymer	Amphomer*	National Starch
E	Octylacrylamide/acrylates/ butylaminoethyl methacrylate copolymer	Amphomer LV-71	National Starch
F	Octylacrylamide/acrylates/ butylaminoethyl methacrylate copolymer	Balance 47	National Starch

*DynamX is a trademark of National Starch Personal Care, Bridgewater, New Jersey. Balance and Amphomer are registered trademarks of National Starch Personal Care.
**Aquaflex is a trademark of ISP Corp., Wayne, New Jersey.
***Luviset is a registered trademark of BASF, Ludwigshafen, Germany.

Hairspray Formula Properties

Viscosity: In order to spray well, hairspray formulas must have a low viscosity. This is applicable to both aerosol and non-aerosol sprays. The low viscosity will allow fine atomization of the formula giving small spray particles, which allow uniform coverage of the hair. These droplets will then quickly flow/wick along the hair, maximizing the number of spot and seam welds and allowing the formula to dry quickly.

Achieving a fast drying 55% VOC hairspray is particularly challenging when high levels of water are present. Because the polymer system is anionic, its surface activity facilitates this process.

Figure 2 shows the very low formulation viscosity that can be achieved using the new technology. Compared with Polymer C (National Starch's first offering for 55% VOC systems) and Polymer D (a well-known industry benchmark for higher alcohol systems), Polymer PA has the lowest solution viscosity at 4% polymer solids. This low viscosity will translate into excellent sprayability. This property is evident across all VOC levels from 4% to 88%. Recent work has shown similar trends up to 93% VOC. Chemists experienced in formulating low VOC hairsprays know very well that a reduction of 2 or 3 cps can make the difference in achieving excellent sprayability.

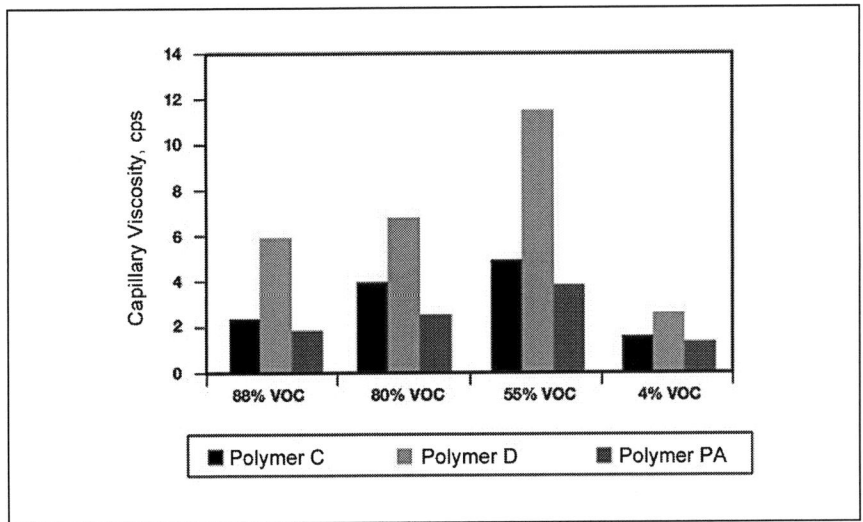

Figure 2. Effect of VOC level and polymer type on viscosity of 4% polymer solutions

Low solids viscosity is not the only challenge to achieving a hairspray of superior performance. Once the spray particles impact the hair, they must be able to flow or wick along the hair to create a maximum amount of well-formed spot or seam welds. These welds are an integral component of style retention and hold.

Our laboratories have determined that spray particles from 55% VOC hairspray (containing 4% polymer solids) increase to about 15% polymer solids when impacting the hair, as solvents evaporate during the spraying process. **Figure 3** indicates that the Polymer PA viscosity is lower than some other commercially available polymer systems at 15% solids. This promotes better hairspray formula flow, wetting and wicking, which lead to better film formation, faster drying and better hold.

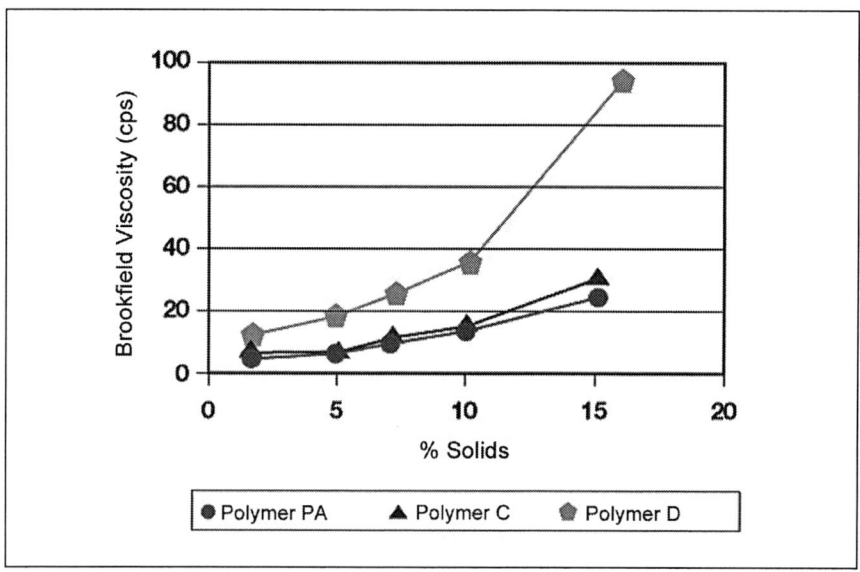

Figure 3. Viscosity of selected styling polymers as a function of polymer concentration (% solids) in a 55% VOC pump hairspray (Brookfield UL adapter, 50 rpm)

Particle size and drying time: We can measure the benefit of particle size and drying time to give a definitive indication of hairspray performance. For example, in our labs we compared three 55% VOC pump hairsprays that differed only in the identity of the styling polymer that was present at 4% in each spray. As shown in **Table 2**, the styling polymers were Polymer PA and two completely different technologies – Polymer A (an imidized isobutylene/maleic anhydride copolymer) and Polymer B (a polyurethane) – available for 55% VOC hairsprays. Particle size was measured instrumentally[b]. Drying time was measured subjectively by a trained group of panelists. After mannequin heads were sprayed 10 times from a distance of 6 inches at 23°C and 50% relative humidity conditions, panelists touched the hair repeatedly until they considered it dry. The overall time was recorded.

When comparing hairspray systems containing similar amounts of water, it is important to keep the spray particle size as small as possible to improve drying time of the formulation. As noted from the data in **Table 2**, Polymers B and PA have smaller particle size, resulting in much faster drying times compared to the formula containing Polymer A.

Table 2
Comparison of sprayability and drying time for selected 55% VOC pump styling polymers

Polymer	Particle size (microns)	Average drying time (seconds)
A	80	429
PA	70	333
B	68	336

Tack: Another aspect of hairspray drying is the amount of tackiness imparted by the formula. Consumers have long desired low levels of tack as the hairspray product dries. This allows consumers to style and work with their hair without the frustration and poor aesthetic feel of hair sticking to hands or styling implements. Short tack times allow the polymer to set quickly and hold the hair.

Figure 4 shows the peak tack of several systems at 5% polymer in a 55% VOC non-aerosol hairspray common in the United States. The Diastron[c] tack and dry method was used at 50% R.H. and 23°C. Polymer PA gives very low tack.

[b]Malvern Particle Size Analyzer (Model #2600), Malvern Instruments Ltd., Malvern, England
[c]Sintech Synergie 200L tensile tester, MTS Systems Corp., Eden Prairie, Minnesota, USA

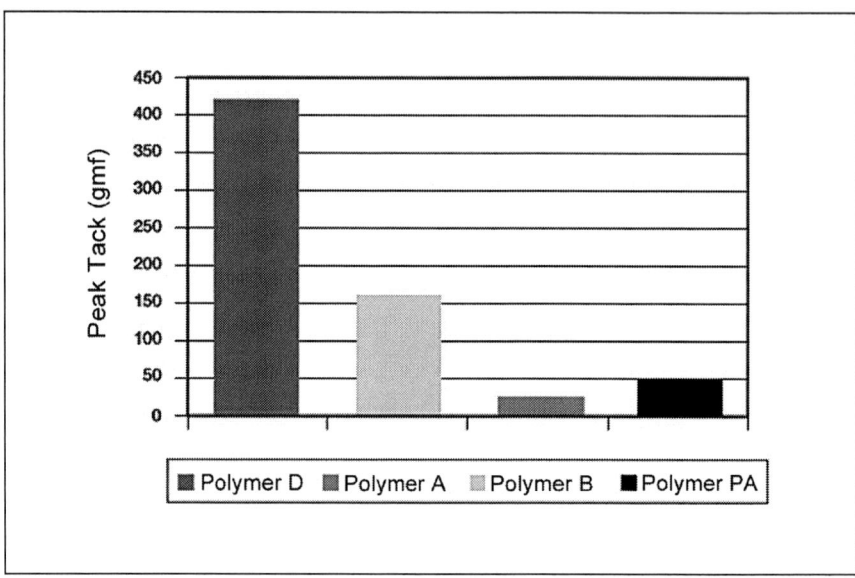

Figure 4. Peak tack of selected styling polymers at 5% in a commercial pump hairspray with 55% ethanol concentrates (measured by the Diastron tack and dry method, 50% R.H., 23°C)

Polymer Film Properties

Toughness: The polymer technology used in the hairspray formulation has a dramatic impact on the final performance of the product. In order to get a durable hold the polymer films must have high levels of elasticity and cohesion; in other words the polymer must be tough. The polymer must have the ability to deform and return to its original shape, thus providing hairstyles with flexibility and memory.

This combination of properties may be the most unique aspect of the new polyurethane and acrylates technology. Prior polymer technologies used in hair styling gave either of two types of films:

- Polymer films that were very brittle, resulting in hairstyles that looked and felt stiff. These hairstyles lacked memory and would lose their shape if moved. If the polymers were plasticized to reduce brittleness, they lost strength due to reduced cohesion.
- Polymer films that were flexible, but weak. This technology allowed the hairstyle to have natural motion, but the weak polymer films were not durable and lacked memory.

Molecular weight versus toughness: By measuring the polymer film toughness (break stress) compared to molecular weight, we can see a unique aspect of this technology. **Figure 5** shows that Polymer PA is able to achieve toughness that is superior to the toughness achieved by polymers using traditional acrylate technology, but it achieves this toughness at a much lower molecular weight.

This property offers several performance advantages. In the past, in order to attain high levels of toughness and hold, the formulator had to choose a high molecular weight polymer. Unfortunately, the high molecular weight also gives higher formulation viscosity, larger spray particle size, and longer drying time. At very high levels of polymer solids, the high molecular weight polymers result in unacceptable spray aesthetics.

Using Polymer PA, formulators can achieve two critical hairspray formulation objectives at the same time – low viscosity for excellent sprayability and fast drying with high toughness for long term hold, flexibility and memory.

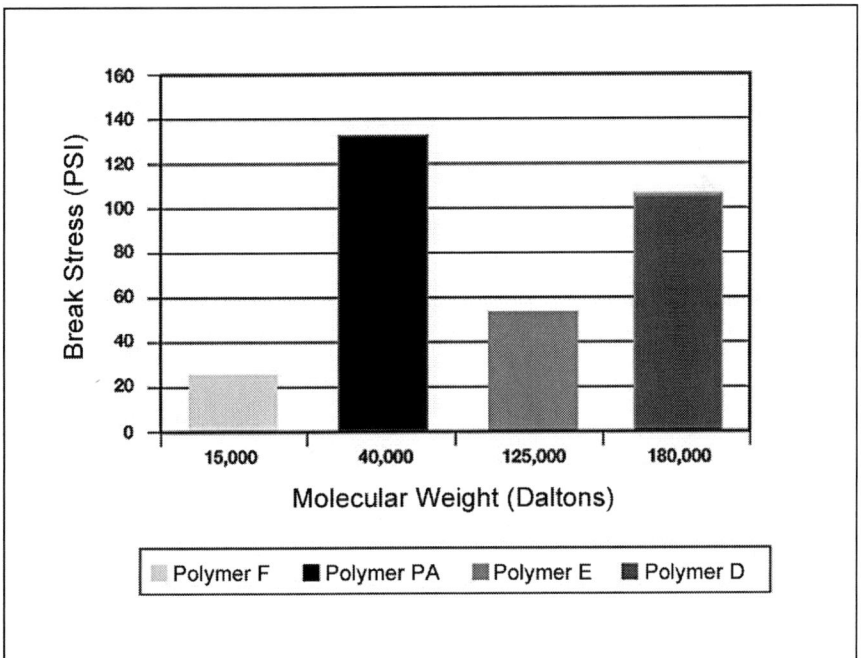

Figure 5. Toughness (break stress) of a 0.25 mm thick film of styling polymers of different molecular weights, delivered in a 55% VOC pump hairspray

Polymer film modulus versus toughness: The polyurethane/polyacrylate components of Polymer PA yield excellent film strength and flexibility. Polymer film properties can be characterized instrumentally. Various solutions containing 15% polymer and 55% ethanol were placed into silicone rubber molds, then dried and equilibrated to form dry polymer films. Each polymer film was placed into a tensile tester[c] and stretched until the film broke.

Figure 6 plots the polymer's film modulus versus the energy required to break the film. The modulus can be correlated to the initial strength, hardness, or stiffness that one would feel on the hair, whereas the energy to break equates to the polymer's toughness and elasticity.

In **Figure 6**, commercial Polymers A and B have high initial strength. However, when enough energy is generated to start stretching the films, they snap instantaneously. Polymer PA provides moderate initial strength, but the film can be stretched for several inches before breaking, as indicated by its high toughness reading. This high toughness value is one of the parameters that indicate Polymer PA's durability and long lasting hold on the hair. The polymer film is able to withstand significant forces without breaking.

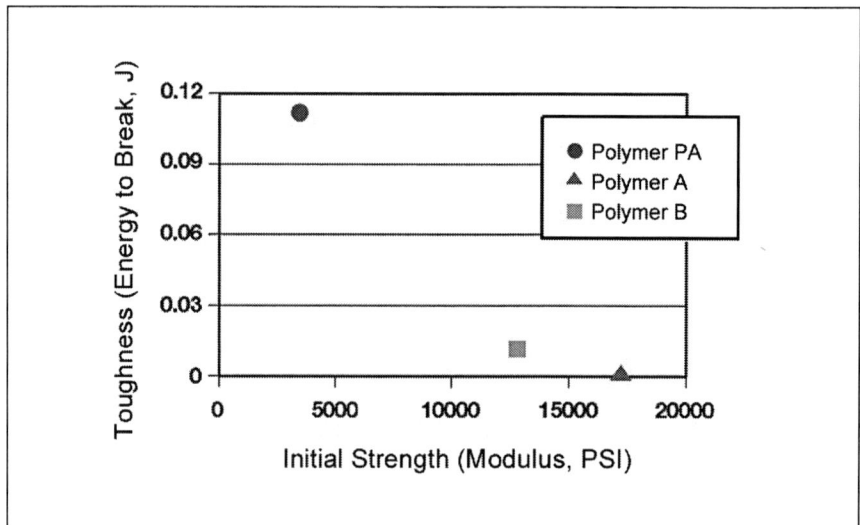

Figure 6. Toughness (energy to break) of a 0.25 mm thick film of styling polymers of different modulus (hardness), delivered in a 55% VOC pump hairspray. (Films were equilibrated at 50% R.H., 23°C.)

Hair-Polymer-Hair Bonding

Once the formulation has been applied to the hair, the properties of the resulting hair-polymer-hair bond formed become important to the overall performance of the hairspray.

The flow and wetting properties of the formula can be qualified by observing spot welds on hair that were formed from traditional 55% VOC hairsprays compared to Polymer PA in the same hairspray system (**Figure 7**). The larger, more uniform spot weld will give a longer lasting hairstyle compared to the smaller, uneven spot weld. This would be true when comparing polymers of similar technology. We have yet to consider the compounded benefits that will be evident using the new technology.

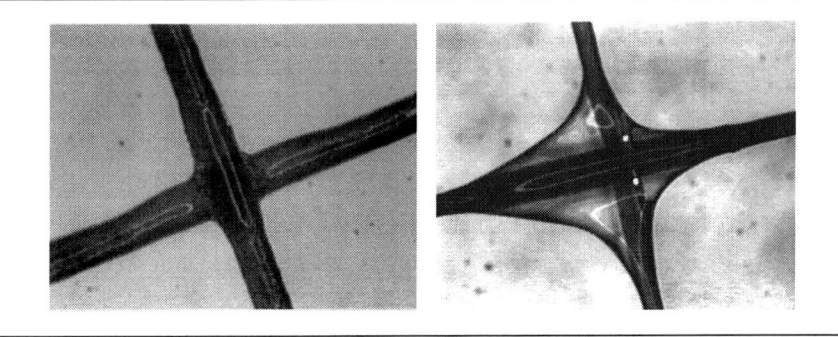

Figure 7. Unstressed spot welds from 55% VOC high water hairsprays with Polymer PA (right) and with traditional technology (left), illustrating the polymer's cohesive forces

Adhesion to hair can be objectively quantified using the Diastron[e] bond strength method. This test measures the force that it takes to break a hair-polymer-hair spot weld. For this particular evaluation, two single hair fibers are placed in a perpendicular fashion, and a fixed amount of hair spray concentrate is applied at the intersection to form a spot weld. All hair spot welds are dried and conditioned appropriately. The Diastron pulls one of the hair fibers until the hair-polymer bond breaks.

Polymers A, B and PA were compared from 55% VOC hair spray concentrates and evaluated for bond strength. The force required to break the spot welds is plotted in **Figure 8**. As expected, the break load for Polymer PA is significantly greater than the force required to break the other bonds.

[e]Diastron MTT670 Tensile Tester, Diastron Ltd., Andover, Hampshire, England

A formula containing Polymer PA provides durability, even when forces are applied to the bond several times. When observing movement of these different spot welds under a microscope, bonds containing Polymers A and B break after pulling the hair fiber once. The durable Polymer PA bond is tough and flexible, and is able to maintain its shape after being pulled in a different direction. **Figure 9** highlights these spot welds.

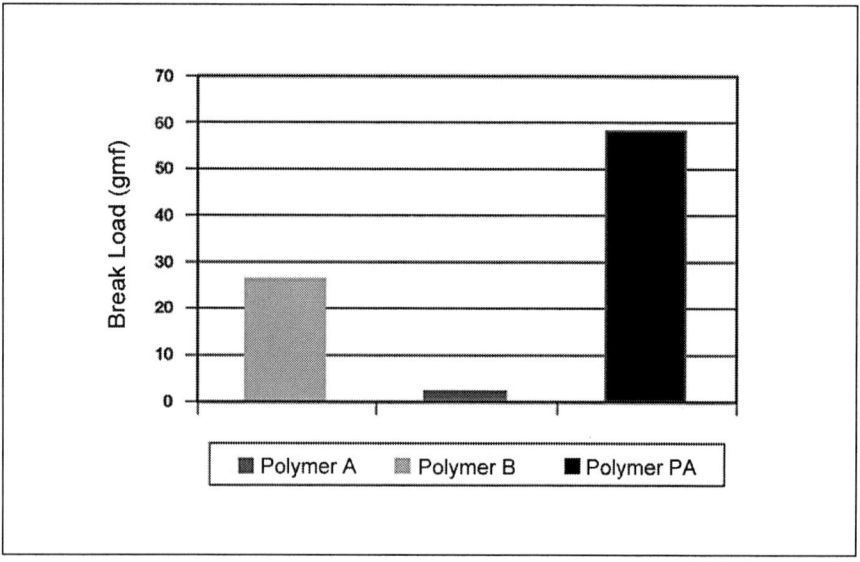

Figure 8. Force (break load) required to break spot welds created by styling polymers at 4% in a pump spray with 55% ethanol concentrates (measured by Diastron bond strength method at 55% R.H.)

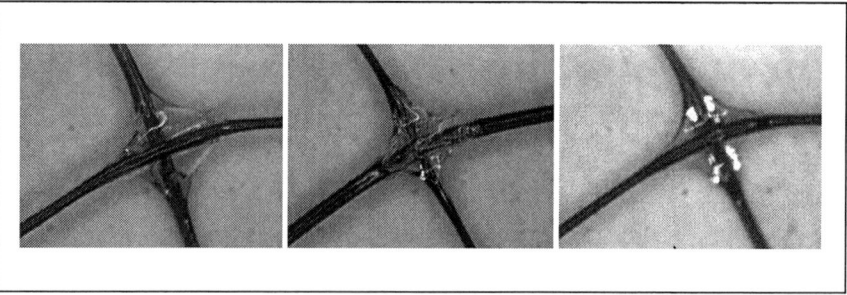

Figure 9. Stretched spot welds from 55% VOC high water hairsprays with Polymer A (left), Polymer B (center) and Polymer PA (right), illustrating both the polymer's cohesive forces and its adhesion to the hair

Summary

In this chapter, we have described "dynamic" style, a new concept in hair styling based on the first truly durable hold. This is a "step change" in formulating ability resulting from a technological advance.

The dynamic style is designed to meet the needs of today's consumer who is active, on the go, and pressed for time, but who still wants to look as good as possible all day. The dynamic style combines the best properties in hold, flexibility and shape memory,' all of which contribute to true durability. Consumer products that offer the dynamic style will help the consumer look and feel great when the hair is first styled each day and stay looking that way, all day.

Beyond these benefits, polyurethane-14 AMP-acrylates copolymer has been "engineered" to offer some features that will make formulations easier to manufacture, and more pleasing to the consumer. Polyurethane-14 AMP-acrylates copolymer technology is pre-neutralized and dissolves readily, making it easy to formulate. It has efficacy in both higher and lower VOC formulas. It has a low viscosity, meaning better sprayability. Because of its solubility and appearance, polyurethane-14 AMP-acrylates copolymer can be used in clear formulations. Finally, the product features a small particle size allowing for fast drying times on hair, and a pronounced reduction in perceivable tack, giving the consumer a more pleasant sensory experience.

Published January 2003 Cosmetics and Toiletries magazine

CHAPTER 17

Using Polyquaternium-64 to Condition Damaged Hair

Kunio Shimada, PhD,
NOF Corporation, Life Science Division, Tokyo, Japan
Kiyoshi Inomata, NOF Corporation,
Tsukuba Research Laboratory, Ibaraki, Japan
Sreekumar Pillai, PhD, and James Hayward, PhD,
Engelhard Corporation, Stony Brook, New York, USA

KEY WORDS: *Polyquaternium-64, MPC, cationic polymer, hair bleach, hair condition, gel, ESCA, fluorescence-labeled polymer, biocompatibility*

ABSTRACT: *Studies reported here show that by forming a gel layer that coats the surfaces of damaged hair fibers, this new, cationic, biomimetic copolymer helps to restore the appearance of healthy hair.*

Products developed to cleanse the skin and bleach the hair also remove fatty acids, lipids, proteins, amino acids and other essential components, leaving the skin and hair rough and dry. Bleaching, for example, removes the fats and proteins that are important for the binding of water to hair.[1] A conditioner is needed to correct these losses.

NOF Corporation has developed a synthetic water-soluble polymer that mimics the structure of skin surface lipid, has the ability to coat the skin and hair surface, and holds moisture.[2] Now from that polymer, NOF Corporation has developed a cationic variant[a], polyquaternium-64, that binds with skin and hair, forms a protective barrier, and helps to prevent the loss of moisture and other components from skin and hair. Its structural similarity to naturally occurring skin phospholipids enables this material to stabilize the lamellar structure of skin and to coat the hair, offering protection from surfactants and harsh chemical treatments.

This chapter reports polyquaternium-64's effect on damaged hair by evaluating moisture retention, combing friction, conditioning efficacy, and tensile strength of damaged hair treated with the copolymer. Other studies report on its ability to form gels on the hair surface and to adhere to that surface. Scanning electron micrographs show its ability to restore moisture to the cuticle and prevent the cuticle from lifting.

Materials

Polyquaternium-64: Polyquaternium-64 is based on the monomer 2-methacryloyl-oxyethyl phosphorylcholine (MPC). The structure of MPC is similar to the polar head group of the phospholipids that compose the extracellular leaflet of human plasma membranes. This chemical moiety is biocompatible, binds copious water, and effectively maintains a quiescent cellular state – qualities that suggest its use in personal care.[3,4]

MPC polymers have the ability to repair the epidermal barrier. They bind water and normalize transepidermal water loss (TEWL).[5] As synthetic monomers, these prosthetic groups can be synthesized into many copolymers, such as polyquaternium-51, which protect human skin cells from detergents or other surfactants, prolong the persistence of perfume, and reduce surface tension.[6,7]

In MPC's zwitterions, the phosphate moiety contributes the anion, while the choline moiety contributes the cation. We have rendered polyquaternium-64 as a cationic polymer by effectively doubling the molar ratio of choline to phosphate.

Polyquaternium-64 (**Figure 1**) is a copolymer of MPC and the cationic monomer, 2-hydroxy-3-methacryloyl-oxypropyltrimethylammonium chloride. The average molecular weight of the polyquaternium-64 was approximately 600,000.

---

[a]Lipidure-C (INCI: polyquaternium-64) is a product of NOF Corporation, Tokyo, Japan.

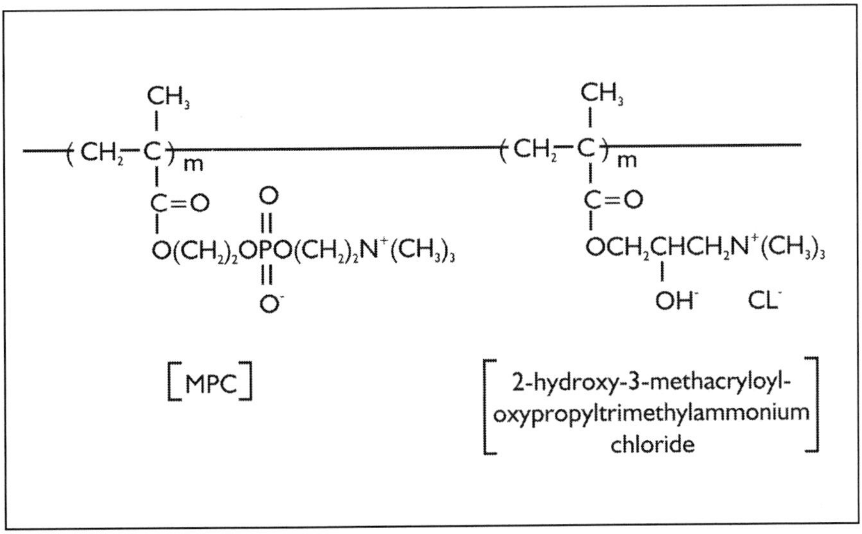

Figure 1. Chemical structure of polyquaternium-64

A 5% polyquaternium-64 solution was used in these studies for evaluating the effects on damaged hair.

Other materials: Samples of normal undamaged black hair that has never been subjected to bleaching or dyeing were obtained[b] from a single donor. Damaged hair was obtained by repeated bleaching as described in the methods section.

Lyophilized porcine skin was obtained[c] and swelled in saline before measurements of frictional coefficients were taken.

Instrumentation

Mean friction coefficient, measured as MIU (a popular term to calibrate friction coefficient in Japan), was measured using a feel tester[d]. MIU is equivalent to the friction factor, μ, the quotient of frictional force and normal force for a sliding body.

Tensile strength was measured using a rheometer[e]. The adhesion of polyquaternium-64 to hair fibers was determined by analysis of phosphorous using ESCA X-ray photoelectron analysis equipment[f]. ESCA stands for Electron Spectroscopy for Chemical Analysis.

---

[b]From Beaulax Co., Ltd, Tokyo, Japan
[c]Alloask S, from Taiho Pharmaceutical Co, Ltd, Tokyo, Japan
[d]KSE-SE friction tester, Kato Tech Corporation, Tokyo, Japan
[e]Reona RE3305 rheometer, Yamaden Corporation, Tokyo, Japan

In Vitro Studies of Polyquaternium-64

Moisture retention by polyquaternium-64: The effect of polyquaternium-64 to retain moisture was compared with two common hair care agents: polyquaternium-7 and dimethicone. While the use percentage for each product was different (polyquaternium-64: 5% solution; polyquaternium-7: 9% solution; dimethicone: 50% emulsified solution), the weight of the polymers used in the studies was kept equal at 0.02 grams each. This was confirmed by measuring the dry weight of the polymer film used in the studies. An aqueous solution of each polymer was poured into a petri dish and dried completely. 20 mg of each of the polymer films formed on the dishes was incubated in 80% relative humidity (RH) for 72 hours and then another 72 hours at 30% relative humidity. The amount of water absorbed by the polymer was determined by weighing the membrane several times during the incubation.

As seen in **Figure 2**, among those three samples, polyquaternium-64 showed the highest degree of water binding, retaining 15-10% water content, even at 30% RH. These results suggest that polyquaternium-64 may have a better ability to form a gel layer on the damaged hair surface when compared to other hydrating agents.

Friction on combing: Generally, hair care products such as shampoos and conditioners are expected to smooth the hair for

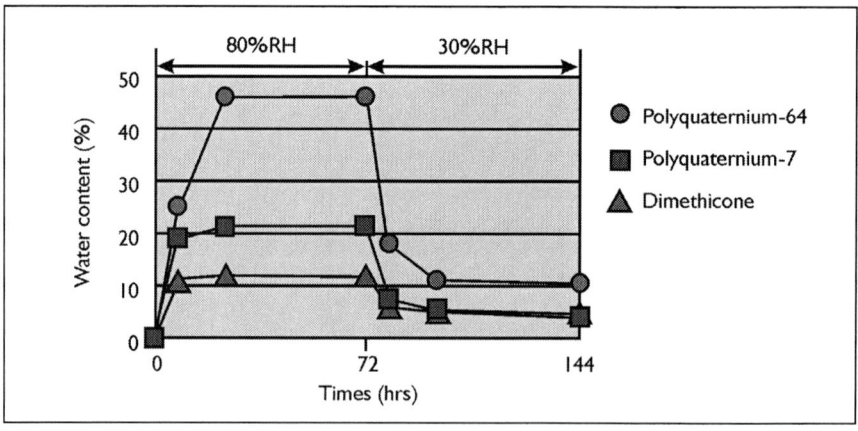

Figure 2. Water holding capacity of polyquaternium-64 (●) in comparison with two other commonly used hair conditioning ingredients, dimethicone (▲) and polyquaternium-7 (■)

---

[f]ESCA-3300 X-ray photoelectron analysis equipment, Shimadzu Corporation, Kyoto, Japan

finger combing. We measured the friction coefficient of polyquaternium-64 on a porcine skin. This test was conducted by swelling a lyophilized porcine skin[c] in saline, dropping 0.5 ml of 1% polymer solution on the skin, and measuring the mean friction coefficient by a friction tester[d] with a silicon adapter.

The observed skin friction coefficient values, measured as MIU and averaged for each tested ingredient, were 1.55, 1.95, 2.85 and 3.60 for polyquaternium-64, dimethicone, polyquaternium-7 and saline solution, respectively. Polyquaternium-64 reduced the skin friction coefficient. The effect was significant compared to skin treated with saline solution only. Polyquaternium-7 and dimethicone were much less effective in reducing friction on skin. Although dimethicone-treated skin also showed significant improvement, the effects were less pronounced than that of polyquaternium-64. Polyquaternium-7 did not demonstrate any significant improvement over control in reducing the friction on porcine skin.

This data clearly suggests not only that polyquaternium-64 binds more water, but also prevents build up of friction on skin surface. The data also suggests that this material would be more effective than polyquaternium-7 or dimethicone in reducing the friction of combing on hair.

Methods for Analysis with Damaged Hair

Preparation of hair: In the washing and drying process, the hair[b] was soaked in 1% aqueous solution of SLES for 1 min at 30-35°C, rinsed, squeezed by a towel, and blow-dried.

In the bleaching process, hair was soaked in 1:1 mixture of 4.5% hydrogen peroxide and 2.5% ammonia solution for 20 min, rinsed, squeezed by a towel, and blow-dried. Each bleaching process was repeated 10 times.

The hair was treated with one of three polymers: polyquaternium-64, dimethicone or polyquaternium-7. Hair was soaked in the specified concentration of polymer for specified time, rinsed in stock water, squeezed by a towel, and blow-dried.

Friction coefficient measurement: The damaged hair and the polymer-treated hair were dried. The hair was kept at 20°C and

40% relative humidity. The hair was fixed on a glass slide using a transparent tape, and the measurement was taken using a silicone attachment that has a friction close to that of human skin. The friction (MIU) was then measured instrumentally[d].

The value for MIU obtained from the instrument indicates the friction of the hair. The lower the MIU, the lower the friction on the hair, and the better the feel of hair and the combability of hair. This reflects better conditioning of hair. A single strand of hair was used to measure frictional coefficient. Measurements were performed at least five times and the average values were obtained.

Tensile strength measurement: Hair tensile strength was measured using a rheometer[e]. Hair was maintained at 20°C and 40% relative humidity during the measurement. Treated hair was compared with untreated damaged hair for tensile strength. Ten strands of hair were tested multiple times for tensile strength and average values were obtained.

ESCA: Electron Spectroscopy to Chemical Analysis (ESCA) involves irradiation of the hair surface with X-rays of known energy that cause core electrons to be ejected from the hair surface. This measuring provides semi-quantitative data for the polymer adhesion volume.

Hair samples were placed on the measuring table of the ESCA equipment and vacuum-dried at 60°C for 12 hrs. The settings used for the various elements were as follows: Carbon – 300-280 eV; Nitrogen – 410-390 eV; Oxygen – 543-523 eV; Phosphorus – 142.9-122.9 eV.

Measurements were taken at intervals of 0.1 eV. Each peak was then quantitated for the respective element concentration (atomic concentration as %). From the data, the ratio of phosphorus to carbon concentration was calculated and expressed as a P/C value.

Statistics: Multiple measurements on single or multiple strands of hair were taken and data was expressed as an average of multiple measurements. Typically, standard deviation did not vary over 5% of the mean values. Wherever the effects were statistically significant, it was indicated in the Results section.

Results of Studies with Damaged Hair

In order to determine the effect of polyquaternium-64 on reducing the level of friction in damaged hair compared to that of healthy hair, damaged hair was prepared according to the procedures described in the Methods section.[8] Unbleached, washed and dried black hair was used as the normal control (healthy hair). The damaged hair was then treated with different polymers by soaking the damaged hair (bleached) in each of the polymer solutions for 20 minutes. The friction coefficient and tensile strength of these polymer-treated hair samples were then measured. In addition, scanning electron micrographs were obtained and the gel-forming ability of polyquaternium-64 was evaluated.

Conditioning efficacy of polyquaternium-64: The friction coefficient of the specimens was measured according to the method of Mastuzawa et al.[9] using a friction tester[d] at 40% RH and 20°C. Resulting MIU values were 2.82, 2.90, 2.79, 2.92 and 2.91 for healthy hair, damaged hair, polyquaternium-64-treated hair, dimethicone-treated hair and polyquaternium-7-treated hair, respectively. Healthy hair shows low frictional coefficient (low MIU value), consistent with no damage. Bleached, damaged hair shows higher MIU values, consistent with increased damage to hair. Both dimethicone and polyquaternium-7 failed to reduce the friction on damaged hair; this indicates that these compounds neither coated the hair nor moisturized it. On the other hand, hair treated with polyquaternium-64 displayed a friction coefficient similar to that of healthy hair, suggesting that polyquaternium-64 coats the hair and binds moisture to make the hair soft and smooth to reduce friction.

From these results, it could be concluded that the hair treated with polyquaternium-64 would be easy to finger comb.

Tensile strength of polymer-treated hair: A rheometer[e] measured the tensile strength at 20°C and 40% RH. Weight at breakage averages (gf/hair) were 120, 87, 110, 110 and 108 for healthy hair, damaged hair, polyquaternium-64-treated hair, dimethicone-treated hair and polyquaternium-7-treated hair, respectively.

As expected, damaged hair showed low tensile strength indicating that hair breakage occurs at low tension. All three hair-conditioning agents increased the strength of hair significantly. Treatment with conditioning agents including polyquaternium-64 restored the tensile strength of the damaged hair to levels closer to that of healthy hair.

SEM comparison: **Figure 3** presents the SEM pictures of the healthy hair, damaged hair and hair treated with polyquaternium-64. As shown in **Figure 3b**, the cuticle is lifted up on the surface of the damaged hair by the repeated bleaching. **Figure 3c** shows that treatment with polyquaternium-64 restored the damaged hair morphology closer to normal hair. The cuticle in the treated hair resembled normal unbleached hair more than it did the bleached hair. This indicates the benefit of polyquaternium-64 in correcting hair cuticle damage caused by hair bleaching. Polyquaternium-64 may bind to the cuticles, restoring the moisture of the cuticle (that is lost during bleaching) and preventing the cuticle from lifting. A lifted hair cuticle is the main reason for damaged hair being "sticky" and brittle.

Gel-forming ability of polyquaternium-64 on hair surface: The cationic polymer conditions the hair effectively by adhering to it. There are detailed reports about the relationship between the adhesion volumes of cationic cellulose and the duration of treatment.[10,11] In view of this, the adhesion of polyquaternium-64 to hair fibers was measured by analysis of phosphorous using ESCA, and based on the fact that polyquaternium-64 contains phosphorous ions that are normally not present in large quantities in normal hair. Any detected presence of phosphorous atoms in treated hair was an indication of adhesion of polyquaternium-64 on hair fibers.

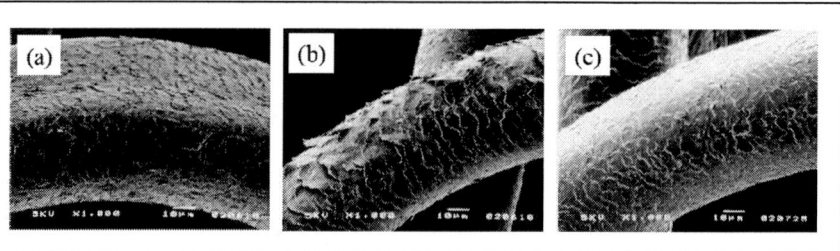

Figure 3. SEM images of hair fibers (X1000)
a = untreated normal hair
b = bleached damaged hair
c = bleached, damaged hair treated with polyquaternium-64

ESCA (XPS) (Electron Spectroscopy for Chemical Analysis by X-ray Photoelectron Spectroscopy) involves irradiation of the hair surface with X-rays of known energy that cause core electrons to be ejected from the hair surface. This measurement provides quantitative data for the polymer adhesion volume.

As seen from **Figure 4**, no peak for phosphorous atoms was observed for the healthy hair or the damaged hair because the chemical structure of human hair consists of mostly water and keratins. On the contrary, damaged hair treated with polyquaternium-64 demonstrated a peak specific for phosphorous (at 135 eV), indicating the presence of phosphorous atoms adhered to the hair. Because the carbon atom is universal to all organic matter, the ratio of P/C was used as a quantitative measure for the adherence of polyquaternium-64 to hair surface.

This novel method can be applied to determine the adhesion volumes of polyquaternium-64 and other phosphorous-containing ingredients on hair or skin surfaces by measuring the volumetric ratio of phosphorous atoms to carbon atoms (P/C values).

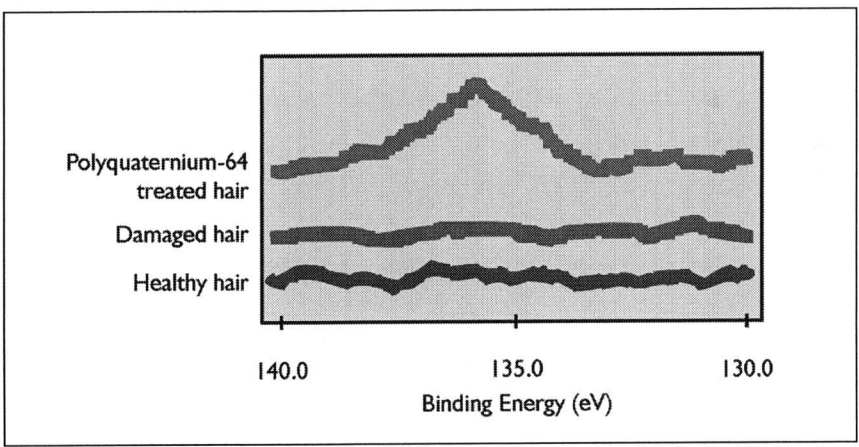

Figure 4. ESCA measurement of phosphorous atoms on hair fiber, showing phosphorous atoms at 135 eV for polyquaternium-64 coated hair

Kinetics of adhesion of polyquaternium-64 to hair surface: Next, we examined the concentration dependence for the adhesion volume of polyquaternium-64 and hair, the time dependence for this adhesion, and resistance to washing on removal of polyquaternium-64 by using the ESCA method.

Concentrations as low as 0.01% of polyquaternium-64 indicated phosphorous association with hair. Increasing the concentration of the active up to 1.00% did not show any significant increase in the association of phosphorous atoms on hair surface, suggesting that even low concentrations of 0.01% of polyquaternium-64 saturate all the binding sites in hair. This indicates that even a small quantity of polyquaternium-64 is enough to form a gel layer on the hair surface.

In the time course study, phosphorous atoms originated by polyquaternium-64 gel are observed on the hair surface within only 30 seconds after the treatment. This indicates that polyquaternium-64 forms a gel layer almost immediately upon contact with hair. These tests demonstrate the high affinity of polyquaternium-64 for damaged hair (a short treatment with a very small quantity).

We evaluated the long-lasting efficacy of polyquaternium-64 after repeated shampooing. Damaged human hair treated with polyquaternium-64 was washed repeatedly using sodium lauryl sulfate solution as shampoo up to 10 times, and the amount of the phosphorous bond to hair was measured. The levels of phosphorous appeared to decrease with repeated washings, but after 10 washings phosphorous could still be detected on the hair fibers.

This series of experiments demonstrates that polyquaternium-64 has high affinity for hair fibers, and that even small quantities applied in short treatments are enough to coat the hair.

Visual images of polyquaternium-64 adhering to hair: In order to confirm the results obtained by ESCA, we carried out a test using a fluorescence indicator, polyquaternium-64-F. It was prepared by co-polymerizing polyquaternium-64 with 5% aminoethylmethacrylate, forming a precursor that was reacted with fluorescein isothiocyanate (FITC) to form the FITC-conjugated polyquaternium-64, which we'll call polyquaternium-64-F. The unreacted FITC was then removed by dialysis.

The damaged hair was treated with 0.5% polyquaternium-64-F, rinsed with water and then blown dry. The fluorescent bond to hair was visualized in **Figure 5** using a fluorescent microscope. **Figure 6** shows the cross section of the hair from the same experiment. Non-treated hair (**Figures 6a and 6b** in a bright field and a dark field,

Using Polyquaternium-64 to Condition Damaged Hair

respectively) showed no fluorescence while the hair treated with polyquaternium-64-F (**Figure 6d**) clearly showed fluorescence in a dark field.

Because only the periphery of the hair fluoresces, as shown in **Figure 6**, we concluded that polyquaternium-64 adheres only to the hair surface and produces the conditioning effect. From this observation and the measurement by ESCA, we concluded that polyquaternium-64 coated the surface of the damaged hair as a gel layer.

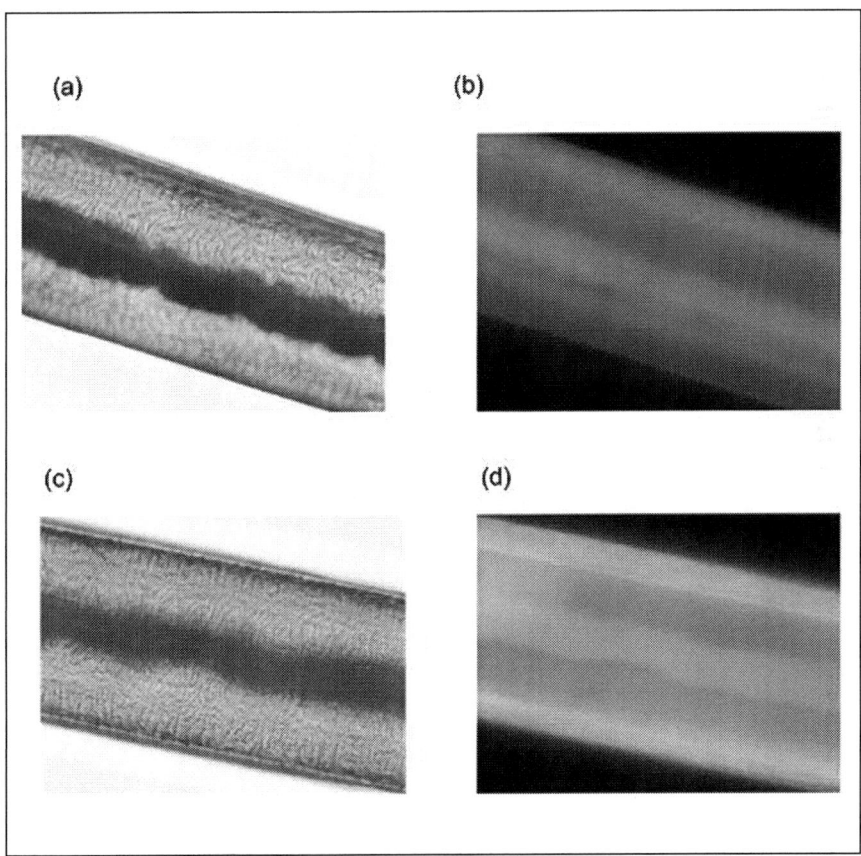

Figure 5. Fluorescence microscopic images of damaged hair fiber
a = non-treated (bright field)
b = non-treated (dark field)
c = FITC-bound polyquaternium-64 treated (bright field)
d = FITC-bound polyquaternium-64 treated (dark field)

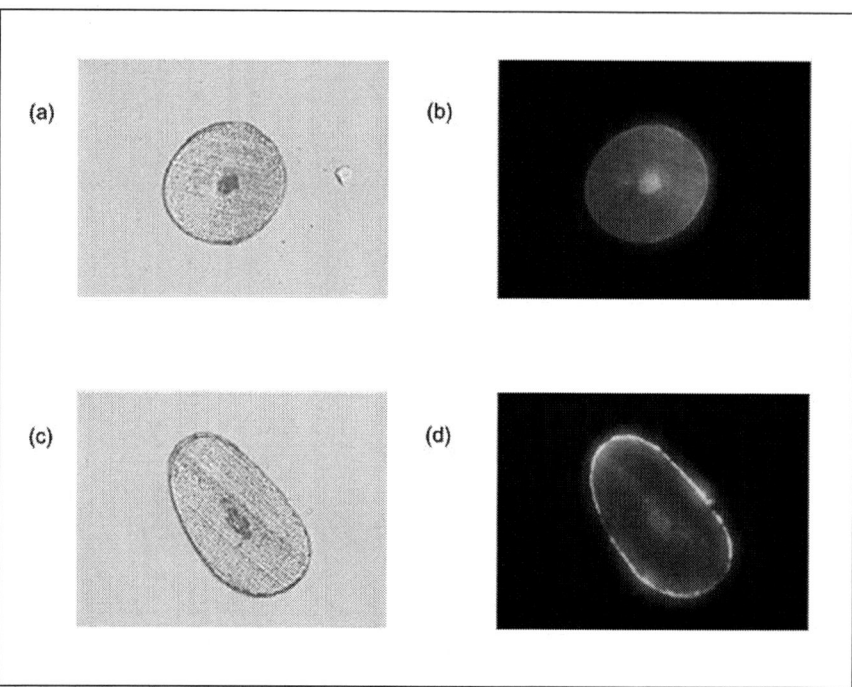

Figure 6. Fluorescence microscopic images of damaged hair cross sections
a = non-treated (bright field)
b = non-treated (dark field)
c = FITC-bound polyquaternium-64 treated (bright field)
d = FITC-bound polyquaternium-64 treated (dark field)

Tips on Formulating with Polyquaternium-64

In working with polyquaternium-64, it is wise to consider the following points:

- Because polyquaternium-64 is a polymer, in an alkaline system with pH>10, its ester bonds will be broken. An amine odor can result.
- Polyquaternium-64 is a cationic polymer. Interaction with an anionic surfactant or polymer may cause precipitation or turbidity.

Discussion and Conclusion

This chapter reports on a newly developed cationic variant of a water-soluble, synthetic polymer that mimics the structure of skin surface lipids, has the ability to coat the skin and hair surface, and holds moisture. The variant, called polyquaternium-64, binds with skin and hair, forms a protective barrier, and helps to prevent the loss of moisture and other components from skin and hair. Its structural similarity to naturally occurring skin phospholipids enables this material to stabilize the lamellar structure of skin and coat the hair, offering protection from surfactants and harsh chemical treatment.

Film formers, such as polyquaternium-64, help protect hair by coating it with a moist gel. As demonstrated in this paper, polyquaternium-64 binds water, reduces the frictional coefficient, improves softness, reduces the surface electrostatic potential, and improves electrical conductivity of hair. ESCA measurements and the fluorescent-labeling method showed that a water gel layer exists on the surface of hair treated with polyquaternium-64. The result is maintenance of moisture, improved smoothness and reduction of damage to hair caused by bleaching and dyeing.

We conclude that polyquaternium-64 is a very effective hair-conditioning ingredient because it combines cationic characteristics with the various functionalities of biocompatible MPC polymer for high affinity binding to hair fibers.

Published November 2004 Cosmetics and Toiletries magazine

References

1. CR Robbins, *Chemical and Physical Behavior of Human Hair*, 4th edn, New York, NY: Springer-Verlag (2001) p 63
2. M Tschudia and K Shimada, An MPC phospholipid polymer with skin protection benefits, *Cosmet Toil* 118(3) 63-68 (2003)
3. M Sakakida, K Nishida, M Shichiri, K Ishihara and N Nakabayashi, Ferrocene-mediated needle-type glucose sensor covered with newly designed biocompatible membrane, *Sensor and Acturators* B 13-14 319-322 (1993)
4. K Ishihara, K Fukumoto, J Aoki and N Nakabayashi, Improvement of blood compatibility on cellulose dialysis membrane. 1. Grafting of 2-methacryloyloxyethyl phosphorylcholine on to a cellulose membrane surface, *Biomaterials* 13(3) 145-149 (1992)
5. M Syaku, H Kuroda, A Ohba, S Ohkura, K Ishihara and N Nakabayashi, Enhancing stratum corneum functions with a bi-functional phospholipid polymer, *J Soc Cosmet Chem Jpn* 30(3) 273-285(1996)
6. K Shimada, H Irie, Y Murata, K Ishihara and N Nakabayashi, Synthesis and application of 2-methacryloyloxyethyl phosphorylcholine copolymer, *Fragrance J* 26(7) 97-104 (1998)

7. M Tsuchida and K Shimada, Development and application of Lipidure-PMB, *Fragrance J* 28(12) 118-121 (2000)
8. H Kouno, K Suganuma and T Hurukawa, Effect of thermal environmental changes on the physical characteristics of human hair, *J Soc Cosmet Chem Jpn* 33(4) 377-385 (1999)
9. S Mastuzawa and N Mikami, PCA-Na smoothing effect on wet hair, *J Soc Cosmet Chem Jpn* 29(3) 227-233 (1995)
10. JA Faucher and EJ Goddard, Sorption and desorption of a cationic polymer by human hair: Effects of salts solution, *Colloid Interface Sci* 55 313 (1976)
11. JA Faucher et al, Influence of surfactants on the sorption of a cationic polymer by keratinous substrates, *Textile Res J* 47 65 (1997)

CHAPTER 18

A New Dimension in Hairstyling – VP/Methacrylamide/Vinyl Imidazole Copolymer

C. Wood, S. Nguyen-Kim and P. Hoessel
BASF AG, Ludwigshafen, Germany

KEY WORDS: *Styling polymer, hair gels, hair mousses, nanoindentation, mechanical measurements*

ABSTRACT: *Data on friction, hardness, tack and other mechanical properties obtained from a nanoindenter on an atomic force microscope combined with conventional stress strain measurements demonstrate the potential of VP/methacrylamide/vinylimadazole copolymer, a new hairstyling polymer.*

Hair gels and mousses have a high rank among styling products. Approximately half of the styling polymers are employed in these application forms, and approximately 25% are used in gel formulations.[1]

Gels are favored for short hairstyles and are particularly used by men. Due to VOC regulations, the trend in the United States is toward water-based styling gels and mousses — away from aerosol hairsprays with propellant and solvent. In Asia, water-based and alcohol-free styling formulations are correlated with purity and traditionally preferred. On strong, dark Asian hair, styling gels and mousses accomplish good setting without flaking.

Most of the hair gels on the market have cross-linked polyacrylic acid as the thickener because it gives them an important advantage: they are thixotropic and have a yield point. This means that they are effortlessly taken from a container, do not flow from the hand, and are easily dispersed on hair. But, only a limited number of setting polymers in these gels are compatible with the thickener. Almost every cationic or anionic setting polymer is incompatible with cross-linked polyacrylic acid, which leads to turbid formulations or precipitation, poor gel rheology, or instability.

Therefore, we set out to create a specialty polymer for clear hair gels. The required properties were excellent clarity in hair gel formulations with cross-linked polyacrylic acid, very low tack, high setting effect and high resistance to humidity. Many of these properties were determined conventionally on human hair as well as with a nanomechanical testing device.

New material development and understanding existing market products requires testing of surfaces or thin films at smaller scales for elastic and friction properties. Nanomechanical testing with a nanoindenter on the atomic force microscope (AFM) provides data with small forces and high lateral resolution, especially thin surface layers down to 100 nm.

Viscoelastic materials such as hair care polymers for styling applications were investigated with this method. These data were compared with data on the sensory assessment of personal care formulations applied to human hair. Subjective manual test results and nanomechanical AFM data of various hair care products evidently correlate to each other. Accordingly, the combability of hair after polymer application is associated to the reduced microscopic friction coefficient determined by a nanoscratching device on polymer films. Polymer raw materials as well as complete cosmetic formulations such as styling gels were tested regarding their performance.

These insights into the mechanical properties of materials were used to create new polymers with defined structures. Nanomechanical testing was recognized as a useful method for the investigation of cosmetic polymers and polymer-containing cosmetic formulations.

The specialty polymer[a] we developed has the INCI name VP/methacrylamide/vinyl imidazole copolymer. In this chapter, we will refer to it as VPMVI copolymer. It is a 20% aqueous solution of a copolymer of N-vinylpyrrolidone, methacrylamide and N-vinylimidazole (**Figure 1**).

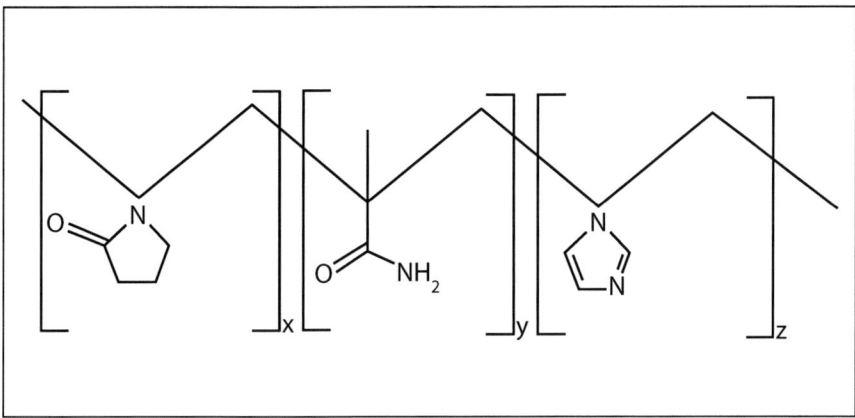

Figure 1. Structure of VPMVI copolymer

Mechanical Properties of Films

The mechanical properties of VPMVI copolymer were optimized during its development. An important requirement for high setting effect is a high tensile strength of the polymer film (**Figure 2**). The mechanical properties of several polymer films (34.5 mm long by 6.0 mm wide by 0.13-0.15 mm thick) were determined with a solids analyzer[b] in a measuring chamber with defined relative humidity of 55%. The VPMVI copolymer was compared to PVP K90 and PVP K30[c] which are the conventional setting polymers used in hair styling gels. The comparison shows the much higher tensile strength of the VPMVI copolymer.

Tack at various humidities: The nanoindentation method is appropriate to study material properties fast and reliably at various relative humidities in a climate chamber. A nanoindenter[d] was used for the nanomechanical measurements (**Figure 3**). During operation, the probe tip is first lowered into contact with the sample,

---

[a]Luviset Clear, BASF, Ludwigshafen, Germany
[b]Rheometric Scientific Solids Analyzer RSA II, New Castle, Delaware, USA
[c]Luviskol K30 and Luviskol K90, BASF Corp., Mt. Olive, New Jersey, USA
[d]Hysitron Nanoindenter, Hysitron, Minneapolis, Minnesota, USA

then indented into the surface, and finally lifted off the sample surface. The indentation depth and the actual force applied to the tip are recorded simultaneously by an electromechanical capacitative 2D-transducer. A plot of the vertical force as a function of indentation depth for one complete indentation and retraction cycle is called a load displacement curve. Such curves were obtained from

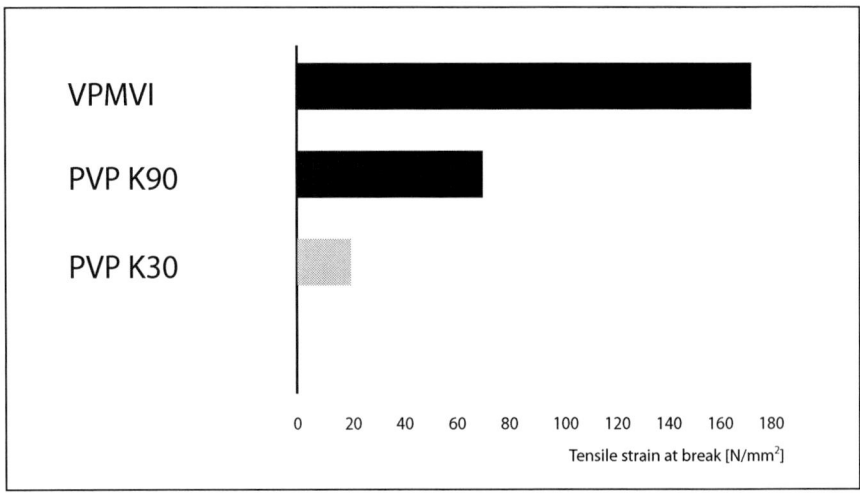

Figure 2. Stress-Strain measurement of polymer films VPMVI, PVP K90 and PVP K30 (250-500 µm; 55% RH)

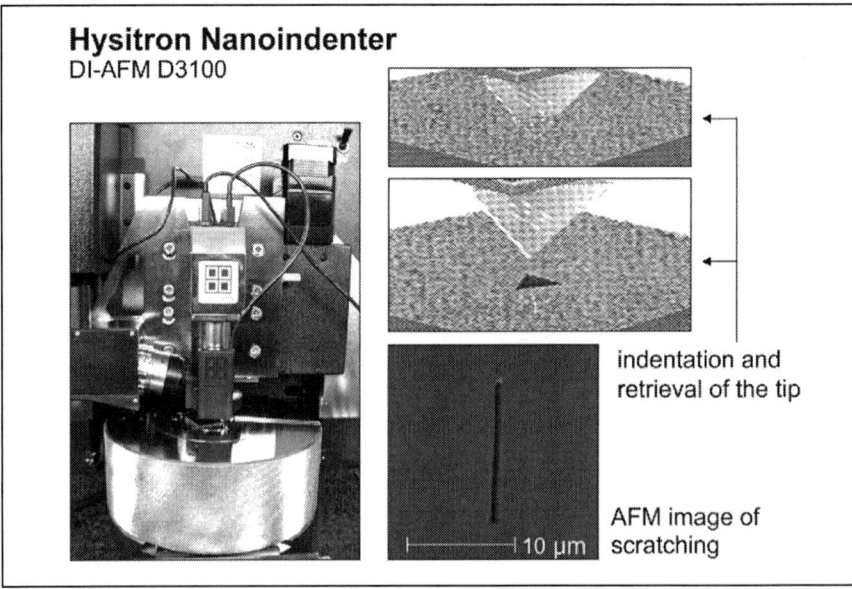

Figure 3. Hysitron nanoindenter (DI-AFM D3100)

about 20 different areas on duplicate surfaces. Hardness and reduced E modulus were calculated from the load displacement curves using an algorithm for an elastic/plastic indentation.[2-5]

The low tackiness of VPMVI copolymer (panel test, subjective and objective tests on glass plates) is supported by the nanoindentation measurements. Contrary to PVP, there is almost no dependence on relative humidity with the new setting polymer (**Figure 4**).

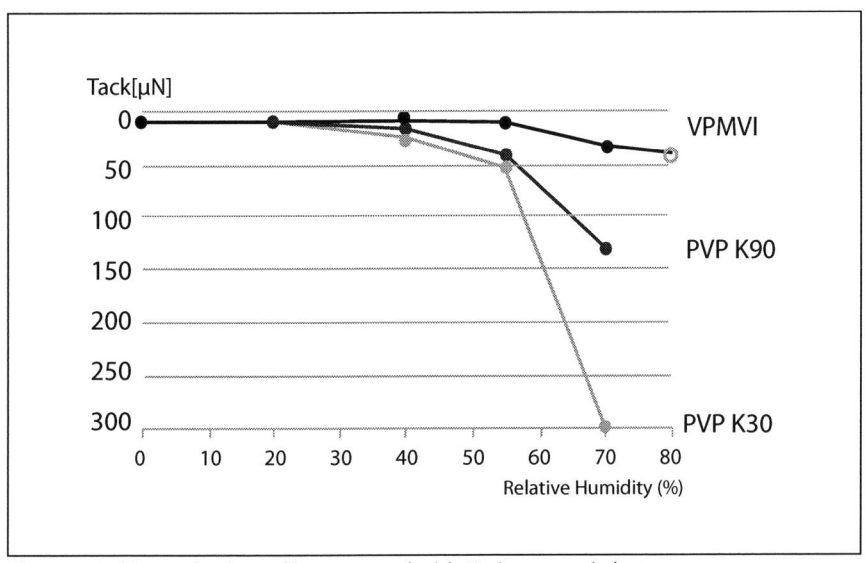

Figure 4. Tackiness of polymer films measured with Hysitron nanoindenter

Friction coefficient: The nanoscratch experiment was performed by applying a constant vertical force of 10 µN and a constant lateral velocity of 500 nm/s. The so-called friction coefficient R from nanoscratching was determined from the ratio of lateral force to normal monitored during scratching. VPMVI copolymer has a strikingly low friction coefficient at high relative humidity (**Figure 5**). The experience with different polymers substantiates a correlation between friction and combability of hair.[6] A low friction coefficient (as in the new setting polymer) goes along with ease of combing.

Tack while drying: A tack tester[e] revealed substantially lower tackiness than PVP during the drying period of the polymer film (**Figure 6**).

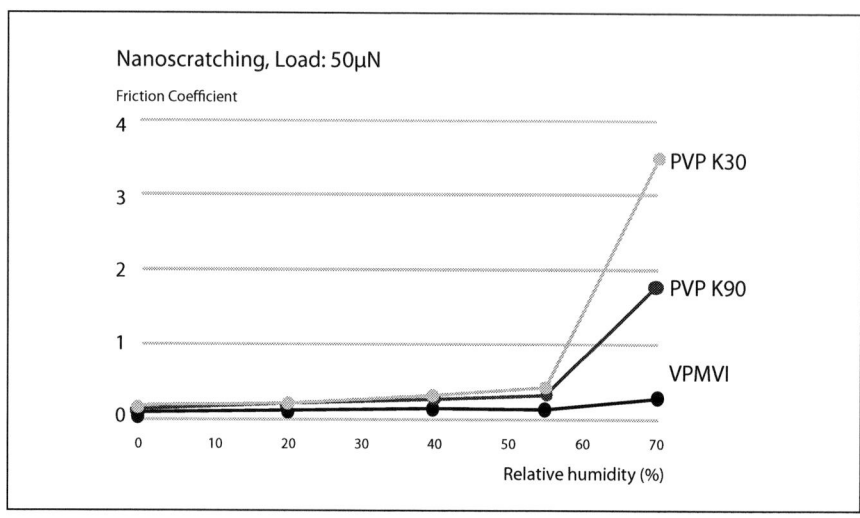

Figure 5. Friction coefficient of polymer films measured by Hysitron nanoindenter (Nanoscratching, load = 50 µN)

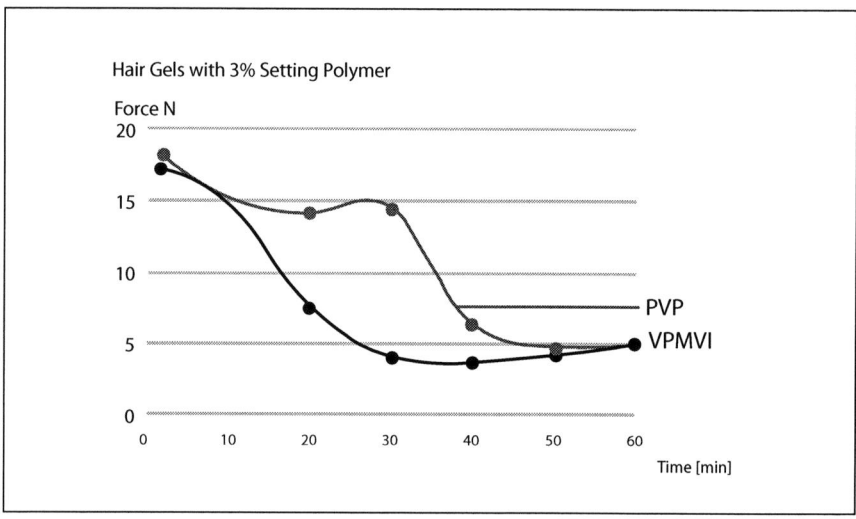

Figure 6. Tackiness of polymer films during drying. Measured by Diastron method. Hair gels with setting polymer at 3%.

Testing the Properties of Gels or Mousses

Tackiness of gels after drying: The tackiness is evaluated with mechanical testing as well as with sensory assessment.

During the mechanical testing, the tested gel is spread with a 120 µm spiral coater on a glass plate. The dry film on the glass plate is put into a climate chamber at 25°C and 90% relative humidity overnight. A rubber stamp presses a carbon band for 10 seconds onto the polymer film. The stickier the polymer surface is, the more printing ink from the carbon band adheres to the polymer film. The print is evaluated to a ranking from 0 (not tacky) to 5 (very strongly tacky).

For the sensory assessment, the tested gel is applied to a hair swatch. After drying, the tackiness is evaluated by at least two persons. They press their hands on a damp cloth and subsequently compress the hair swatch for 10 seconds in their hands. At release, the stickiness is evaluated with a ranking from 0 (not tacky) to 3 (strongly tacky). For comparison, always a standard should be used in parallel.

Tackiness of gels during drying: With a tensile tester[f], the force until separation (given in Newtons) of a metal stamp pressed on a drying polymer film is measured as a function of drying time. The measurement is performed in a climate chamber at 20°C and 65% relative humidity.

Stiffness test: The stiffness test is the determination of the bending stiffness of a gel. The tested gel is diluted until a low viscous mass is formed. Hair tresses are dipped repeatedly into the diluted gel. Excess gel is wiped off and formed by hand to a round cross-section. At 20°C and 65% relative humidity, the tresses are dried overnight. The measurement of the bending stiffness is performed with a tensile tester. During testing, the gel film breaks, and the needed force in Newtons is monitored. Each sample of diluted gel is tested with at least five different hair tresses for its bending stiffness.

With mousses, the wet hair tresses are dipped into the solution of the mousse formulation containing setting polymer and prepared as described above. The measurement of the bending stiffness is performed as described above.

Curl retention of a gel or a mousse: A sufficient amount of the tested gel is spread on a glass plate, and the gel is applied with a scoop evenly on a hair tress. Excess gel is squeezed off and the hair tress is coiled around a Teflon curler. After that, the prepared tresses are dried overnight at 70°C. After 30 minutes of cooling to room temperature, the curl is carefully removed from the curler. The curls are hung up

---

[e]Tack Tester, A. Coesfeld Ltd., Dortmund, Germany
[f]Tensile Tester, A. Coesfeld Ltd., Dortmund, Germany

at one end, and their starting length is recorded. The determination of the curl retention is performed at 25°C and 90% relative humidity. After 5 hours, the final length of the curls is recorded. The stability of the curls in the particular climate is calculated and given in percent.

With mousses, the wet hair tresses are dipped into the solution of the mousse formulation containing setting polymer and prepared as already described. The determination of the curl retention is performed at 25°C and 75% relative humidity and determined as already described.

Combing force measurement for mousse application: The mousse is dispersed into the wet hair swatch. Prior to measurement, the hair swatch is detangled until no loops or coils remain. Next, the swatch is positioned into a clamp and combed into the testing comb that is part of the tensile tester. The combing force reduction is given in percent and calculated from the force ratio between treated swatch value and blank value (untreated swatch).

Light transmittance of gels (clarity measurements): The measurement of the transmittance is carried out with a UV/VIS spectrometer. Macro cuvettes with layer thickness of 1 cm were used. The transmittance value is determined at a wavelength of 600 nm. For comparison, the transmittance of distilled water is measured.

Results: Excellently transparent hair gels were made with VPMVI copolymer as the setting polymer. The precondition is a transparent thickener base, such as acrylates / C10-C30 alkyl acrylate crosspolymer[g]. **Figure 7** shows the clarity of a formulation consisting of this thickener at 0.4% and VPMVI copolymer at 3.0% in distilled water. The light transmission of the gel base with 0.4% thickener is 97.4% (middle image). The addition of VPMVI copolymer enhances transparency to more than 99% (right image).

With 3% content of the setting polymer, one can achieve a very strong setting that outperforms most of the commercially available gels on the market. As shown in **Table 1**, VPMVI copolymer is recommended at levels between 1% and 5% with the commonly used thickeners for the manufacture of clear gels. The details of formulation procedure vary from one formulation to the next, but in general the recommended procedure requires these steps:

---

[g]Ultrez 21, Noveon, Cleveland, USA

- Making of a diluted solution of the thickener;
- 100% neutralization of the thickener solution and formation of the gel;
- Addition of the 20% VPMVI copolymer solution

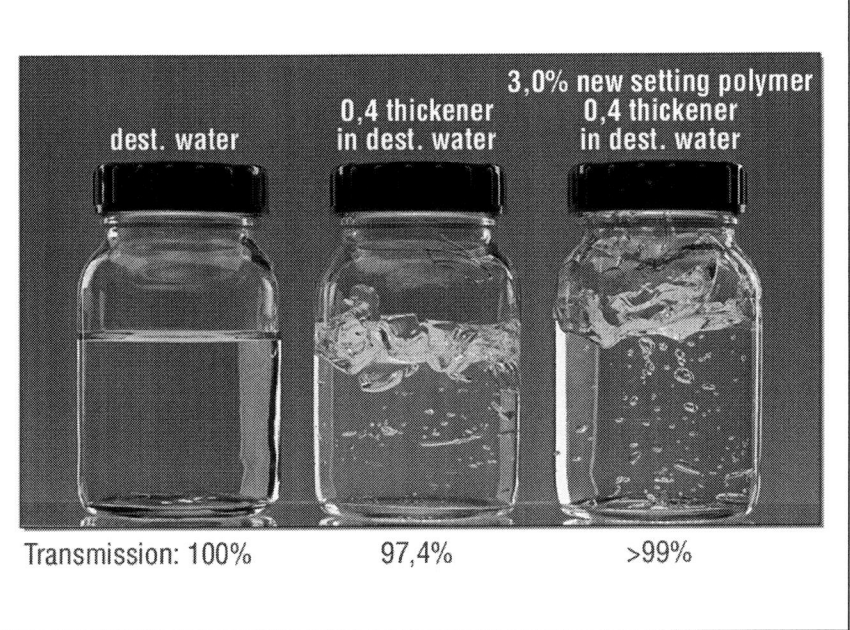

Figure 7. Clarity of a hair gel with VPMVI copolymer

In **Table 2**, the properties of VPMVI copolymer in hair gels are pointed out. The clarity of certain formulations is even better than that of polyvinylpyrrolidone formulations. The setting effect is high. The curl retention is above 90%.

As **Table 3** shows, VPMVI copolymer is appropriate in hair mousses also. It can be used as a single setting polymer or in combination with various polyquaterniums. For example, the combination with polyquaternium-46[h] is recommended for extra strong hold and high humidity resistance. Combined with polyquaternium-16[i], it achieves high conditioning performance and better curl retention than with conventional VP/VA copolymers.

Sample formulations are shown in **Formulas 1, 2 and 3**.

---

[h]Luviquat Hold, BASF Corp., Mt. Olive, New Jersey, USA
[i]Luviquat Style, BASF Corp., Mt. Olive, New Jersey, USA

Table 1
Recommended percentages of some common thickeners used with VPMVI copolymer

INCI name	Trade name	Supplier	Solid content (%)
Acrylates / C10-C30 alkyl acrylate crosspolymer	Ultrez 21	Noveon	0.4-0.5
Acrylates beheneth – 25 methacrylate copolymer	Aculyn 28	Rohm & Haas	ca. 1.0
Carbomer	Carbopol 940	Noveon	0.4-0.5

Table 2
Properties of 3.0% VPMVI copolymer in hair gels thickened with 0.5% acrylates / C10-C30 alkyl acrylate crosspolymer

	VPMVI	PVP K90	PVP K30
Clarity*	crystal clear	clear	clear
Transmission* (%)	99.2	96.8	98.8
Tackiness at 90% RH (rating)	0-1	3	3
Stiffness test (cN)	190-200	125-145	70-80
Curl retention at 90% RH (%)	>90	61	47

*Visually in 250 ml glass tubes; Transmission T at 600 nm

Table 3
Properties of 3.0% VPMVI copolymer in hair mousses

	Setting (cN)*	Curl retention (%)**	Combability (%)***
VPMVI (3%)	217	81	70
VPMI (2%) and PQ-46 (1%)	299	66	72
VPMVI (2%) and PQ-16 (1%)	295	24	78
VP/VA 64 (3%)	67	2	62

* Stiffness Test in Newtons
** measured at 75% RH
*** Combing Force Reduction in %

Formula 1
Spiky hair gel for very strong hold

A. Water (*aqua*), deionized	48.95% w/w
Preservative	qs
B. Acrylates/C10-30 alkyl acrylate crosspolymer	
(Ultrez 21, Noveon)	0.5
Triethanolamine	0.75
C. Water (aqua), distilled	22.00
PEG-40 hydrogenated castor oil	
(Cremophor CO 40, BASF)	0.10
Fragrance (*parfum*)	qs
D. PEG-8 (Pluracare E 400, BASF)	2.00
Panthenol	0.50
PEG-25 PABA (Uvinul P25, BASF)	0.10
Dimethicone copolyol (DC190, Dow Corning)	0.10
VP/methacryamide/vinyl imidazole copolymer	
(Luviset Clear, BASF)	25.00

Procedure: Put A into a beaker, stir and disperse B into it until the particles sink to the bottom. Then add C and stir until a homogeneous gel has been formed. Prepare D and stir until dissolved. Then add D to the gel.
pH value: 7.2
viscosity (Brookfield): 30500 mPas
transmission: 97% (600 nm)

Summary

VPMVI copolymer is an innovative ingredient for clear hair gels, hair mousses and other styling products. New is the combination of the ability to formulate clear hair gels based on cross-linked polyacrylic acid with improved properties during application and after drying on hair. The new setting polymer can be employed as single polymer or in combination together with other styling polymers. VPMVI copolymer provides low polymer film tackiness. The values of curl retention at 90% relative humidity (values above 90%) and the setting effect are high. The advantages of the new setting polymer over conventional setting polymers are demonstrated by application assessments and conventional mechanical studies.

In particular, nanomechanical measurements are well suited to differentiate between polymer film properties on substrates. This

Formula 2
Shiny hair gel

A. Water (*aqua*), distilled	74.10% w/w
PEG-40 hydrogenated castor oil (Cremophor CO 40, BASF)	0.10
Fragrance (*parfum*)	qs
B. VP/methacryamide/vinyl imidazole copolymer (Luviset Clear, BASF)	15.00
Acrylates beheneth-25 methacrylate copolymer (Aculyn 28, Rohm & Haas)	5.00
Glycerol 87%	5.00
Dimethicone copolyol (SF 1288, GE Silicones)	0.10
PEG-25 PABA (Uvinul P25, BASF)	0.10
Preservative	qs
C. Triethanolamine	0.60

Procedure: Solubilize A. Weigh the components of B into A and stir until homogeneous. Neutralize AB with C and stir until homogeneous.
pH value: 7.0
viscosity: 90200 mPas
transmission: 97.0% (600 nm)

Formula 3
Volumizing aerosol mousse 6% VOC

A. Water–(*aqua*), distilled	47.10% w/w
VP/methacryamide/vinyl imidazole copolymer (Luviset Clear, BASF)	10.00
Polyquaternium-46 (Luviquat Hold, BASF)	5.00
Preservative	qs
B. Water (*aqua*), distilled	30.00
Ceteareth-25 (Cremophor A-25, BASF)	0.20
Cocotrimonium methosulfate (Luviquat Mono LS, BASF)	0.40
Laureth-3 (Rhodasurf L-3, Rhodia)	0.70
Fragrance (*parfum*)	qs
C. Propellant A70 (propane/isobutane)	6.00

Procedure: Add ingredients of A in order listed with adequate agitation, making sure all components are completely dissolved before adding the next. Premix ingredients of B until homogeneous. Add B to A with adequate agitation. Fill into appropriate containers and charge with C.

method of nanoindentation and nanoscratching was introduced into the material science for cosmetics for the first time. It is can be applied to polymer films as well as films of complete cosmetic formulations. Tack, hardness and friction of the VPMVI copolymer films correlate with important application properties on hair, such as tackiness, setting effect and combability. These insights into the mechanical properties of materials were used to tailor the new polymer, which takes formulations to a higher level of product performance.

Published February 2004 Cosmetics and Toiletries magazine

References

1. P Hoessel, Hair styling gels and alternative styling products – Market trends and polymer formulation concepts, Euro Cosmetics 3 40-45 (2001).
2. GM Pharr, Measurement of mechanical properties by ultra-low load indentation, Mat Sci Eng A 253 151 (1998).
3. GM Pharr, WC Oliver, FR Brotzen, On the generality of the relationship between contact stiffness, contact area, and elastic modulus during indentation, J Mater Res 7(3) 613 (1992).
4. WC Oliver, GM Pharr, An improved technique for determining hardness and elastic modulus using load and displacement sensing indentation, J Mater Res 7(6) 1564 (1992).
5. WC Oliver, Alternative technique for analyzing instrumented indentation data, J Mater Res 16(11) 3202 (2001).
6. C Wood, Nanomechanical Measurements in Hair Care, PCIA Conference, 5-7 March 2003, Manila, The Philippines

CHAPTER 19

Testing Polysilicone-19 for Claims of Hair Conditioning and UV Protection

Sascha Herrwerth, Holger I. Leidreiter, Uta Kortemeier, Christian Hartung and Burghard Grüning,
Evonik Goldschmidt GmbH, Essen, Germany

Sahar Fakhry-Smith,
Evonik Goldschmidt Corp., Hopewell, N.J., USA

KEY WORDS: *UV protection, color protection, hair dye protection, cationic siloxane copolymer, conditioning*

ABSTRACT: *Polysilicone-19, a new cationic siloxane copolymer for rinse-off shampoos and conditioners, protects dyed hair against UV fading by sunlight. The polymer also protects hair from sunlight damage and provides a conditioning effect.*

Modern hair treatments have to fulfill technical requirements and high emotional demands. While data on combing work, tensile strength or fatigue testing are common to support technical claims, the market success of a product is essentially determined by fulfilling those emotional characteristics that are claimed in the advertisement.

In hair care these emotional aspects are determined mainly by feel and appearance. Both of these parameters are hard to assay directly by objective methods. They have to be scored by sensory assessment and can be supported by a combination of various technical investigations.

In this study the appearance of hair tresses has been evaluated by color measurements of hair tresses, fiber tensile strength and a keratin degradation parameter. The type of damage selected was irradiation by ultraviolet/visible (UV/VIS) light simulating the sun.

Materials

UV absorbers: The UV absorber investigated in this study was polysilicone-19 (PS-19), a substantive siloxane copolymer grafted with 4-methoxycinnamic acid ester and cationic alkoylamidopropyl dimethyl ammonium groups. PS-19 is shown graphically in **Figure 1**. PS-19 has a silicone backbone for soft feel and silky appearance. It has cationic centers for substantivity on hair and other surfaces. Finally, it has methoxycinnamic acid residue for UV absorption. Earlier studies[1] have described the principal structural features of this product[a].

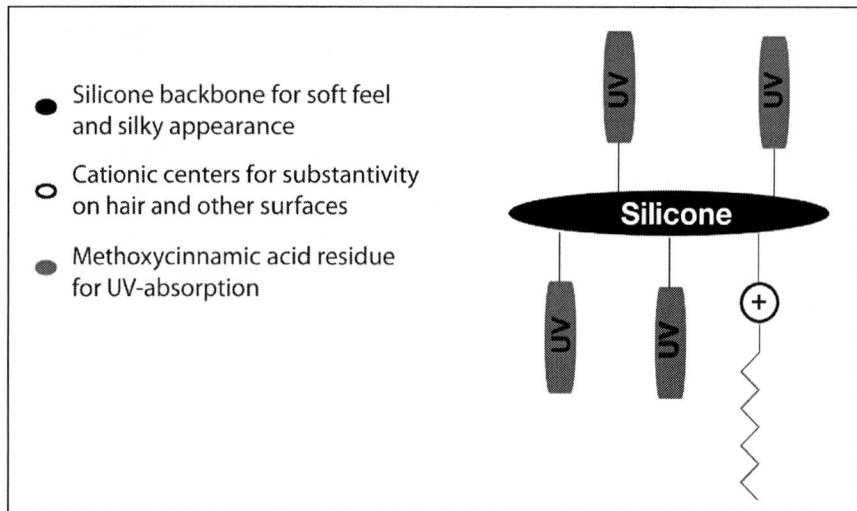

Figure 1. Schematic structure of polysilicone-19

The substantivity on hair of PS-19 out of shampoos and conditioners was proven by confocal laser scanning microscopy (CLSM).2 For this purpose a special derivative of PS-19 with a covalently bound fluorescent marker was prepared without significantly changing the molecular structure and surface interaction. The PS-19 modified with fluorescent marker was

---

[a] ABIL UV Quat 50 (INCI: Polysilicone-19) is a product of Evonik Goldschmidt GmbH, Essen, Germany. ABIL is a registered trademark.

incorporated into shampoo and rinse-off conditioner test formulations (**Formulas 1** and **2**). After this treatment, single hair fibers were investigated with CLSM (**Figure 2**). The reflection mode shows the topography of the hair fiber investigated. The image in fluorescence mode shows the localization of the labeled material on the same fiber area. It demonstrates that the PS-19 material is substantive out of a rinse-off conditioner application to hair. Similar results were received out of a rinse-off shampoo application. Untreated hair as a control does not show any fluorescence effect.

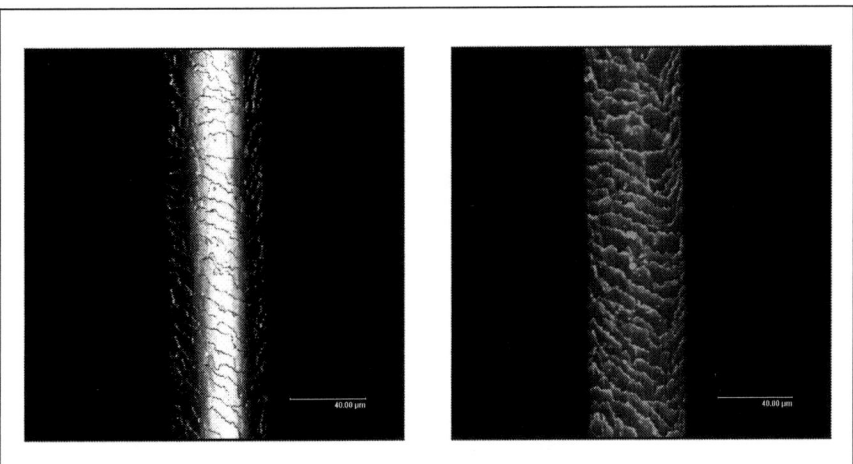

Figure 2. Confocal laser scanning microscopy showing substantivity of polysilicone-19 by a) reflection and b) fluorescence

In this study PS-19 was compared with four other commercially available cationic and neutral UV screens. These four products were selected for this study because of their claimed ability to protect the hair fiber against UV irradiation. The tested cationic UV absorbers were dimethylpabamidopropyl laurdimonium tosylate (DMPLT)[b], polyquaternium-59 (PQ-59)[c] and polyamide-2 (PA-2)[d]. The tested neutral silicone-based material was polysilicone-15 (PS-15), also known as diethylbenzylidene malonate dimethicone[e].

[b]Escalol HP-619 (INCI: Dimethypabamidopropyl laurdimonium tosylate (and) propylene glycol stearate) is a product of International Specialty Products.
[c]Crodasorb UV-HPP (INCI: Polyquaternium-59 (and) butylene glycol) is a product of Croda International Plc.
[d]Solamer GR 8 (INCI: Polyamide-2) is a product of Nalco Co.
[e]Parsol SLX (INCI: Polysilicone-15) is a product of DSM Co.

Formula 1
Shampoo

Test material†	0.5% w/w
Sodium laureth sulfate (Texapon NSO, Cognis)	32.0
Cocamidopropyl betaine (Tego Betain F, Evonik Goldschmidt)	7.9
Hydroxypropyl guar hydroxypropyltrimonium chloride (Jaguar C-162, Rhodia)	0.3
Citric acid, to pH 5.5	qs
Water (*aqua*)	qs to 100.0

† *The tested material incorporated one of the following:*
Polysilicone-19 (ABIL UV Quat, Evonik Goldschmidt)
Dimethypabamidopropyl laurdimonium tosylate (and) propylene glycol stearate
 (Escalol HP-619, ISP)
Polyquaternium-59 (and) butylene glycol (Crodasorb UV-HPP, Croda)
Polyamide-2 (Solamer GR 8, Nalco)
Polysilicone-15 (Parsol SLX, DSM)

Formula 2
Rinse-off conditioner

Test material†	2.0% w/w
Cetrimonium chloride (Varisoft 300, Evonik Goldschmidt)	1.0*
Ceteareth-25 (Teginacid C, Evonik Goldschmidt)	0.5
Cetyl alcohol (Tego Alkanol 16, Evonik Goldschmidt)	2.0
Citric acid, to pH 4.0–4.3	qs
Water (*aqua*)	qs to 100.0

*1.0% in irradiation tests; 0% in conditioning tests
† *The tested material incorporated one of the following:*
Polysilicone-19 (ABIL UV Quat, Evonik Goldschmidt)
Dimethypabamidopropyl laurdimonium tosylate (and) propylene glycol stearate
 (Escalol HP-619, ISP)
Polyquaternium-59 (and) butylene glycol (Crodasorb UV-HPP, Croda)
Polyamide-2 (Solamer GR 8, Nalco)
Polysilicone-15 (Parsol SLX, DSM)

The absorption spectra of all investigated materials are shown in **Figure 3**. The data were obtained with concentrations of 50 mg/L in ethanol. Strongest UVB absorption was observed with DMPLT. This material is a monomeric quat without any polymeric backbone; therefore it is the material with the highest density of chromophores, i.e., the absorbers of UV light at special wavelengths. Among the polymeric test products, PS-19 shows the strongest and widest absorption in the UVA and UVB range.

Hair treatments: Two types of cosmetic treatments have been applied as model systems. One was a standard shampoo (Formula 1) based on sodium laureth sulfate (SLES) and cocamidopropyl betaine (CAPB) as one surfactant system and the other formulation was a conditioner rinse (Formula 2) based on fatty alcohol and cetrimonium chloride (CTAC). The test compounds were incorporated into these base formulations.

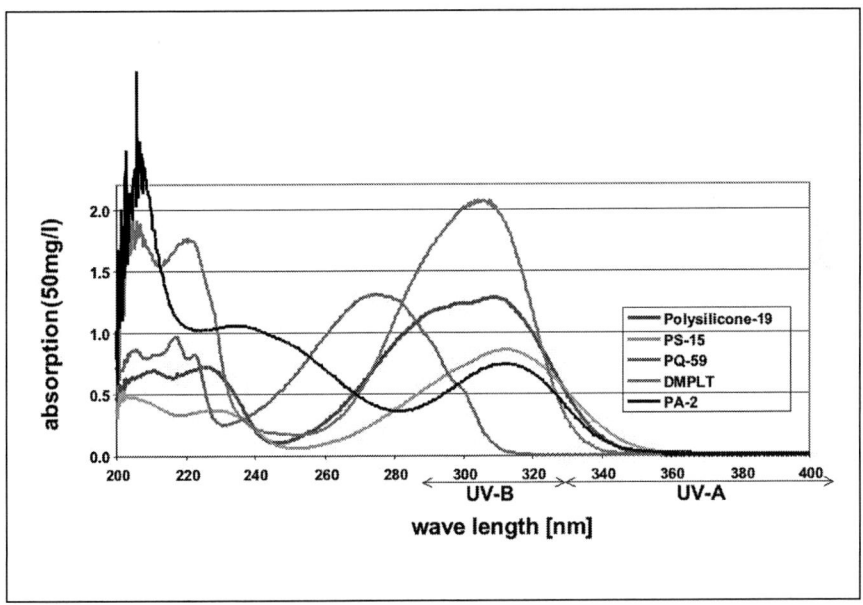

Figure 3. Traces of tested UV absorbers

The evaluation was conducted using European hair. The hair tresses used in this investigation had been pretreated by a bleaching process. This pretreatment damages the hair fiber in a way that simulates the damage typically caused when consumers perm, bleach or dye the hair. For color fading tests, hair tresses were dyed using commercially available coloration kits purchased from retailers. Both permanent (level 3)[f] and demipermanent (level 2)[g] dyes were applied (see **Semi-, Demi- and Permanent**).

Red shades of hair color were chosen because they are the most likely to fade when exposed to UV.

UV/VIS-irradiation: UV/VIS irradiation was induced using a sunlight simulator[h]. The sunlight simulator was used to provide light spectrum D65. Within 4 hr, this spectrum simulates the dose rate of one day of sunlight at 50° northern latitude (e.g., Frankfurt, Germany). The irradiation time between single test treatments and measurements corresponded to twice a natural daily dose. All measurements were calibrated by pairwise comparison of the values before and after irradiation.

Methods

Hair fiber tensile strength, fiber keratin integrity and hair color were measured instrumentally. Conditioning properties were subjected to a sensory assessment.

Tensile strength: The tensile strength of single hair fibers with and without UV irradiation was tested to detect damage from exposure to UV light. The hair fibers were European virgin brown hair, pre-damaged by bleaching (10% H_2O_2, 30 min, 22°C). The test products were incorporated into the conditioner formulation at a level of 2% active (**Formula 2**). As control, the same formulation was used without test material. The fibers (30 per test formula) went through four treatment cycles including: soaking in conditioner (10 min), rinsing under tap water (6 sec, 38°C), drying (12 hr, 22°C, 50% RH) and irradiation for 7 hr.

Data of tensile strength were obtained as start and end values. The start value was the tensile strength of the pretreated fiber. The end value was the tensile strength of the fiber after four test cycles. The tensile strength value was taken as "load 15%" (mN/mm^2), i.e.,

---

[f]Poly Brillance, number 868, grenadine, Schwarzkopf&Henkel
[g]Garnier Movida, number 27, grenadine, L'Oréal
[h]Hoenle sun simulator SOL2, Dr. Hoenle AG, Graefelfing, Germany

the force value at 15% elongation measured instrumentally[k]. The value of ΔLoad is the difference before and after the treatment procedure. After measurement of the start value the hair fibers had to be relaxed by soaking in water for 2 hr.

Keratin integrity: The hair fiber keratin integrity was investigated using differential scanning calorimetry (DSC).[13] This method delivers information about the degree of damage to the fiber's keratin structure.

In the test setup flat tresses (European human hair, single bleached) of 0.5 cm width were used. The tresses underwent four treatment cycles, including a shampooing step (0.5 g/tress for 30 sec, 1 min residence, 1 min rinsing) followed by conditioning (0.5 g/tress, 2 min residence, 2 min rinsing). In the shampoo tests the application was repeated once in each cycle without applying any conditioner. In the conditioner tests both the control shampoo and the test formulation were applied only once per cycle. **Formula 1** was again used as the text formulation, and the control was **Formula 1** without the test material.

After drying at room temperature, the tresses were irradiated for 4.25 hr (dose rate of approximately one day of sunlight). To maintain homogeneous irradiation, the hair tresses were spread to single fibers. Finally the hair tips were cut to the required amount for the DSC determination. Each test product was run in triplicate.

Color measurement: Hair color was measured using a CIE-$L^*a^*b^*$ color meter[m] to detect fading due to UV exposure. The color variations are expressed as integral difference, ΔE, based on changes of brightness (L^*), red-green (a^*) and blue-yellow (b^*) shift.

Application of shampoo or rinse conditioner or both can lead to fading of hair dye; this fading may overlie the effect of the UV/VIS light. In the case of hair that has been exposed to both treatments (i.e., shampoo and/or conditioner) and UV/VIS light, interpretation of color measurements would not be accurate. Best differentiation with good reproducibility was obtained when conducting the measurement directly before and after irradiation, without any intermediate treatment.

---

[k]MTT670, Diastron, Andover, UK
[m]CIE-$L^*a^*b^*$ Colorimeter, Dr. Lange, Dusseldorf, Germany

The selected procedure used flat-glued tresses of single-bleached European human hair, 4 g in weight, 16 cm long and 2 cm wide. The dye was applied according to the operating guidelines delivered with the product. Eleven tresses were treated with a single coloration. After a drying time of at least 24 hr, the tresses were treated with the test formulations (**Formula 1** and **2**) or the control formulation (**Formula 1** and **2** without the test material). The tresses were dried again. The color value was determined by 12 single measurements of the CIE-L*a*b* color values on one tress. An irradiation period of 7 hr was chosen to apply a dose rate approximating two days of sunlight. After treatment the color values were determined again and the change in color (ΔE) was calculated using the following equation:

$$\Delta E = \sqrt{(\Delta L^*)^2 + (\Delta a^*)^2 + (\Delta b^*)^2}$$

Conditioning evaluation: The conditioning performance of the five UV absorbers in **Formula 2** without cetrimonium chloride was assessed by a sensory hair swatch test done by experts using a standardized scale. Detangling, wet comb and wet feel were rated by sensory assessment on a scale in which "5" means "excellent" and "1" means "poor". As control a conditioner rinse (**Formula 2**) without test material and cetrimonium chloride was applied.

Results

Protecting hair fiber tensile strength: Sunlight, especially the UV fraction, can cause a reduction of the tensile strength of hair fibers. The test conditions in this study for unprotected hair fibers resulted in a reduction of the force measured at 15% extension by about 5 mN per fiber. This is a reduction of about 3% relative to the starting value.

Some of the UV-absorbing products provided protection when used in a conditioner formulation. The best performance was observed with PS-19, PA-2 and PS-15, with more than 40% less reduction of the tensile strength. The PQ-59 and DMPLT evaluated in this study scored protection values that were not significantly different from the control formulation containing only cetrimonium chloride. **Figure 4** shows the data in comparison.

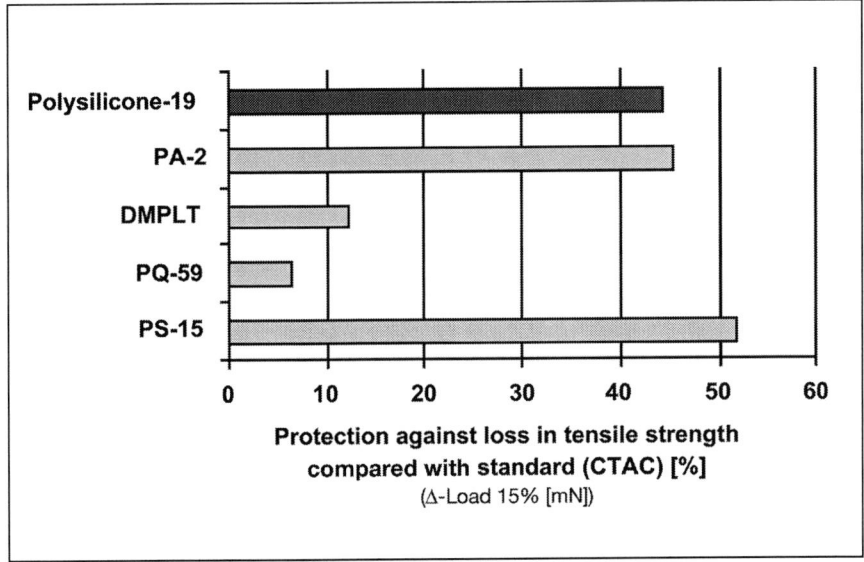

Figure 4. Protection offered by tested UV absorbers against hair fiber tensile strength loss caused by UV irradiation, as a percentage of the loss suffered by a cetrimonium chloride standard (Load 15% mN)

Protecting hair fiber keratin integrity: The DSC data exhibit high reproducibility and small standard deviation. Non-irradiated hair shows a DSC signal at about 154°C, while the treatment without protection reduces the decomposition temperature to about 142°C. The standard deviation in the data of this evaluation is below ±0.5°C. The best protection of the keratinous structure according to DSC measurement was the 12% provided by PS-19 out of conditioner application. In a shampoo application PS-19 provided approximately 10% protection. No DSC measurements with the other four materials were performed.

Protecting dyed hair against fading: The color change (ΔE) generated by the equivalent of approximately two days sunlight in the control **Formulas 1 or 2** without test material was 2.8 and 2.6 units, respectively, for a permanent dye, and 3.9 and 3.3 units, respectively, for a demipermanent dye, as shown in **Figure 5**. These data show that the use of a UV-absorbing material in a rinse-off formulation leads to an improved preservation of the color. This was observed out of both conditioner and shampoo applications.

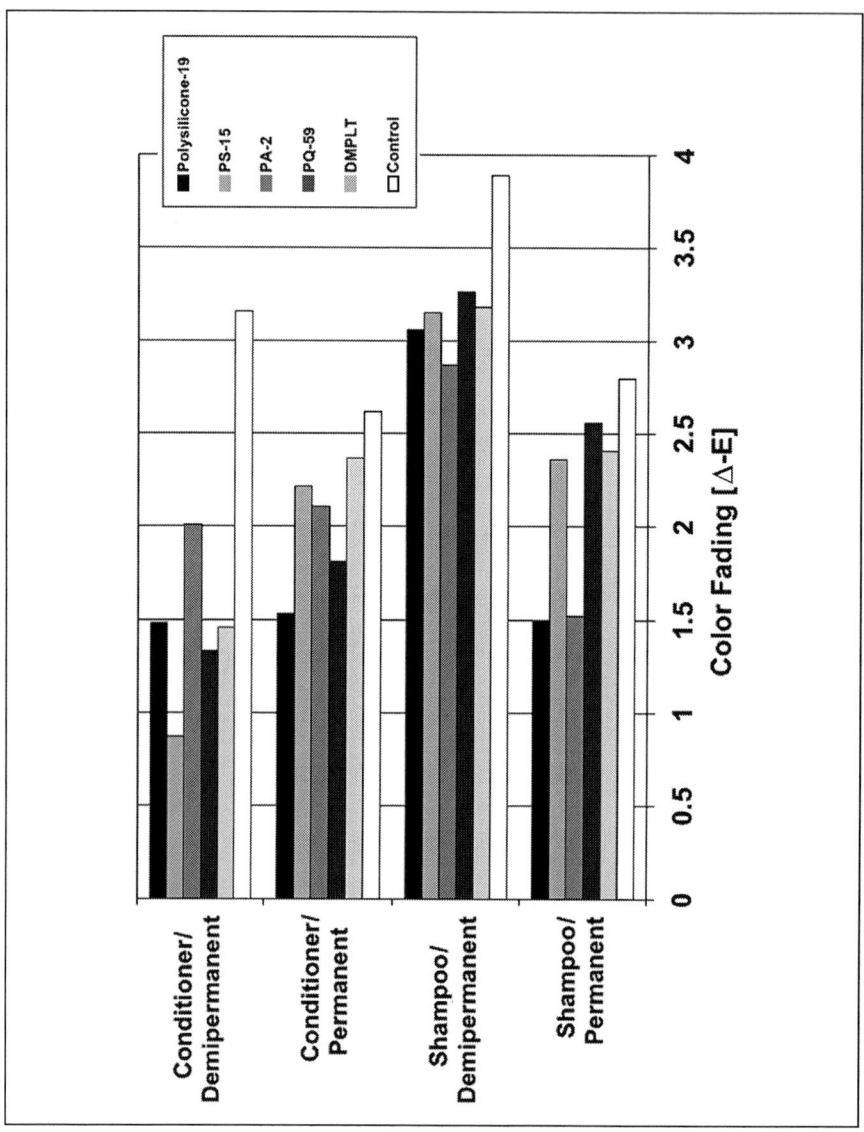

Figure 5. Color fading of hair tresses colored by permanent dye or demipermanent dye and protected by selected UV absorbers in a shampoo (0.5% actives) or rinse-off conditioner (2% actives)

In both shampoo and conditioner, PS-19 provided the best protection effect for the permanent coloration. The color fading was reduced by more than 40% both in the shampoo and conditioner application on permanent-dyed hair. Besides PS-19, PA-2 also performed well in the shampoo application, while PQ-59 provided a good performance in the conditioner formulation.

The protection effect from shampoo application for the demipermanent coloration was difficult to differentiate. In this application the protection of the demipermanent dye was approximately 20%.

In the conditioner application with demipermanent dye, PS-19 reduced the fading by more than 50%. In this comparison a maximum effect of about 65% protection was obtained with PS-15.

Conditioning application properties: The findings of the sensory assessment for detangling, wet comb and wet feel as the most important sensory parameters are shown in **Figure 6**. No cetrimonium chloride was used in the tested conditioning rinse formulation. The best conditioning effect was observed with PS-19 even as a single ingredient in conditioner applications. Only DMPLT showed almost similar results. The other products and the control scored significantly lower.

SEMI-, DEMI- AND PERMANENT

The hair coloring industry describes its products using one of three terms: permanent, demipermanent or semipermanent. They differ in terms of mechanism, damage and color durability.

Semipermanent color delivers tiny color molecules to the cuticle and the cortex. The molecules are small, so they wash out during repeated shampooing. No ammonia or peroxide is used in this process, so damage is minimal.

Demipermanent color delivers pre-color molecules to the cortex, where they partner to form medium-sized color molecules that take longer to wash out. These products contain a small amount of peroxide.

Permanent color uses both ammonia and peroxide in a process that delivers tiny color molecules to the cortex and expands them there so they are too large to wash out. The color is durable but the process can be damaging.

—From the editors

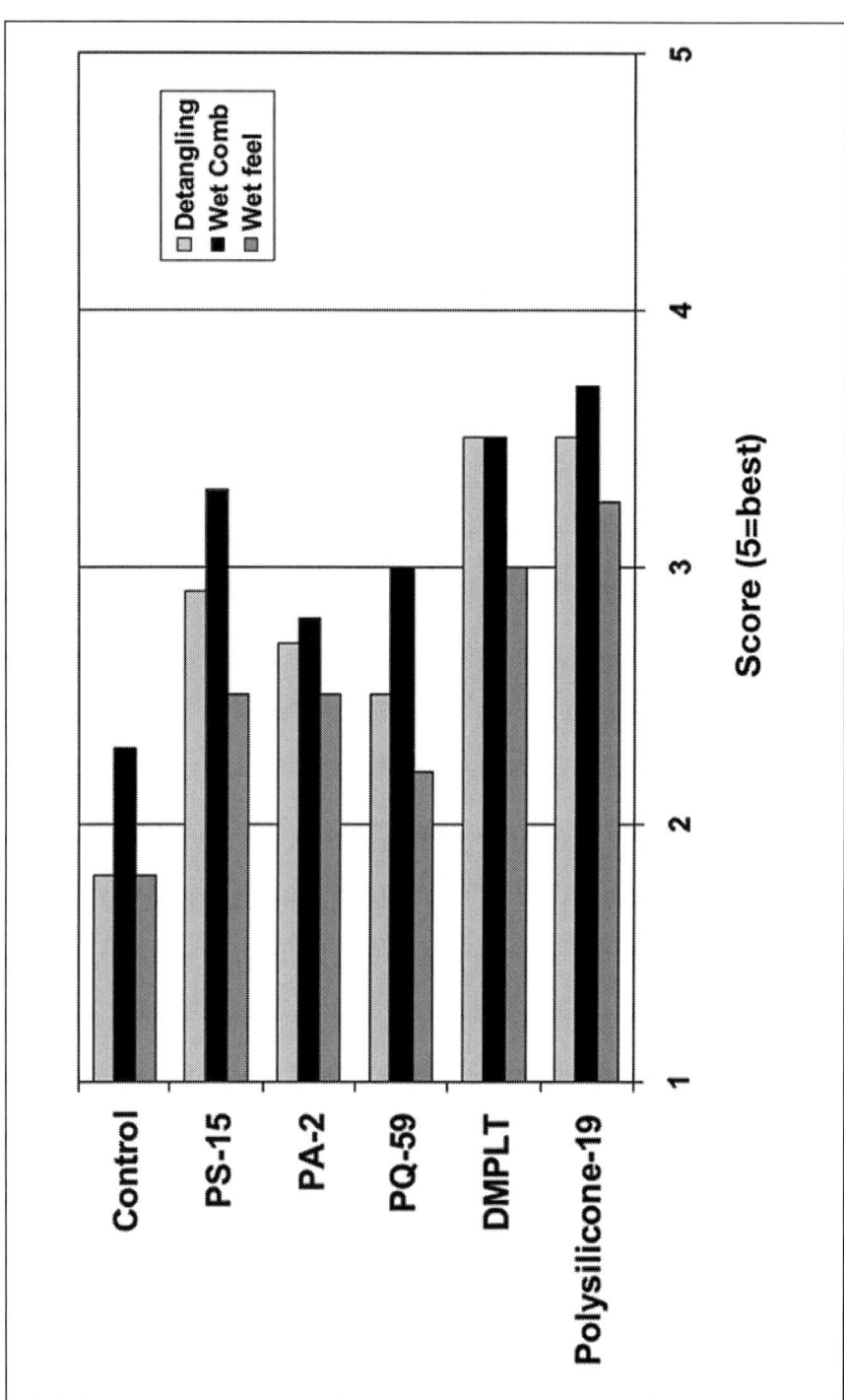

Figure 6. Sensory scores of hair tresses treated with one of five selected UV absorbers in a rinse-off conditioner formulation (Formula 2)

Conclusion

Tensile strength and DSC measurements were shown as a useful and highly reproducible tool for the determination of hair fiber damage by UV light. Both test methods can be used for the claim substantiation of UV protection of hair fibers, whereas the tensile strength measurement leads to more significant differentiations.

The protection of dyed hair against UV fading could be clearly demonstrated and measured with a CIE-L*a*b* color meter. Compared to the integrity measurement by DSC or tensile strength, the hair color is more easily perceived by consumers and therefore of high interest for claim substantiation of raw materials and consumer products.

In order to achieve best performance, a UV-protecting agent should combine UV absorption (by UV-absorbing groups), substantivity (by cationic groups) and conditioning (by silicone character). The new material polysilicone-19 combines these three features. In tests against four other commonly used UV absorbers, polysilicone-19 was found to perform best out of both shampoo and conditioner types of rinse-off hair care formulations.

Published May 2008 Cosmetics and Toiletries magazine

References

1. HI Leidreiter, U Kortemeier, U Maczkiewitz and M Pascaly, Protection of hair fiber appearance and strength against UV damage, *Proceedings of the 23rd IFSCC Congress, Orlando, Florida, USA, 2004*, New York: The Society of Cosmetic Chemists (2004)
2. M Minsky, Memoir on inventing the confocal scanning microscope, *Scanning* 10 128–138 (1988)
3. FJ Wortmann, C Springob and G Sendelbach, Investigations of cosmetically treated human hair by differential scanning calorimetry in water, *J Cosmet Sci* 53 219–228 (2002)

CHAPTER 20

New Hybrid Polymer for Hair Spray Formulations

Claudius Schwarzwälder, Jean Verlinden, Heidemarie Aigner, Christina Ecker and Roswitha Lang
Wacker Chemie AG, Munich, Germany

KEY WORDS: *Hair styling polymer, silicone/vinyl acetate copolymer, hold, feel, low VOC hair spray*

ABSTRACT: *Crotonic acid/vinyl C8–12 isoalkyl esters/VA/bis-vinyldimethicone crosspolymer is a new hybrid polymer for use in hair sprays. This highly branched block copolymer gives hair a firm hold and a soft, natural feel. It is recommended for use in quick-drying, low-tack hair sprays with high water content.*

When choosing a hair spray, consumers are often guided by the degree of hold the product offers.[1] However, surveys and market studies show that most respondents consider a pleasant touch to be just as important as good hold.[2]

These contradictory goals present formulators with a challenge:[3] a hair spray that gives a very firm hold has poor tactile properties—the hair feels unnaturally stiff, hard, inflexible and rough. Conversely, if a hair spray is to impart a pleasant, soft and natural feel, the hold will inevitably be reduced.

Other requirements, too, are contradictory.[4,5] For example, the polymer film that forms on the hair must be readily soluble or dispersible in water so it can be washed out with water and shampoo, but it must not be hygroscopic or the hair will become tacky in humid air and lose its hold. Various desirable mechanical properties—failure stress and shear strength; elasticity and hardness—are likewise contradictory, as are the polymer film's cohesive and adhesive properties.

For environmental reasons, hair spray manufacturers also seek significant reductions in the content of volatile organic compounds (VOC).[3,6] If this involves substituting water for a considerable proportion of the ethanol, a highly volatile solvent, and if conventional polymer systems are used, both the formulations' technical quality and the useful properties of hair spray products will be degraded. One of the consequences is an increase in the polymer solution's viscosity and surface tension, which leads to the formation of large aerosol particles and prevents uniform distribution of the solution on the hair. In addition, a higher water content in organic polymers typically results in longer drying times and a more tacky film.

Modifying Properties by Copolymerization

Today, the principal styling ingredient in hair sprays is usually a copolymer. Block and comb polymers are still used relatively infrequently. Many polymer properties can be customized by judicious selection of the monomers or—in the case of block and comb polymers—of the polymer segments used. For example, a balance can be achieved between the hydrophilic and hydrophobic properties as well as between conflicting mechanical properties.[4] Nevertheless, the authors' experience in testing commercially used products indicates that the conflict between hold and feel remains if the polymer contains only purely organic building blocks.

One approach to resolving the feel-versus-hold conflict uses silicones. Silicones are known for their friction-lowering and hence feel-enhancing effect.[7] The friction-lowering effect is a result of the flexible molecular skeleton that characterizes the silicones. The polysiloxane chains are highly mobile and thus enable silicone-treated hair or textile fibers to slip past each other very easily; friction between the treated fibers and other materials is likewise reduced. Silicone products improve the feel of hair and its combability. Furthermore, silicones have a low surface tension as well as a hydrophobic effect. The low surface tension increases the wetting and spreading behavior. The hydrophobicity helps to maintain the hold properties even at high humidity. Therefore, hybrid polymers combining organic and silicone building blocks in a copolymer should, in theory, be able to reconcile the contradictory requirements of good hold and natural feel.

A New Hair Styling Product

Wacker Silicones product developers created and screened several different hybrid polymers made up of organic and silicone segments ("blocks"). The starting point for selecting the organic building blocks was a group of monomers that had already proven successful in conventional hair styling polymers. The silicone blocks were selected from divinylpolydimethylsiloxanes. The hybrid polymers were tested principally for styling performance and ease of handling. Among the polymers tested, crotonic acid/vinyl C8–12 isoalkyl esters/VA/bis-vinyldimethicone crosspolymer proved the most suitable for use as a hair styling polymer. For convenience in this chapter, this new polymer[a] will be referred to as the silicone/vinyl acetate copolymer or SVAC.

Structure: The structure of this highly branched block copolymer is illustrated schematically in **Figure 1**. The macromolecules consist of two different building blocks: an organic polymer segment and a silicone block. Branching is effected by the silicone blocks. The chain lengths of the two blocks and the molecular weight of SVAC have been optimized.

The organic block is mostly vinyl acetate with a sprinkling of crotonic acid and vinyl-C8–12-isoalkyl ester. The silicone block consists of polydimethylsiloxane. The silicone blocks have reactive terminal groups to which the organic polymer segments bond during production.

The organic polymer segments impart the required hold. They not only provide the necessary adhesion to the surface of the hair fibers, but also make it possible to wash out the polymer. The silicone blocks improve the feel (see **Bereck Model**) and prevent the polymer film from becoming tacky due to water absorption. Thus, they enhance the hydrophobic property already conferred on the polymer by the polyvinyl acetate chains. Furthermore, they keep the polymer's surface tension low.

Physical properties: SVAC is a practically colorless, nonhygroscopic solid that dissolves completely in ethanol or in ethanol/water

---

[a]Wacker-Belsil P101 (INCI: Crotonic Acid/Vinyl C8–12 Isoalkyl Esters/VA/Bis-Vinyldimethicone Crosspolymer) is a product of Wacker Chemie AG. Wacker-Belsil is a registered trademark of Wacker Chemie AG.

mixtures, but also disperses in water. Even after a freeze/thaw cycle in which an aqueous ethanolic solution of polymer was cooled to −20°C, the polymer remained fully dissolved. This is important for applications in spray cans because the temperature in the spray head is apt to drop abruptly during spraying. If polymer were to precipitate out, it could block the valve. In this case, however, there is no risk that SVAC will block the valve.

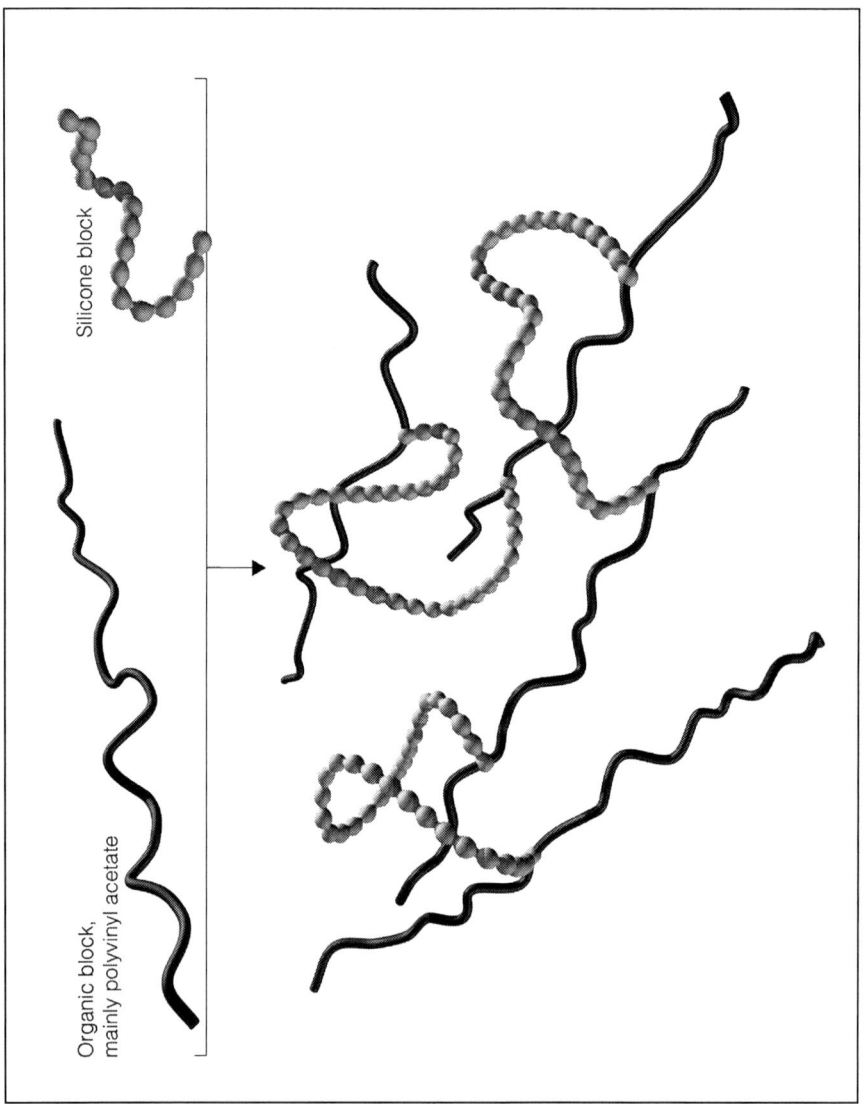

Figure 1. Schematic structural model of crotonic acid/vinyl C8–12 isoalkyl esters/VA/bis-vinyldimethicone crosspolymer

BERECK MODEL

To understand the silicone/vinyl acetate copolymer, or SVAC, discussed in this chapter, and in particular to understand how it works, consider the Bereck model originally used in textile engineering to describe the interaction between an aminofunctional silicone and a cotton fiber.[10] In this model, the silicone is anchored via its amino groups to the fiber such that the unsubstituted polydimethylsiloxane chain segments between the amino groups are in the form of loops directed away from the fiber surface. These flexible and hydrophobic loops, which are typical of silicones, have a lubricating effect. They are responsible for the pleasant tactile properties, such as soft feel, of silicone-treated textiles.

This model helps to illustrate how the SVAC works. The macromolecules are anchored to the surface of the hair fibers via the crotonic acid in the organic blocks. The polymer chain between two points of anchorage resembles a loop. It consists predominantly of polydimethylsiloxane, which forms the long, central part of the loop. The surface of the hair fiber is thus covered with movable silicone loops
(**Figure 7**), and these strongly reduce interfiber friction, friction between fiber and skin and friction between fiber and comb. The hair accordingly feels pleasantly silky and soft, and is easy to comb.

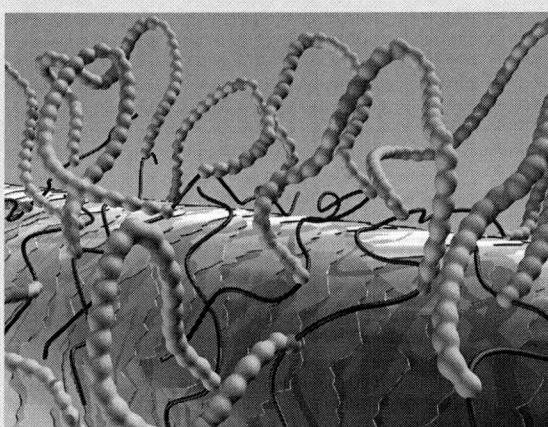

Figure 7. Silicone loops reduce interfiber friction between hair fibers, explaining the soft feel of hair styled with the organic-silicone hybrid polymer.

Electron micrographs of cast samples and sprayed films (**Figure 2**) show that the silicone blocks in the SVAC are arranged in small domains. Material with a higher atomic number has a higher scattering cross section and therefore leads to stronger scattering.

For this reason, the silicone domains appear black. With the help of energy dispersive X-ray spectroscopy (EDX), it is possible to show that the black areas—i.e. the domains—consist mainly of silicon atoms. However, because these domains are mostly smaller than 50 nanometers, SVAC films are transparent.

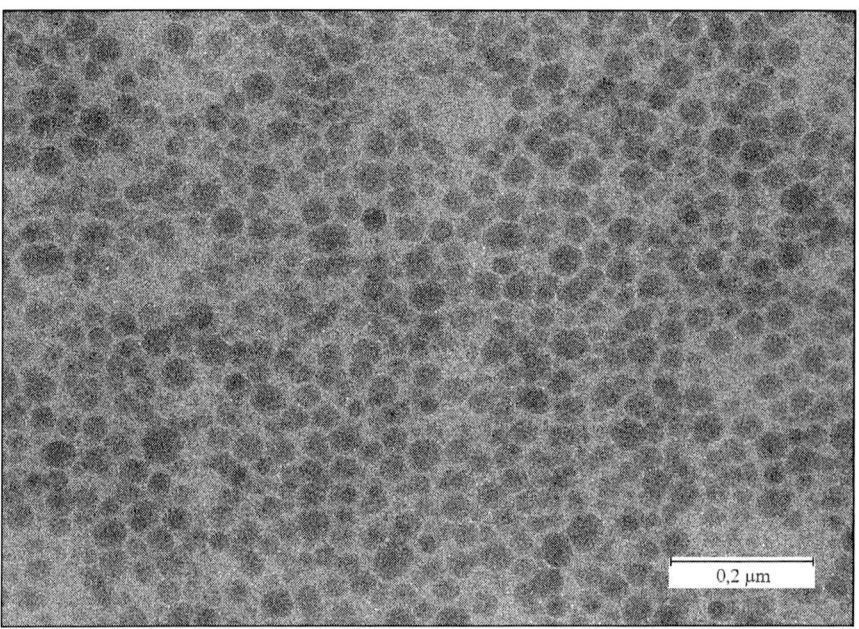

Figure 2. TEM micrograph of a sprayed film of crotonic acid/vinyl C8–12 isoalkyl esters/VA/bis-vinyldimethicone crosspolymer

The glass transition temperature was determined by differential scanning calorimetry (DSC). It is slightly below 40°C and thus a good 10 degrees lower than the glass transition temperature of comparable silicone-free copolymers. The low glass transition temperature shows SVAC to be a relatively soft, flexible material with no tendency to form polymer flakes on the hair.

Technical properties: SVAC's technical properties were investigated using test formulations that differed in their polymer and water contents. The formulations were limited to the essential components, as shown in **Formula 1** and **Formula 2** for two different, typical polymer contents.

The viscosity of solutions of SVAC, unlike that of most organic polymers, is low even when the proportion of water is high. This was shown in tests performed on formulations that contained no propellant, but did contain 35% w/w water; this corresponds to 20% w/w water in a propellant-containing final formulation. The polymer content was varied between 5% and 15%, equivalent to 3–9% polymer in spray with propellant. These test formulations proved to be only half as viscous as reference formulations in which the hybrid polymer had been replaced by a vinyl acetate-crotonate-neodecanoate copolymer (**Figure 3**). SVAC is miscible with organic polymers. The viscosity of the solution can be adjusted as required by adding an organic polymer.

Formula 1
Hair spray test formulation with 4.5% hybrid polymer

A. Ethanol	33.33% w/w
Aminomethylpropanol, 30%	0.68
Water *(aqua)*	21.50
B. Crotonic acid/vinyl C8–12 isoalkyl esters/VA/bis-vinyldimethicone crosspolymer (Wacker-Belsil P101, Wacker)	4.50
C. Dimethyl ether	<u>40.00</u>
	100.00

Procedure: Mix A. Dissolve B into A. Fill the solution into aluminum cans and charge with propellant C. Physical properties: Appearance: transparent; pH ~ 7; viscosity: 8.9 cst.

Formula 2
Hair spray test formulation with 6.0% hybrid polymer

A. Ethanol	32.21% w/w
Aminomethylpropanol, 30%	0.90
Water *(aqua)*	20.89
B. Crotonic acid/vinyl C8–12 isoalkyl esters/VA/bis-vinyldimethicone crosspolymer (Wacker-Belsil P101, Wacker)	4.50
C. Dimethyl ether	<u>40.00</u>
	100.00

Procedure: Mix A. Dissolve B in A. Fill the solution into aluminum cans and charge with propellant C. Physical properties: Appearance: transparent; pH ~ 7; viscosity: 8.9 cst.

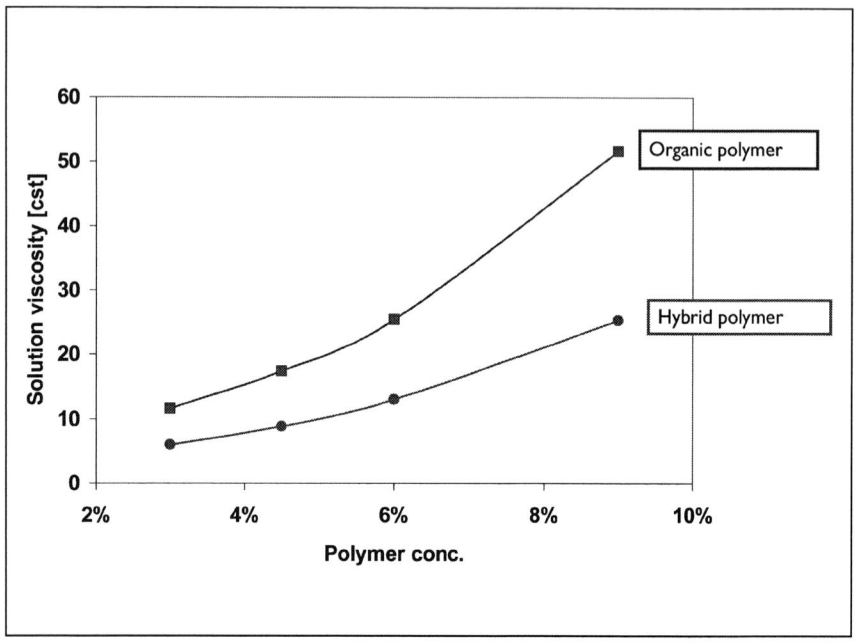

Figure 3. Viscosity of aqueous ethanol formulations of an organic-silicone hybrid polymer and a comparable organic polymer
Organic polymer = vinyl acetate-crotonate-neodecanoate copolymer
Hybrid polymer = crotonic acid/vinyl C8–12 isoalkyl esters/VA/bis-vinyldimethicone crosspolymer

Because formulations containing SVAC have low viscosity, they can be sprayed as a fine aerosol. Spray[b] from the test formulations (40% w/w dimethyl ether as propellant) contained aerosol particles ranging in size from 52 μm to 85 μm. Particle size was measured with a laser particle size analyzer[c] by means of light diffraction at a wavelength of 632.8 nm.

Aqueous ethanolic formulations based on the new hybrid polymer dry quickly. In panel tests, the participants judged hair tresses treated with the **Formula 2** test formulation (6% w/w polymer content) as being tacky for only 23 sec and dry just 40 sec after they had been sprayed. Tresses treated with polymer blends of the hybrid polymer and vinyl acetate-crotonate-neodecanoate copolymer took longer to dry.

---

[b]The spray was generated with ST300T spray head and LI valve (with aluminum Microflex mounting cup, Perbunan outer gasket, Butyl U-133 G-1978 inner gasket, 1 ́ 0.33-mm stem and LI-98 RTP 0.5-mm housing. All equipment was obtained from Lindal, Bad Oldesloe, Germany.
[c]Helos laser particle size analyzer, Sympatec GmbH, Clausthal-Zellerfeld, Germany

To ensure that the hair style returns to its original shape after mechanical loading such as gusts of wind, the sprayed hair must remain elastic. The three-point bending test[8] showed that hair tresses treated with SVAC retained their elasticity even after repeated mechanical loading. **Figure 4** shows the results for the test formulation with a polymer content of 4.5%. The bending tests were carried out at 65% relative humidity and 23°C.

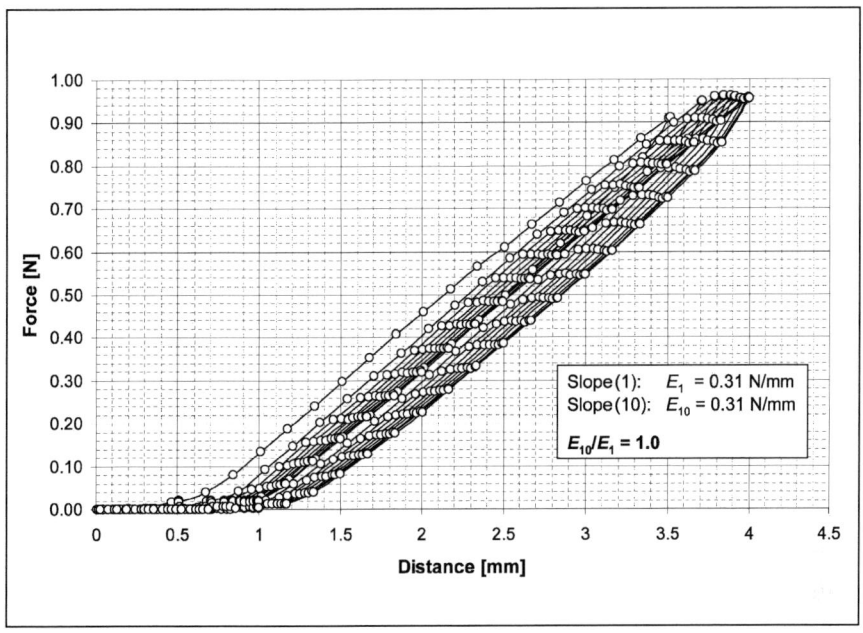

Figure 4. Results of the three-point bending test (10 cycles, 65% RH, 23°C) using hair tresses treated with the Formula 1

The new hybrid polymer absorbs only a very small amount of water and is thus only slightly softened by water. The hold imparted by the polymer is thus retained in humid air. Proof of this was provided by curl retention tests (**Figure 5**) that were carried out at 90% relative humidity and 23°C. The curl retention values measured under these conditions ranged from 85% to 95% depending on the hybrid polymer content. The tests were performed on tresses of brown European hair (3.5–4 g per 15-cm strand of hair). The tresses were wound around a polyvinyl chloride rod of 11 mm diameter and then, when dry, sprayed with the test hair spray formulations.

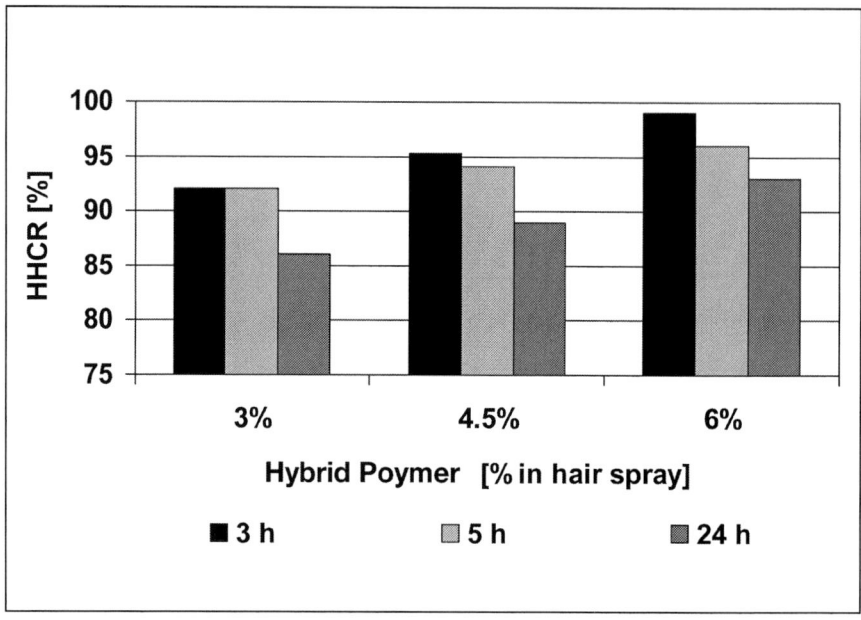

Figure 5. High humidity curl retention (HHCR) (90% RH, 23°C) of the organic-silicone hybrid polymer crotonic acid/vinyl C8–12 isoalkyl esters/VA/bis-vinyldimethicone crosspolymer

Effectiveness: In panel tests, all the participants rated the SVAC positively and thought it well-balanced. They were asked in a number of trials to compare the effects of SVAC-based test formulations (**Formulas 1 and 2**) with those of commercially available hair sprays (**Figure 6**).

The first comparative product (Benchmark 1) claimed to impart a "firm hold." The testers judged the effect of the test formulations (**Formulas 1 and 2**) as being somewhat more balanced than the comparative product. They found only a small or no difference in hold with **Formula 1** and **Formula 2**, respectively, but confirmed that the SVAC-treated hair tresses had more pleasant tactile properties, such as softness, smoothness and flexibility before and after combing.

For the second benchmark test, a product was used that promised a high level of flexibility. This time, the testers considered the SVAC-containing formulations to be superior with respect to softness, hold and combability.

285
New Hybrid Polymer for Hair Spray Formulations

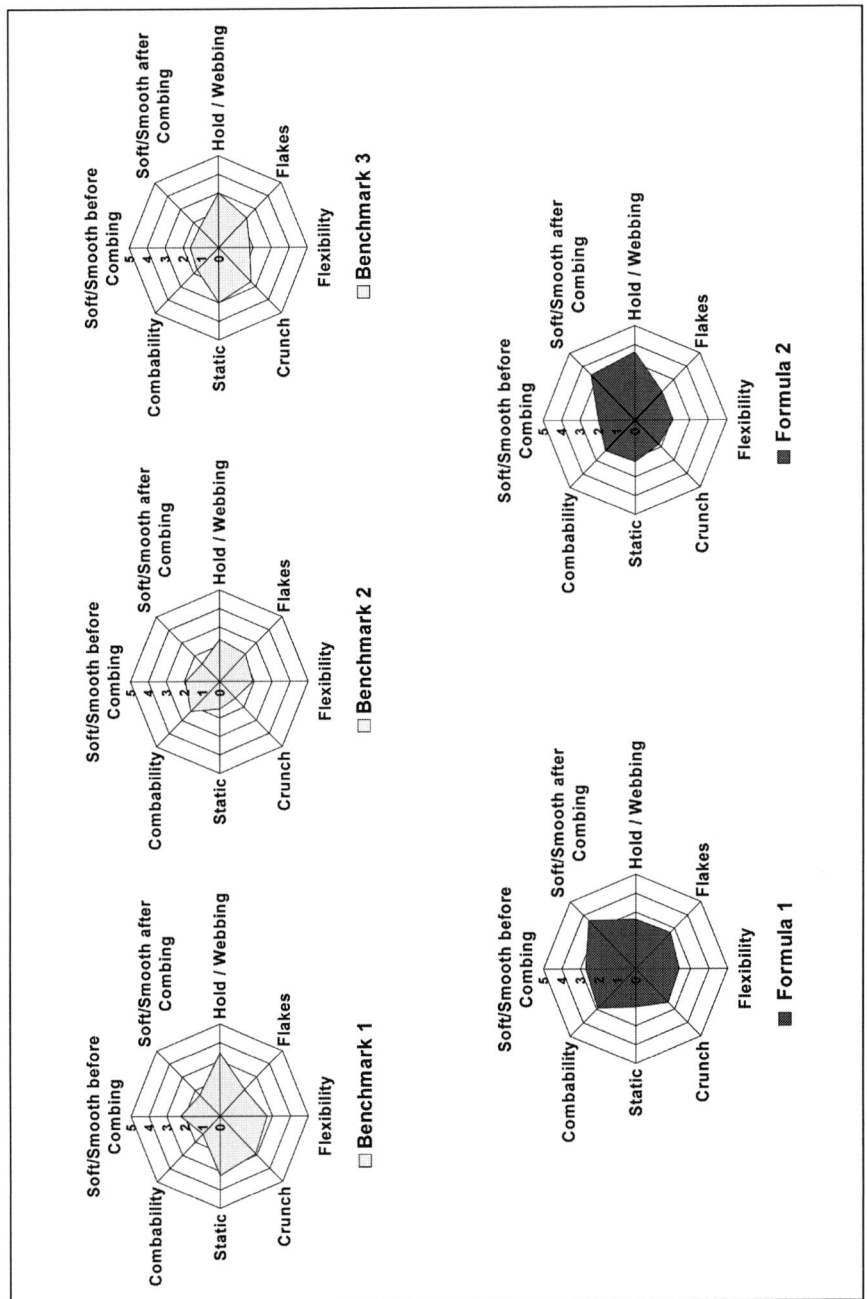

Figure 6. Specific properties of hair tresses treated with Formula 1 (organic-silicone hybrid polymer at 4.5% w/w) and Formula 2 (organic-silicone hybrid polymer at 6% w/w) compared with commercially available hair spray products that claim to offer "strong hold" (Benchmark 1), "flexibility" (Benchmark 2) or "extra-strong hold" (Benchmark 3). Each graphic represents poor performance at the center and improving performance at increasing distances from the center.

In the third comparative test (Benchmark 3), the effects of the test formulations were compared with those of a hair spray that boasted an "extra-strong hold." Here, the panel participants rated the test formulations as imparting clearly superior softness and flexibility to the hair. The test formulation containing 6% w/w SVAC was considered to impart a slightly better hold than the comparative product.

Summary and Outlook

The test results show that crotonic acid/vinyl C8–12 isoalkyl esters/VA/bis-vinyldimethicone crosspolymer, called SVAC in this chapter, combines the useful properties of organic polymers with those of silicones. Because this new hybrid polymer is not hygroscopic, even formulations with a high proportion of water do not produce a tacky film. Thus, SVAC allows hair sprays to be formulated with a high proportion of water.

Formulated in a hair spray, SVAC was tested in accordance with the Organisation for Economic Cooperation and Development (OECD) guideline[9] for its aerosol inhalation toxicity. No relevant effects were produced in this test, which means the product is classified as "non-dangerous" according to hazardous substances legislation.

Used as a hair styling polymer, SVAC can combine the hitherto conflicting properties of good hold and natural feel. The hybrid polymer thus paves the way to a new generation of hair sprays. Hair treated with a spray based on SVAC dries quickly, feels silky-soft and pleasant, is held well, retains its shape even in humid air, does not become tacky and is easy to comb. SVAC is also suitable for pump-spray formulations. Its use in mousses is currently under test. Initial results are promising. Additional tests are currently underway on variants that impart a firmer hold.

Published December 2007 Cosmetics and Toiletries magazine

References

1. CM Rocafort, Global hair styling and fixative overview, *SÖFW-Journal* 131(9) 26–33 (2005)
2. V Rudd, Hair styling sales don't hold up in western Europe, *Happi* 43(10) 35–36 (2006)

3. M Ashton, Hairspray, In *The Chemistry and Manufacture of Cosmetics*, vol 2, chap 13, ML Schlossmann, ed, Carol Stream, Illinois, USA: Allured Publishing (2000) p 327
4. G Müller and M Kutschera, Polymere für die Haarkosmetik – Haarfestiger und Haarconditioner, *Bunsenmagazin* 7(4) 94–100 (2005)
5. RY Lochhead and LR Huisinga, Advances in polymers for hair styling, *Cosmet Toil* 120(5) 59–68 (2005)
6. JA Dallal and CM Rocafort, Hair styling/fixative products, In *Hair and Hairsprays*, chap 5, DH Johnson, ed, New York: Marcel Dekker (1997) pp 105–165
7. S Mitra, Recent developments in silicone technology for hair care, In *Cosmetics and Toiletries Manufacturer Worldwide*, S Bond and M Caine, eds, Hemel Hempstead, Hertfordshire, UK: Aston Publishing Group (1995) pp 177–179
8. J Jachowicz and R McMullen, Mechanical analysis of elasticity and flexibility of virgin polymer-treated hair fiber assemblies, *J Cosmet Sci* 53(6) 345–361 (2002)
9. Organisation for Economic Cooperation and Development Guideline 403, *www.oecd.org* (Accessed Oct 16, 2007)
10. A Bereck, B Weber, D Riegel, J Mosel, J Bindl, P Habereder, KG Huhn, H-J Lautenschlager and G Preiner, Einfluß von Siliconweichmachern auf Griff und mechanische Eigenschaften von textilen Flächengebilden, Teil 4: Wechselwirkung zwischen Siliconen und Fasersubstrat, *Textilveredlung* 32 158–163 (1997)

CHAPTER 21

Peptides, Amino Acids and Proteins in Skin Care?

Karl Lintner, PhD
Sederma/Croda

It is difficult today to find a cosmetic or personal care brand that does not claim that at least some of its SKUs contain one or more peptides in their formulas. The concept of using active peptides in skin and hair care was slow to catch on but has gained considerable momentum over the last five years in all branches of the industry. It would thus be useful to clarify some of the concepts, ingredients and claims in connection with peptides in cosmetics. The relationship of peptides to amino acids and proteins, as indicated by the curious and specifically chosen title of this column, will become evident throughout this explanation.

Definitions

Confusion reigns in regard to the use of some technical terms in this field. Because any discussion of cosmetic activities, benefits and claims must be based on precise language, this chapter will begin with some definitions with which readers having chemical and biochemical backgrounds may already be familiar.

Amino acids: Amino acids are the building blocks of peptides and proteins. Their molecules have one thing in common: a carbon backbone with at least one amino ($-NH_2$) and at least one carboxyl ($-COOH$) group attached. This confers specific electrochemical or charge-related behavior to them, as well as the useful functionality of being able to link into chains; furthermore, the various amino acids are distinguished by the nature of their carbon backbone and the side chains that, in turn, confer additional functions, solubility and linking capabilities to these entities.

Peptides: Peptides are chains of at least two amino acids linked by the eponymous "peptide bond" between the carboxyl group of one and the amide group of the following amino acid. Oligopeptides are chains generally understood to be composed of less than approximately 20 amino acids. Polypeptides have longer chains; for example, insulin has approximately 50 amino acids.

Although no precise cut-off point has ever been agreed upon in scientific nomenclature, most scientists would agree that beyond 100 amino acids and a molecular weight of approximately 10,000 Daltons, the term protein is preferred over peptide. *Proteins:* Thus, proteins are long, usually linear chains of amino acids that can reach 1,000 or more links; collagen for example is approximately that size; fibronectin has a MW of approximately 400 kDaltons (approximately 4,000 amino acids). Unfortunately, the term protein is often used for raw materials that are totally or partially hydrolyzed proteins, or to blends of peptides and/or amino acids. To prevent confusion, this imprecise use of the term clearly should be avoided.

Origin and Manufacturing

A few words should be stated about origin and manufacturing.

Amino acids: Amino acids can be synthesized according to the Strecker method[1] and subsequent improvements, which yields amino acids in a racemic mixture of L- and D-stereoisomers; the separation into the biologically predominant and active L-form is possible but costly. Industrial production of amino acids uses either total protein hydrolysis followed by chromatographic separation, or biotechnology processes whereby specific microorganisms are solicited to manufacture a chosen amino acid in high yield.

Peptides: Peptides come in two forms: either they are synthesized as undefined mixtures of protein fragments obtained by partial hydrolysis of collagen, elastin, keratin, wheat or other plant proteins; or they are synthesized one peptide link at a time until a well-defined and well-chosen amino acid sequence is achieved. This latter method, albeit tedious and expensive, leads to reproducible, analytically defined and well characterized entities with chosen biological activity and usually extremely high potency.

Proteins: Proteins are practically impossible to synthesize by these methods in the laboratory and even less so in industrial scale. They are either carefully extracted from natural sources such as cow hide, bird feathers, human or animal hair, fish muscle or various plants, or produced by specifically chosen, sometimes engineered, microorganisms.

Amino Acids and Cosmetics

Amino acids have the general chemical formula: H-NH-CHR-CO-OH; R being a side chain of variable nature (see **Figure 1**).

Yet too often in the literature, certain amino acid terms are used without being clearly defined. Examples include: the 20 amino acids, "essential" amino acids, and natural and non-natural amino acids.

In fact, the number of possible amino acids is much higher than 20. It is theoretically infinite and practically quite large because one can always invent or imagine a new side chain, R, obtained by chemical means.

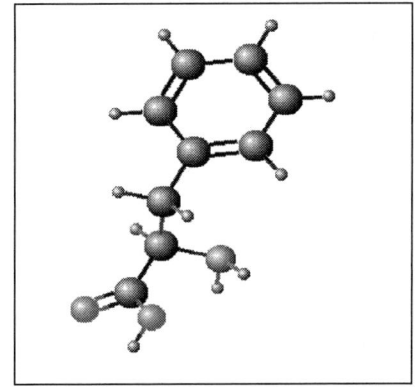

Figure 1. The amino acid phenylalanine

The so-called "natural" amino acids—those that have been identified in living organisms—number less than 35, of which 20 are particularly important to know. Only those 20 amino acids are coded for in human DNA and used by human cells to build proteins such as enzymes, collagen, elastin, keratin, muscle myosin and actin (see **Proteins and Cosmetics** later in the text).

Finally, within those 20 coded amino acids, six are called essential amino acids because humans, contrary to other species, are not able to synthesize these six molecules from simpler building blocks. Therefore, humans must ingest these molecules in one way or another in order to survive.

Amino Acids in Cosmetics

Amino acids have been used in cosmetics for many decades, either as rather undefined mixtures of fully hydrolyzed proteins obtained from collagen, elastin, keratin, wheat gluten or milk casein, or as specifically chosen individual amino acids in pure, isolated form.

In skin care, specifically chosen, purified, amino acids such as serine, threonine, alanine and pyroglutamic acid are popular ingredients because they are key components of the natural moisturizing factor (NMF); although, given their zwitterionic charged nature and low lipophilicity, they tend to remain at the surface of the stratum corneum and act only as water-binding molecules. Tyrosine and its derivatives such as acetyl-tyrosine or oleoyl-tyrosine[a] are used as melanin precursors in tanning accelerators.

Carnitine, creatine and taurine—all naturally occurring but not part of the coded 20 amino acids—are promoted as energy stimulating factors, co-factors or precursors, often in analogy to nutritional supplement claims.

Peptides and Cosmetics

Far more interesting, from a cosmetic science point of view, are the peptides, especially those with defined sequence and structure possessing specific biological activity. It is not excluded that partial protein hydrolysates that are "rich in peptides" show some cosmetic activity at sufficiently high concentration; however, their chain length, molecular weight, chemical composition, charge distribution and mechanism of action, if any, are unknown factors.

In contrast to these hydrolysates, synthetic peptides of defined chemical structure—those presently en vogue—have quite a different history and use. Glutathione, a tripeptide with important biological function in humans as an antioxidant and in the transport of amino acids, was discovered in 1921. Since then, hundreds of oligopeptides have been isolated from biological material, identified, synthesized and studied for biological activity. Among the better-known examples are oxytocin, vasopressin, angiotensin and bradykinin that release

---

[a]Tyr-ol (INCI: Oleoyl tyrosine (and) butylene glycol (and) oleic acid) is a product of Sederma, France. Ty-rol is a trademark of Sederma.

hormones such as TRH, ACTH, MSH, LHRH, substance P, rigin, enkephalin and endorphins.

The one important concept to understand is the strong correlation that exists between the specific amino acid sequence in the peptide chain and the resulting bio-activity. Most of these peptides act at precise cell receptors and trigger physiological responses in various cells and organs. Changes in the amino acids composing the peptide almost always lead to changes in the potency, type or duration of the activity. An example of this high selectivity is the tripeptides composed of the amino acids glycine, histidine and lysine (Gly-His-Lys) (see **Figure 2**). In the Gly-His-Lys sequence, wound-healing properties are observed through the stimulation of collagen synthesis in fibroblasts.[2] In contrast, the Gly-Lys-His structure has lipolytic activity on adipocytes.[3]

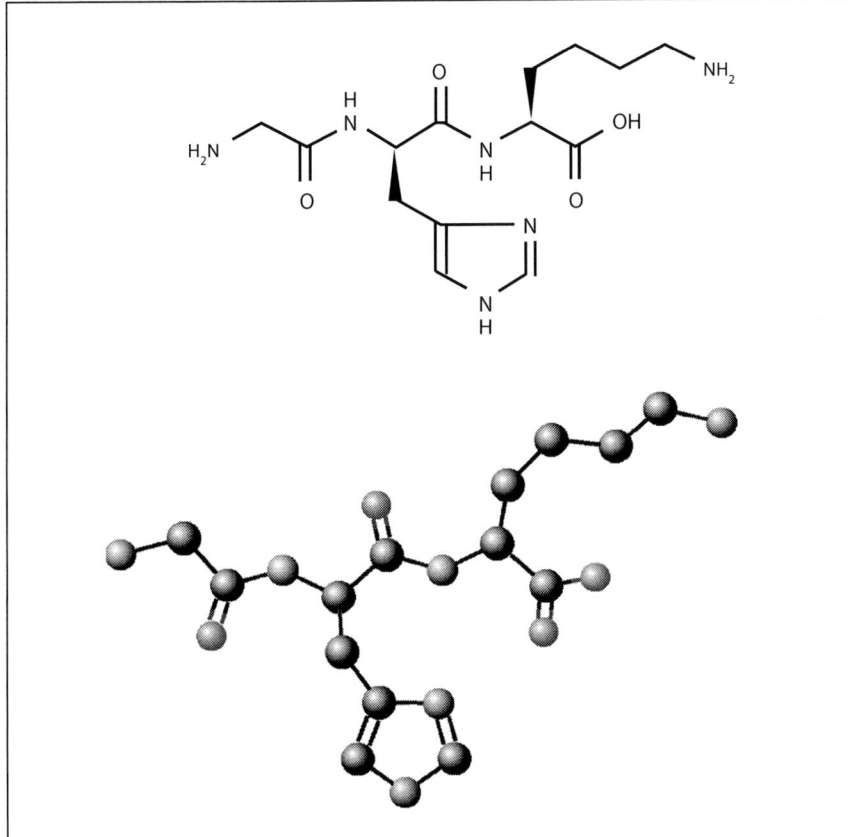

Figure 2. Th tripeptide Gly-His-Lys

The fabulous thing about peptides of this nature is the fact that they act at nano- to micromolar concentration, so long as they reach their target cells.

How peptides work: Before looking more closely at the cosmetic aspects of peptide use, consider how these peptides work. The general scheme evokes a "key and lock" model whereby a peptide, arriving from blood, lymph, tissue diffusion or some other external source is recognized by a specific receptor molecule or protein at the cell membrane surface. The recognition is due to complementary three-dimensional structures, such as amino acid side chain entities, that fit into pockets of the receptor molecule like a key into a lock. The binding of the peptide to the receptor then triggers conformational changes in this transmembrane structure, which leads to further cascade events in the cell's interior biochemistry. The receptor thus acts like a transistor in electronics: a tiny amount of signal, i.e., the peptide, can lead to macroscopic events including collagen synthesis, lipid metabolism and nerve signal transmission within the cells.

Fundamental peptide biology research and pharmacological investigations into these mechanisms have in many cases confirmed the basic tenets of this model. A variant of the mode of peptide activity is found when the peptide seems to enter the target cell and then interacts with the cell nucleus directly, triggering genetic reactions (DNA transcription) and the like. Because of the signaling nature of the peptides, they are often called "messengers" of biological information.

Where peptides come from: With Nature being economical, most of the peptides described in the scientific literature are actually breakdown fragments of larger molecules. For instance, keratinocytes and certain other cells produce a protein molecule called pro-opiomelanocortin (POMC) that consists of 241 amino acids. Depending on the organism's needs, POMC is cleaved by enzymes into one of three peptides: ACTH, MSH and ß-endorphin. ACTH (adrenocorticotropine), consisting of 34 amino acids, acts at surrenal glands in case of stress. MSH (melanocortin), a fragment of 13 amino acids found within the ACTH sequence, leads to increased tanning in melanocytes. ß-endorphin, containing 31 amino acids, controls breathing, digestion and other activities; it in turn can be cleaved to release the pentapeptide enkephalin or natural pain killer.

The "natural" origin of peptides and their high potency at low concentration, coupled to the rapid clearing of peptides in the bloodstream, are of great importance for their use in human applications: low dosage, little remanence and identity to endogenous molecules make peptides a very safe and effective family of active ingredients, especially for cosmetics. Of course, any change in amino acid sequence from its original one, designed perhaps to enhance or modify activity, might require more detailed investigation on potential side effects. In the field of skin care, this aspect is particularly crucial.

Cosmetic aspects of peptide usage: The challenges to using peptides in cosmetic formulas are not negligible, however. The foremost is targeting and bioavailability (i.e., skin penetration): oligopeptides of the nature and structure described do not easily reach their targets. Although low use concentrations of the usually expensive synthetic peptides allow the economic equation to work out for most skin care uses, detection of ppm levels of peptides in complex cream matrices is a challenge. Nevertheless, as stated in the introduction, peptides have become a main staple in skin care formulations because it has been made possible to overcome these hurdles.

Lintner and Peschard[2] have shown that palmitoylation of short peptides improves the skin penetration behavior by a factor 100 to 1000, thus making it possible to achieve wrinkle reduction and other cosmetic effects even at 10 µM concentration.[4–5] Fluorescent tagging coupled to high performance liquid chromatography allows the detection of these milligram (ppm) quantities even in rich cosmetic textures.

What cosmetic activities, properties and claims could then be based on peptides? Foremost, the peptides derived from wound-healing research are targeted for matrix regeneration because they stimulate collagen, fibronectin, GAG synthesis and allow for wrinkle repair, skin thickening and skin firming. A well-known example is the family of matrikines, peptides that are released by the breakdown of structural proteins such as collagen, elastin and fibronectin, of which the pentapeptide Pal-KTTKS[b],[4–5] the

---

[b]Matrixyl (INCI: Palmitoyl-pentapeptide 4) is a product of Sederma. Matrixyl is a trademark of Sederma.

tripeptide Pal-GHK, and the hexapeptide Pal-Val-Gly-Val-Ala-Pro-Gly are prominent representatives.

Other interesting cosmetic activities include the modulation of melanin synthesis in melanocytes, either by stimulating or inhibiting the melanin production for accelerated tanning or so-called skin lightening/toning; the stimulation of lipolysis for "slimming" and anti-cellulite claims;[3] and anti-inflammatory properties produced by reducing interleukin secretion and even neuronal activity that lends soothing, calming properties to the finished cosmetic formula.[2] Hair growth stimulation and/or hair loss prevention can also be effected with peptides such as Biotinoyl-Gly-His-Lys, which has been demonstrated to stimulate the synthesis of collagen IV and laminin 5.[6]

Small peptides have gained prominence in skin care because they constitute a novel and highly effective approach to today's sophisticated skin care market that is at the same time generally risk-free. Peptides are highly versatile molecules and even by staying within the restriction of approximately dekapeptides (chains containing 10 amino acids), the number of possible peptide sequences based on only the 20 coded amino acids is 20^{10} or 200 billion. Although most of these sequences will likely have no activity, there is still room for research and innovation.

How does one choose the right peptide? It will be a peptide known to the fundamental peptide research community, or it will be a peptide selected from a library of peptides created by efficient, rapid, parallel synthesis coupled to more or less rapid screening methods. Peptide design from molecular modeling is an attractive alternative but would require more knowledge about the structural features of the cellular surface, the receptors or other interactions governing peptide activity. In this author's opinion, there is as of yet little to go on to achieve this.

Limitations of peptide use in skin care may arise from solubility, bio-availability and penetration characteristics, potential toxicological problems (although they should be rare), stability parameters and formulation compatibilities, economic considerations and, last but not least, intellectual property issues because the number of nonpatented oligopeptide sequences is shrinking fast.

Proteins and Cosmetics

Categories of proteins: The intention of this chapter was to focus on peptides; proteins and their use in cosmetic skin care applications would need at least as much space to be discussed in detail. Briefly, proteins can be placed into four main categories: structural, functional, signal or defense molecules:

- Larger **structural** entities such as collagen, elastin, fibronectin, laminin, myosin, actin and many others participate in the building and maintenance of connective tissue of the three-dimensional arrangement of the organs that constitute the human body, including muscles and skin layers.
- **Functional** proteins, such as enzymes, of which thousands are present in low concentration within cells and the blood stream, can act as chemical catalysts that initiate, regulate and modulate all biochemical processes. Other functional proteins include transport molecules such as transferrine, hemoglobin, myoglobin (**Figure 3**) and lipoproteins.
- Cytokines, chemokines, interferon and interleukins are smaller proteins that possess, like the oligopeptides, a **signaling** function, triggering a downstream cascade of events.

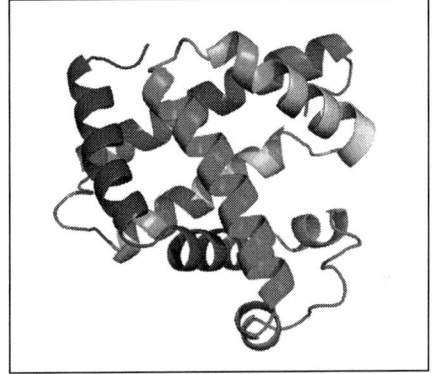

Figure 3. Representation of myoglobin, a functional protein with a chain of 153 amino acids, presented to show the difference in size and structure of a protein as compared to an amino acid or a peptide.

- Finally, antibodies are large protein structures with the specific function of **defending** the organism against invasion by foreign matter such as bacteria or viruses, allergens and the like.

Cosmetic applications of proteins: Are any of these protein categories useful for skin care applications? Collagen can be extracted in its native, non-hydrolyzed form from cow hide or fish skin and employed as a natural film former and water-binding molecule. Fibronectin, isolated from horse serum, was used for some time for similar purposes. Proteins of high molecular weight also can be obtained from wheat, rice, potatoes and other plants; they are used, for instance, as skin-tightening actives.

Certain enzymes have found some use in cosmetic formulas. The lactoperoxidase/glucose oxidase system, with its antimicrobial activity, was used as an aid in fighting acne-type symptoms on the skin but could also, at higher concentrations, be used in helping to preserve finished products against spoilage. Because of stability concerns, the technology did not find widespread application.

Proteolytic enzymes[c], lipolytic enzymes[d] and more recently, heat- and UV-stable protective antioxidant enzymes[e][7–8] have found acceptance in skin care.

The other two categories, cytokines and antibodies, present too many challenges in relation to synthesis or extraction from animal tissue, toxicological and pharmacological concerns, to have made an impact in the field of skin care. Cytokines are often mentioned as being the mediators of certain cosmetic activities; however, they are not used as ingredients.

Conclusion

In numerous articles, advertising copy and general media jargon, amino acids, peptides and proteins are too often bunched together as if they were a single entity of cosmetic ingredients with similar activity and usefulness. The present introduction aims to clarify the clear differences between these categories of chemicals, whatever their origin. Over the last few years, it has become evident that peptides, if designed well, correctly chosen and intelligently employed, possess by far the greatest potential for beneficial cosmetic use because they have unambiguous, clearly-defined specific activity. In addition they are analytically pure, biomimetic, biodegradable, nontoxic and nevertheless highly innovative. Most individual amino acids are too small and simple to show specific

---

[c] Keratoline (INCI: Bacillus subtilis ferment) is a product and trademark of Sederma, France.
[d] Cyclolipase (INCI: lipase) is a product and trademark of Sederma.
[e] Venuceane (INCI: Thermus thermophilus ferment) is a product and trademark of Sederma.

biological activity, and most proteins are too big, unwieldy and difficult to obtain to be considered as major players in the field of skin care ingredients.

Published October 2007 Cosmetics and Toiletries magazine

References

1. A Strecker, Annalen der Chemie und Pharmacie, 75 27 (1850)
2. K Lintner and O Peschard, Biologically active peptides: from a lab bench curiosity to a functional skin care product, Int J Cosm Sci 22 207–218 (2000)
3. R Leroux, O Peschard, C Mas-Chamberlin, K Lintner, A Guezennec and J Guesnet, Shaping up, Soap, Perfumery & Cosmetics 73(12) 22–24 (Dec 2000)
4. K Lintner, Promoting production in the extracellular matrix without compromising barrier, Cutis 70 6S (suppl) 13–16 (2002)
5. LR Robinson, NC Fitzgerald, DG Doughty, NC Dawes, CA Berge and DL Bissett, Topical palmitoyl pentapeptide provides improvement in photo aged human facial skin, Int J Cosm Sci 27(3) 155–160 (2005)
6. C Mas-Chamberlin, P Mondon, F Lamy, O Peschard and K Lintner, Reduction of hair-loss: Matrikines and plant molecules to the rescue, Proceedings ASCS Conference Bangkok (2005)
7. C Mas-Chamberlin, F Lamy, P Mondon, S Scocci, L de Givry, F Vissac and K Lintner, Heat- and UV-stable cosmetic enzymes from deep sea bacteria, Cosmet Toil 117(4) 22–30 (2002)
8. K Lintner, F Lamy, C Mas-Chamberlin, P Mondon, S Scocci, P Buche and F Girard, Heat-stable enzymes from deep sea bacteria: A key tool for skin protection against UV-A induced free radicals, IFSCC Mag 5(3) 195–200 (2002)

CHAPTER 22

Hyperbranched Polyalphaolefins Enhance Anhydrous Stick Formulations

Florence Nicholas and Jeff Brooks
New Phase Technologies, a Division of Baker Petrolite Corp., Sugar Land, Texas USA

KEY WORDS: *Pouring temperature, stick, synthetic wax*

ABSTRACT: *Hyperbranched polyalphaolefins offer distinctive functional and aesthetic properties due to their branch-on-branch configuration. In anhydrous stick formulations containing polyethylene or other crystalline waxes, the addition of hyperbranched polyalphaolefins is shown in this chapter to lower pour points by as much as 10C, increase gloss, modify structure and improve formula stability.*

In today's global personal care marketplace, consumers have specialized needs based on function as well as fashion. In response, formulators strive to develop unique, high-performance products to meet rapidly evolving trends. Ingredients that combine multiple benefits offer potential for differentiated solutions while making formulation simple and more cost-effective. Among the array of product forms, cosmetic sticks are practical and easy to use. However, they can also present formulation challenges in terms of structure, stability and aesthetics.

A Multifunctional Solution

Hyperbranched polyalphaolefins (HBPs) commonly are used to form flexible films and impart gloss. Known by their INCI designation as *synthetic wax*, HBPs also have film-forming properties that allow them to act as conditioners and moisturizers.

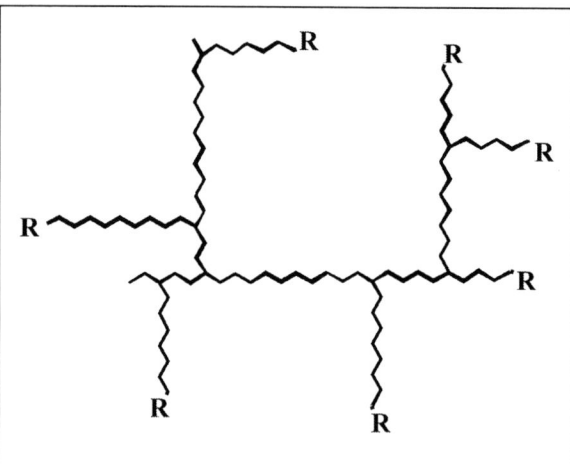

Figure 1. Structure of hyperbranched polyalphaolefins

Their distinctive branch-on-branch structure enables them to lower pour points, modifies structure and improves formula stability, making HBPs useful for a number of personal care applications ranging from lipsticks to lotions. **Figure 1** illustrates the structure of these materials, which can be designed in numerous branch lengths.

Depending on branch length and associated molecular weight, HBPs exist as low-melting solids or as liquids, which have the added advantage of making them cold-processable.

Polyethylene and other highly crystalline waxes typically are used in stick formulations to provide efficient structuring and to prevent syneresis that can be associated with natural materials such as beeswax, carnauba wax and candelilla wax. However, the use of polyethylene results in high pour points and a matte finish—issues that can be resolved by adding HBPs.

Four HBP products[a], designated in this chapter as HBP-1 through HBP-4 according to their branch lengths from longest to shortest, were evaluated in anhydrous stick formulations where polyethylene was the main structurant for commonly used oils. The oils were

---

[a]Performa V 103 polymer (designated here as HBP-1), Performa V 260 polymer (HBP-2), Performa V 343 polymer (HBP-3) and Performa V 825 polymer (HBP-4) (all INCI: Synthetic wax) are products of New Phase Technologies, a division of Baker Petrolite Corp., Sugar Land, TX USA.

mineral oil, isododecane, isopropyl palmitate, C12-C15 alkyl benzoate and safflower oil. In addition to their wide use in personal care formulations, these five materials were chosen to illustrate polar and nonpolar examples, and to include one natural ingredient. **Table 1** summarizes the properties of these HBPs.

Table 1
Physical properties of tested HBPs

HBP	Branch Length	Molecular Weight (Mn)	Melting Point (°C)	Viscosity (cP, 99°C)	Refractive Index
HBP-1	Longest	2900	74	350	1.510
HBP-2	Long	1900	54	300	1.506
HBP-3	Short	1800	41	130	1.486
HBP-4	Shortest	1200	Liquid	1200 (RT)	1.473

*Refractive indices for the solid synthetic waxes HBP-1, HBP-2 and HBP-3 were measured via the Becke line method (589.3 nm at 25°C) by Cargille Laboratories Inc., Cedar Grove, NJ USA. For the liquid HBP-4, the refractive index was measured according to the ASTM D542-00 (2006) Standard Test Method for Index of Refraction of Transparent Organic Plastics, by Plastics Technology Laboratories Inc., Pittsfield, MA USA.

In the tests described here, the control in each case was a polyethylene/oil base (**Formulas 1 and 2**). If the oil was isopropyl palmitate, C12-C15 alkyl benzoate, mineral oil or safflower oil, polyethylene was added at 12%. In the case of isododecane, 30% polyethylene was added to achieve an appropriate stick structure. The various HBPs were added at 5%, which is an average level used in the industry. In actual personal care formulations, use levels for the solid HBPs -1, -2 and -3 are typically less than 10%. In the case of HBP-4, use levels may be 5% or higher because of the liquid nature of the material.

Lowering Pour Point

Research has shown that polyalphaolefins can act as pour point depressants by modifying crystal shape and size, as well as flow characteristics.[1-2] This attribute can also provide advantages in personal care applications, including safer handling, easier mixing and lower energy costs.

Formula 1
Anhydrous stick base

	Control	Test
Mineral oil or safflower oil or isopropyl palmitate or C12-C15 alkyl benzoate	87%w/w	83%w/w
Polyethylene	12	12
HBP	-	5
	100	100

Formula 2
Anhydrous stick base

	Control	Test
Isododecane	70%w/w	65%w/w
Polyethylene	30	30
HBP	-	5
	100	100

Pouring temperature is the lowest temperature at which a molten wax mixture can be easily dispensed. Blends of polyethylene in various oils were tested as controls and the impact of adding 5% of the HBPs was evaluated. The test was conducted by solubilizing the waxes in the oil and slowly cooling the specimen under observation. The pouring temperature was recorded at the point where the mixture was still homogeneous and fluid, but the authors observed a sharp increase in viscosity. Thereafter, viscosity continues to increase until the specimen reaches the congealing point, or "no flow" condition.

In this study, HBPs were found to depress the pour points for high-melting crystalline waxes (**Figure 2**).

In combination with mineral oil, HBP-1 depressed the pouring temperature by a full 10C, to 62C. Although, as described later, this combination is not stable on a long-term basis, the addition of HBP-3 and HBP-4 at 5% lowered the pouring temperature nearly as much, to 63C and 64C respectively, in mineral oil; both combinations were found to be stable. In the case of isopropyl palmitate, HBP-3 lowered the pouring temperature by 9C.

The present studies on HBPs as well as research noted in the literature[1–2] suggest the pour point depressant mechanism of HBPs is influenced by the average side chain length, the distribution of side chains and the characteristics of the oil in the mixture. The HBPs modify the shape and size of the waxy hydrocarbon crystal to slow agglomeration and lower the effective pouring temperature. SEM photos (**Figure 3**) illustrate the changes in the wax crystals formed.

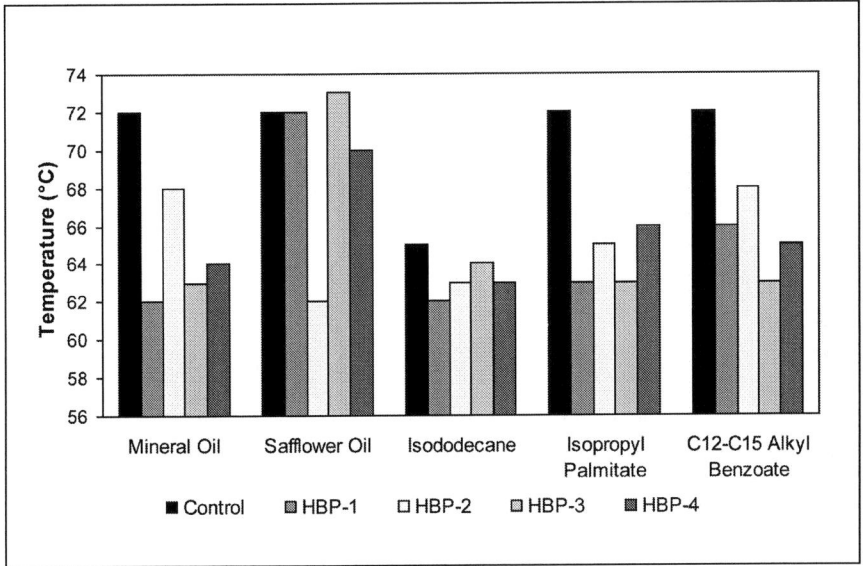

Figure 2. Pouring temperature of polyethylene/oil bases with 5% addition of several HBPs

Lowering pouring temperature adds another dimension of formulating flexibility by offering greater protection for volatile ingredients such as fragrance, isododecane, volatile active ingredients or combinations of ingredients that may be sensitive to heat.

Gloss Improvement

HBPs can enhance gloss in anhydrous systems. To evaluate this effect, gloss measurements of the samples were conducted using a glossmeter[b] and following a standard method[3] for specular gloss.

A specimen of each test formula (**Formulas 1 and 2**) weighing 0.5 g was applied to a 4.5 x 5.5-inch test surface[c] with a circular motion for 1 to 2 min, and a minimum of three gloss readings were taken at an angle of 60 degrees.

---

[b]The D48-7 Glossmeter is a product of Hunter Associates Laboratory, Reston, VA USA.
[c]Leneta card, a product of the Leneta Company Inc., Mahwah, NJ USA

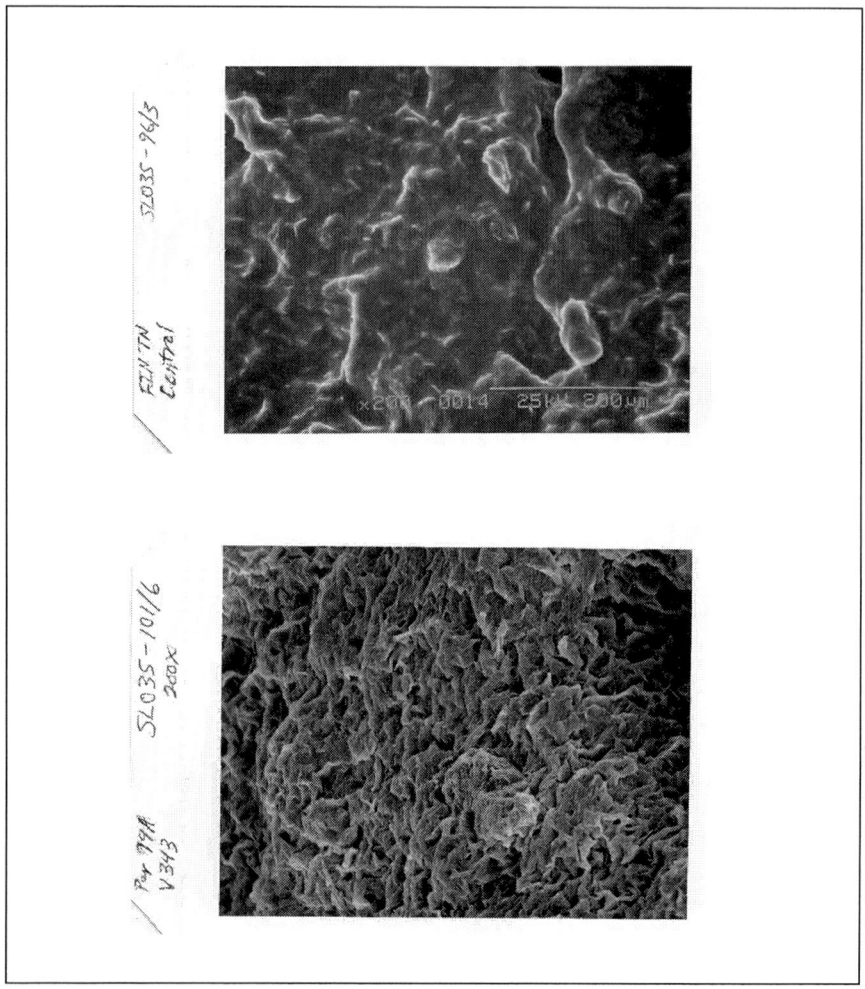

Figure 3. SEM of stick base structures of polyethylene/isododecane (left) and polyethylene/isododecane/HBP-3 (right)

Polyethylene typically imparts a matte appearance. However, in anhydrous systems, HBPs provide gloss even in matte bases. Enhanced gloss primarily is the result of the highly branched characteristics of the HBP. This structure results in high refractive indexes (RIs). For example, the tested HBPs all showed RIs in the range of 1.473 to 1.510 (Table 1), comparing favorably with the 1.46 and 1.497 RI values achieved, respectively, by the widely used cosmetic industry glossing agents[d] phenyltrimethicone and polyisobutene.

---

[d]Examples are DC556 (INCI: Phenyltrimethicone) from Dow Corning, Midland, Michigan USA, and Indopol H (INCI: Polyisobutene) from Ineos Olefins & Polymers USA, League City, Texas USA.

In most cases, gloss measurements based on the addition of various HBPs to the polyethylene/oil blends showed noticeable improvement versus the blends alone (**Figure 4**).

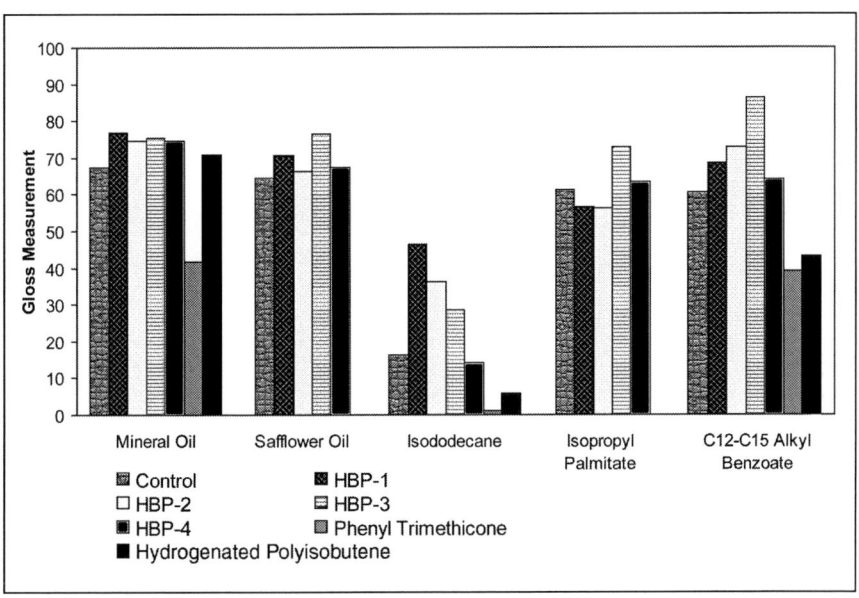

Figure 4. Gloss of polyethylene/oil bases with 5% addition of several HBPs

In additional studies[4] with prototype formulations, the HBP allowed greater pigment loading and aided wetting and dispersion, resulting in highly stable systems. Micronized pigments and organic lakes dispersed in HBPs also imparted higher gloss and color strength without change of hue compared to nondispersed pigments and lakes.

Structuring and Stability

Evaluations of the structuring capability and stability of the HBPs were conducted, again using **Formulas 1 and 2**. In these evaluations, stability is defined as the lack of syneresis—i.e., no oil bleed—in the mixture.

The HBPs were evaluated for structuring capability and stability. The anhydrous systems of **Formulas 1 and 2** were cooled overnight in covered containers. On the following day, a minimum of three penetration values were recorded using a 35 g cone needle and a penetrometer[e]. This approach measures the distance a cone penetrates into the test material in five seconds; thus, the lower the measurement, the harder the material. Measurements of hardness were recorded in decimillimeters (dmm) at various sections within the sample using a standard protocol.[5] **Figure 5** illustrates the results of this test.

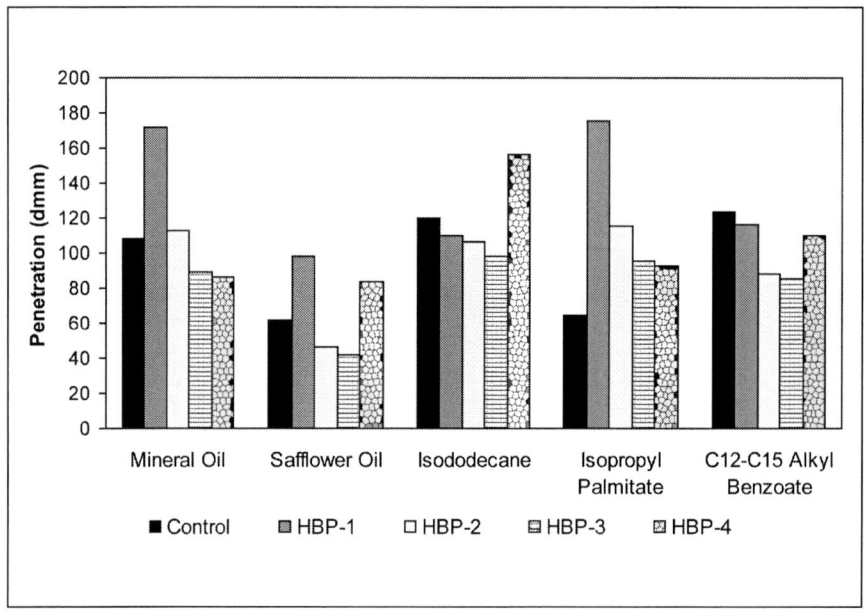

Figure 5. Hardness of polyethylene/oil bases with 5% addition of several HBPs

Overall, HBP-2 and HBP-3 performed best in the systems that were identified as stable, i.e., without syneresis for more than six weeks (**Table 2**). Each sample was evaluated for six weeks at room temperature, at 49°C and through three freeze-thaw cycles.

In some cases, the addition of HBP softened the sample. For example, the two HBPs with the long branch length (HBP-1 and HBP-2) softened the systems with mineral oil, safflower oil and isopropyl palmitate and made them unstable, an effect not seen in these same systems when the two HBPs with short branch lengths were added. It is important to select the correct branch length of HBP for specific formulation types or requirements. In general,

---

[e]The K19500 penetrometer is a product of Koehler Instrument Company Inc., Bohemia, NY USA

HBPs with shorter branch lengths result in greater stability, while longer branch lengths tend to reduce structuring effects.

Table 2
Effect of 5% HBP on oil bleed stability of prototype stick bases

S = Stable after six weeks; no syneresis
NS = Not stable

Oil	Control	HBP-1	HBP-2	HBP-3	HBP-4
Mineral oil	S	NS	NS	S	S
Safflower oil	S	NS	NS	S	S
Isododecane	S	S	S	S	S
Isopropyl palmitate	S	NS	NS	S	S
C12-C15 alkylm benzoate	NS	NS	S	NS	S

The SEM photographs in **Figure 3** show that the addition of an HBP creates a structure that is more uniform with smaller wax domains. This effect suggests the HBP acts as a compatibilizer between the oil and polyethylene to help disperse the polyethylene in the oil, with the result being a smaller crystal size and the entrapment of oil within the crystalline matrix.

With its longest branch length, HBP-1 is effective at low levels for modifying the crystalline characteristics of the polyethylene/oil system; however, it has an optimum use level. In contrast, the SEM photographs in **Figure 6** illustrate how an excess of the HBP can affect the crystalline matrix of polyethylene. Here, the compatibilizing effect is too great, resulting in a crystal size that is too small and not stable. In this example, decreasing the level of HBP-1 from 5% to a level less than 5% might improve its oil-binding capabilities, resulting in a more stable system.

In general, the degree of compatibilization is related to both branch length and type of oil. The longer the chain length of an HBP, the more it typically decreases structuring capabilities. However, oil binding may also be affected depending on branch length. For this reason, it is important to assess these parameters with the specific ingredients used in individual applications.

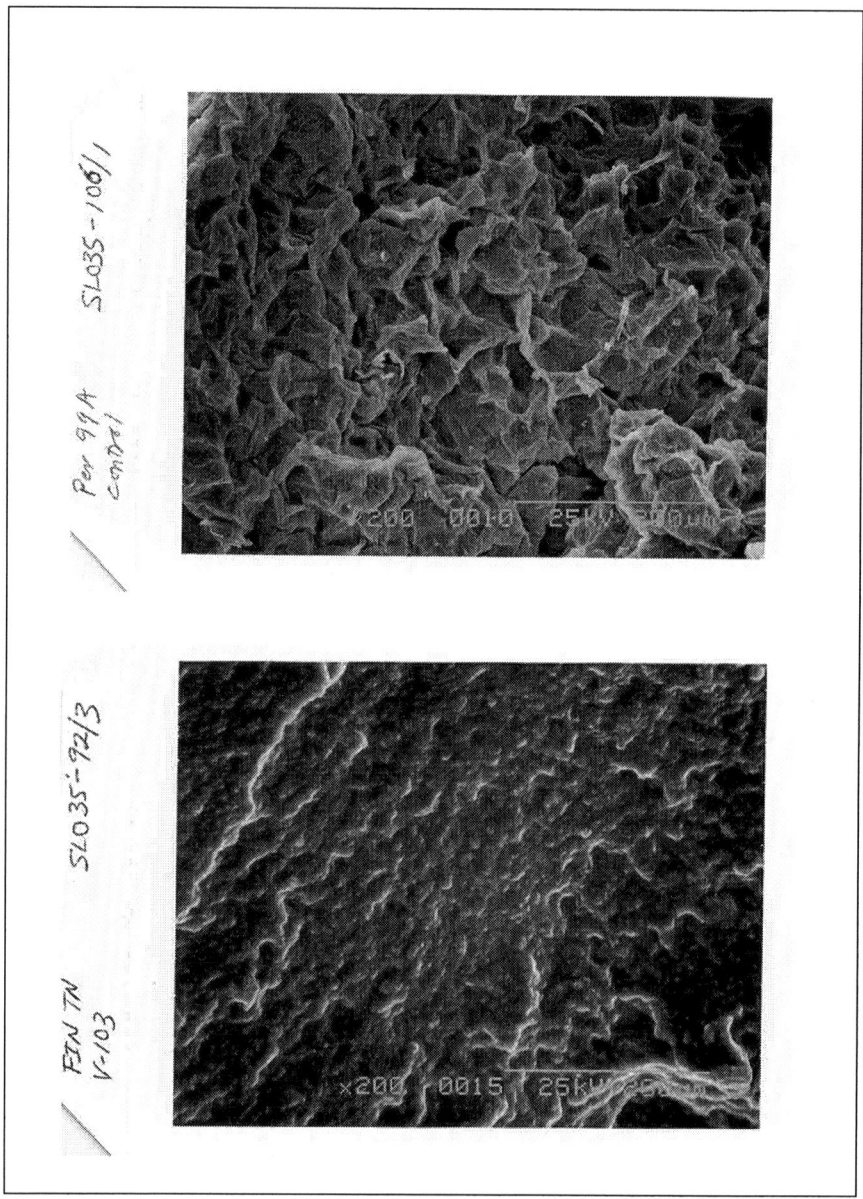

Figure 6. SEM of stick base structures of polyethylene/C12-C15 alkyl benzoate (left) and polyethylene/C12-C15 alkyl benzoate/HBP-1 (right)

Summary

Given the specific concentrations of polyethylene and HBPs in the present studies, it is possible to make some general statements related to pouring temperature, gloss and stick structure. These results may help to serve as a screening tool during ingredient selection. However, formulators should carefully evaluate ingredients based on their specific formulations and applications.

Mineral oil: Among the stable systems shown, HBP-3 and HBP-4 were best for depressing pouring temperature and increasing gloss in mineral oil. They were also best for increasing hardness, with improvements of 19 and 22 dmm, respectively.

Safflower oil: HBP-2 was found to be the most effective for reducing pouring temperature—from 72C to 62C—although this system did not show long-term stability. Among the stable systems, the HBP-4 wax performed best. The best material for enhancing gloss and hardness was HBP-3, with an increase of 12 points for gloss and a 20 dmm improvement in hardness.

Isododecane: All four HBPs reduced pouring temperature slightly, with HBP-1 performing best for a drop in temperature of 3C. In terms of gloss, HBP-1 again was best, raising gloss by nearly 30 points. The addition of HBP-4 resulted in a slight decrease of gloss; HBP-3 was best for enhancing hardness, with a decrease of 22 dmm.

Isopropyl palmitate: Among the stable systems, HBP-3 performed the best for reducing pouring temperature, with an improvement of 9C. This wax also showed the best enhancement for gloss. All HBPs softened the stick base containing isopropyl palmitate.

C12-C15 alkyl benzoate: Among the systems showing long-term stability, HBP-4 was shown as the best for lowering pouring temperature. HBP-2 was best for enhancing gloss and hardness in the stable systems.

Conclusions

The results of several evaluations indicated that HBPs can lower pour points, with chain length and oil type as factors that resulted in different performance. The results also indicate that stick stability is more likely to be compromised by the incorporation of longer branch length HBPs—in these tests, HBP-1 and HBP-2. HBPs can also increase gloss and improve formula stability. Two of the polymers tested also improved hardness in most of the oils tested. While demonstrating new benefits, the results of this study have potential as a screening tool to help formulators focus on useful combinations of materials for specific applications. This approach may help reduce development time and cost.

Formula 3.
Lip moisturizer stick

A. Polyethylene (Performalene 400 Polyethylene, New Phase Technologies)	9.00% w/w
C20-40 alcohols (Performacol 425 Alcohol, New Phase Technologies)	10.00
Cetyl lactate	4.00
Theobroma cacao (cocoa) seed butter	5.00
Di-C12-15 alkyl fumarate	3.00
Hexyl decanol	48.90
Synthetic wax (Performa V 343 Polymer, New Phase Technologies)	8.00
B. Mica (and) titanium dioxide (and) tin oxide	5.00
C. *Carthamus tinctorius* (safflower) oil	3.00
Simmondsia chinensis (jojoba) seed oil	3.00
Mineral oil (and) *Cocos nucifera* (coconut oil) (and) *Aloe barbadensis* leaf extract	1.00
Tocopheryl acetate	0.10
D. Fragrance (parfum)	qs

Procedure: Heat A to 94–99°C with propeller mixing until dispersed and uniform. Reduce temperature to 85–90°C. Add B and continue propeller mixing until dispersed and uniform. Reduce temperature to 80–85°C and add C. Add D at 75–80°C; continue mixing until uniform. Pour into lipstick molds.

The anhydrous sticks discussed in this chapter and illustrated in **Formula 3** have obvious applications in the color arena in product forms such as lipsticks, lip balms, foundation sticks, concealers and eye shadow sticks. It should be noted that the applications extend to other areas of personal care, such as sunscreen sticks, AP sticks and facial sticks, and beyond to laundry sticks for the household and acne control stick products in the pharmaceutical area. Overall,

HBPs can be valuable ingredients to help formulators create novel, high-performance personal care, household and pharmaceutical products that meet changing global needs.

Published February 2008 Cosmetics and Toiletries magazine

References

1. US Pat 5,641,736, Synergistic pour point depressant combinations and hydrocarbon lube mixtures, TR Forbus, assigned to Mobil Oil Corp. (Jun 24, 1997)
2. C-X Xiong, The structure and activity of poly-alphaolefins as pour point depressants, Lubric Eng 196-200 (March 1993)
3. ASTM D 523-89, Standard Method for Specular Gloss (1999)
4. Unpublished data supplied by Kobo Products, South Plainfield, NJ USA (2007)
5. ASTM D 937-77, Standard Test Method for Cone Penetration of Petrolatum (2004)

CHAPTER 23

Enhancing the Feel of Vegetable Oils with Silicone

Anne-Lise Girboux and Emilie Courbon
Dow Corning SA, Seneffe, Belgium

KEY WORDS: Borago officinalis *seed oil, sensory, silicone, surface tension, triglycerides, vegetable oil*

ABSTRACT: *Adding silicone to natural oils can reduce surface tension thus improving their spreading characteristics. This results in finished formulations with improved sensory profiles and in addition, it expands on the opportunities for using these natural ingredients.*

As consumer interest in natural ingredients continues to grow, along with the demand for novel textures and product forms, the use of vegetable oils in personal care formulations is increasing. In fact, the consumption of natural oils in Europe is forecasted to grow at about 5% over the next five years.[1] Although these natural ingredients offer distinct benefits including emolliency, gloss and lubricity,[2] they also challenge formulators to provide easy application and pleasant aesthetics without a greasy or oily feel.

Lipids and silicones can act as complementary ingredients in finished formulations.[3] This chapter illustrates how silicones such as caprylyl methicone, phenyl trimethicone, cetyl dimethicone and cyclopentasiloxane can enhance the feel of natural lipids, allowing formulators greater flexibility to expand the use of natural ingredients in their products. Even at low use levels, silicones can decrease the surface tension of vegetable oils, improve their spreading characteristics and offer a wider range of sensory profiles.

The Source for Vegetable Oils

Vegetable oils, also referred to as natural lipids, are oily substances derived from plant sources. They have a variety of chemical compositions but most used in personal care are rich in triglycerides that are mechanically extracted from the seeds of plants. The non-triglyceride components are referred to as the unsaponifiable fraction and this typically consists of tocopherols, sterols, free fatty alcohols and triterpenes.

Triglycerides are esters composed of one glycerin molecule bonded to three fatty acids—long-chain carboxylic acids in which the alkyl chain normally contains ten or more carbons. This structure is depicted in **Figure 1**, where R1 R2 and R3 are fatty acids.

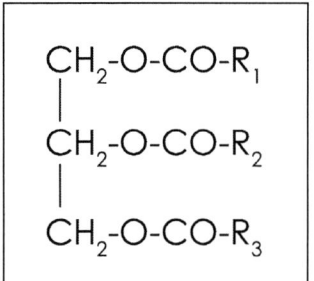

Figure 1. Triglycerides are esters composed of one glycerin molecule bonded to three fatty acids.

The three fatty acids can have equal or different chain lengths and their carbon chains can be saturated or unsaturated. The fatty acid composition of triglycerides varies according to their source. For example, triglycerides derived from coconut are rich in lauric acid (saturated C12 fatty acid), and in many cases, materials such as sodium lauryl sulfate still retain a slight odor of coconut oil from which this surfactant is derived.

Based on the International Nomenclature Cosmetic Ingredient (INCI) system, natural lipids are named according to the genus and species of the plant. For example, the INCI name for borage oil is *Borago officinalis* seed oil.

Complementary Silicones

Silicones are synthetic polymers made from quartz, a natural form of crystalline silicon dioxide, and methanol. These materials have been used in personal care products for more than 50 years. Most silicones for personal care applications are based on polydimethylsiloxane or dimethicone. This linear polymer is available in a range of molecular weights, with the molecular weight for a particular dimethicone determining its viscosity. Volatile silicones such as cyclopentasiloxane are short-chain cyclic polydimethylsiloxanes. Another commonly used silicone is phenyl trimethicone, a highly branched phenyl-functional silicone.

Silicones are good emollients that improve the feel of formulations, while lipids act as moisturizers and can also restore the barrier function of skin.

Two vegetable oils were evaluated in this study: borage oil[a] and a vegetable oil blend[b] composed of Brassica campestris (rapeseed) seed oil and Elaeis guineensis (palm) oil.

These oils were blended with four compatible silicones:

- Caprylyl methicone, a caprylyl-branched liquid trisiloxane;
- Phenyl trimethicone, a highly-branched, liquid phenyl-functional silicone;
- Cetyl dimethicone, a linear liquid polysiloxane with alkyl chains randomly distributed. It is highly compatible with organic ingredients; and
- Cyclopentasiloxane, a cyclic molecule that provides transient emolliency because of its volatility.

Lowering Surface Tension

Surface tension is a measure of the work needed to create a new surface area. High surface tension, together with high viscosity, can contribute to tackiness.[4] A bubble pressure tensiometer[c] was used in the present study to measure dynamic and static surface tension.

Gas bubbles were produced in the sample liquids at an exactly defined bubble generation rate. As the dynamic surface tension is recorded as a function of bubble life time, the rate decreases while the bubble life time increases. The bubbles enter the liquid through a tube of known radius, calibrated prior to taking measurements, and the pressure reaches a maximum that is recorded by the instrument.

---

[a]Cosmosil B (INCI: Borago officinalis seed oil) is a product of International Cosmetic Science Centre, Lystrup, Denmark.
[b]Dow Corning HY4008 Vegetable Oil Blend (INCI: Brassica campestris (rapeseed) seed oil (and) Elaeis guineensis (palm) oil) is a product of Dow Corning Corp., Midland, MI USA.
[c]The Science Line T60 tensiometer is a product of SITA Messtechnik GmbH, Dresden, Germany.

Silicones have an inherent low surface tension (see **Table 1**) due to the methyl groups attached to the backbone.

Figure 2 shows the decrease of dynamic surface tension of borage oil with the addition of phenyl trimethicone. **Figure 3** shows the decrease of static surface tension of borage oil with the addition of cyclopentasiloxane, phenyl trimethicone, caprylyl methicone or cetyl dimethicone. Similar results were obtained with the vegetable oil blend.

Table 1
Static Surface Tension Data

Silicone	Static Surface Tension (mN/m)
Caprylyl methicone	20.34
Phenyl trimethicone	21.76
Cetyl dimethicone	26.62
Cyclopentasiloxane	19.00

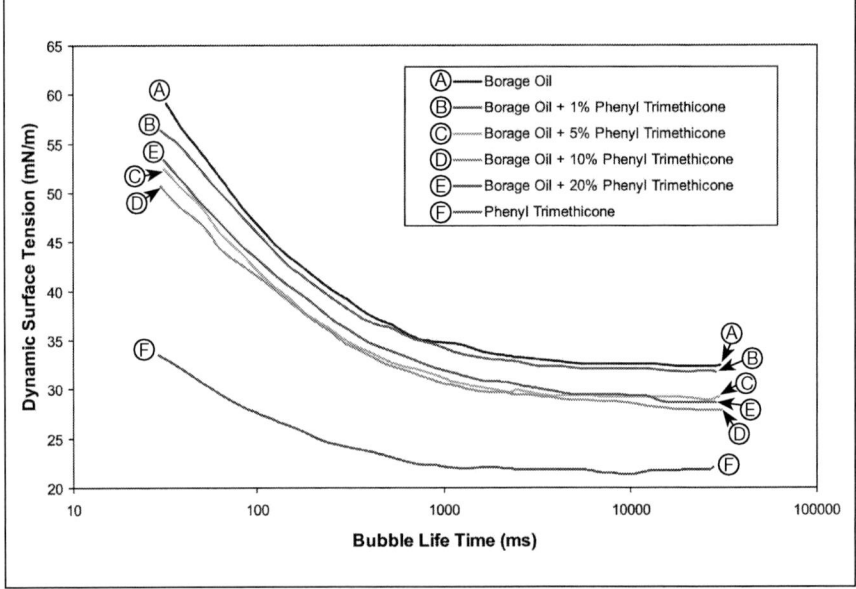

Figure 2. Effect of the addition of phenyl trimethicone on the dynamic surface tension of borage oil

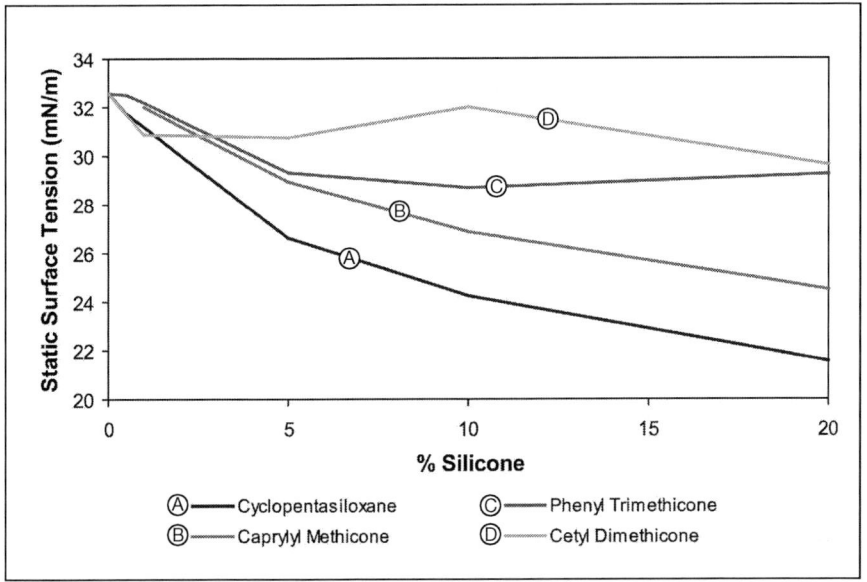

Figure 3. Effect of the addition of cyclopentasiloxane, phenyl trimethicone, caprylyl methicone or cetyl dimethicone on the static surface tension of borage oil

Enhanced Spreading

The spreading characteristics of cosmetic oils determine how easily they can be applied and how well they will be distributed onto the skin. In general, the more readily the oil spreads, the more pleasant it will feel on the skin. A gelatin test is a common in vitro method for measuring the spreadability of cosmetic oils because gelatin is a fairly representative model of the human skin surface. To conduct this test, a gelatin film is applied to polystyrene plates (Petri dishes) and a 5-μL sample of the cosmetic oil is applied onto the film. A stereomicroscope is used to measure the diameter of the oil droplet at time zero and after 10 min. **Equation 1** shows how spreadability is calculated.

$$\text{Oil Spreadability} = \frac{\left(\begin{array}{c}\text{Droplet size} \\ \text{at 10 min}\end{array}\right) - \left(\begin{array}{c}\text{Droplet size} \\ \text{at time zero}\end{array}\right)}{\text{Droplet size at time zero}} \qquad \text{Eq. 1}$$

Values can be compared only when they have been determined under identical humidity and temperature conditions, and the average of at least three measurements should be used. Results are expressed as an enhanced spreadability factor (see **Equation 2**).

$$\text{Enhanced Spreadability Factor} = \frac{\text{Spreadability of oil with additive}}{\text{Spreadability of pure oil}} \qquad \text{Eq. 2}$$

This method was used to determine the effect of silicone on the spreadability of vegetable oils. If the enhanced spreadability factor is found to be greater than 1, the additive improves spreadability; if it is less than 1, the additive decreases spreadability.

Figure 4 shows how the spreadability and surface tension of borage oil can be influenced by the addition of silicone. The improvement of spreadability depends upon the type and level of silicone used.

The effect of silicone on viscosity also was studied using a rheometer and a stress ramp procedure (see **Table 2 and Figure 5**).

Results demonstrated that borage oil and its blends with silicone are Newtonian liquids. The addition of cyclopentasiloxane,

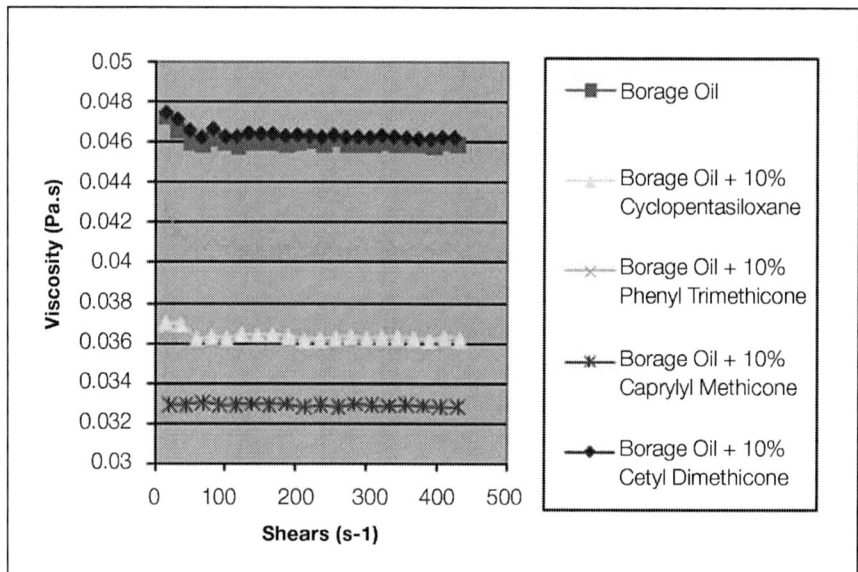

Figure 4. Effect of the addition of cyclopentasiloxane, phenyl trimethicone, caprylyl methicone or cetyl dimethicone on the viscosity of borage oil

Enhancing the Feel of Vegetable Oils with Silicone

Table 2 The Effect of Silicone on Viscosity of Test Samples

Borage oil		Borage oil + 10% Cyclopentasiloxane		Borage Oil + 10% Phenyl trimethicone		Borage oil + 10% Cetyl dimethicone		Borage oil + 10% Caprylyl methicone	
Shear rate 1/s	Vis. Pa.s	Shear rate 1/s	Vis. Pa.s	Shear rate 1/s	Vis. Pa.s	Shear rate 1/s	Vis. Pa.s	Shear rate 1/s	Vis. Pa.s
15.86	0.04715	17.54	0.03694	14.76	0.04260	15.81	0.04740	22.52	0.03292
33.04	0.04653	39.09	0.03685	34.20	0.04153	32.62	0.04708	46.36	0.03293
50.78	0.04587	61.56	0.03619	54.24	0.04078	49.87	0.04654	70.05	0.03303
68.27	0.04581	83.41	0.03628	73.73	0.04082	67.25	0.04621	94.23	0.03290
85.01	0.04611	105.30	0.03620	92.88	0.04086	83.66	0.04662	118.00	0.03293
102.70	0.04590	126.70	0.03638	112.40	0.04085	101.20	0.04624	141.80	0.03295
120.30	0.04569	148.60	0.03635	132.50	0.04059	118.20	0.04625	165.70	0.03293
137.10	0.04590	170.30	0.03636	151.90	0.04055	134.80	0.04641	189.60	0.03294
154.40	0.04591	192.50	0.03629	171.60	0.04055	152.00	0.04637	213.90	0.03281
171.60	0.04592	214.70	0.03614	190.60	0.04068	168.90	0.04637	237.30	0.03291
189.40	0.04576	236.60	0.03616	209.90	0.04077	186.30	0.04627	261.90	0.03282
206.30	0.04586	258.20	0.03624	229.50	0.04068	203.10	0.04633	285.10	0.03295
223.20	0.04598	279.90	0.03628	248.70	0.04075	220.20	0.04628	309.30	0.03288
241.40	0.04574	302.10	0.03620	269.00	0.04057	237.50	0.04622	333.60	0.03284
257.60	0.04605	323.60	0.03625	287.80	0.04074	254.10	0.04632	357.10	0.03291
275.50	0.04582	345.60	0.03624	307.20	0.04075	271.50	0.04621	381.20	0.03285
293.30	0.04575	368.10	0.03618	326.90	0.04071	288.70	0.04623	405.50	0.03282
310.80	0.04574	390.30	0.03609	346.90	0.04064	305.90	0.04620	429.90	0.03278
327.40	0.04584	411.40	0.03625	365.60	0.04069	322.30	0.04630		
345.00	0.04576	433.40	0.03616	385.00	0.04072	339.60	0.04623		
362.20	0.04580			405.10	0.04065	357.10	0.04618		
379.80	0.04581			424.60	0.04067	374.30	0.04614		
397.70	0.04567					391.60	0.04613		
413.90	0.04586					407.80	0.04621		
431.20	0.04581					425.20	0.04619		

phenyl trimethicone or caprylyl methicone decreases the viscosity of borage oil, while the addition of cetyl dimethicone increases its viscosity slightly. The greatest reduction in viscosity was obtained with caprylyl dimethicone.

Additional trials were carried out with the vegetable oil blend (**Figure 6**).

These results show that spreadability improvement can be achieved for more than one type of vegetable oil with the addition of silicone.

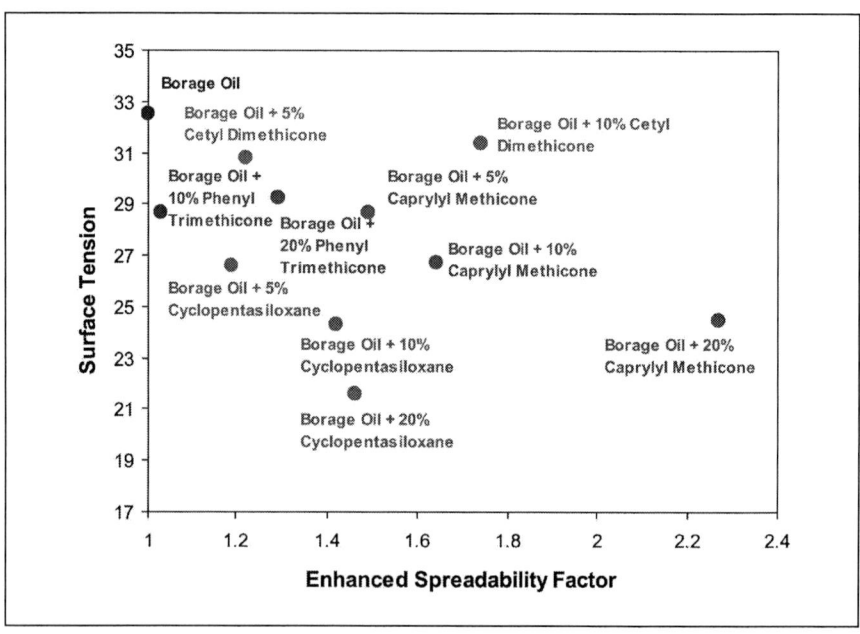

Figure 5. Relationship between surface tension and spreadability results for borage oil

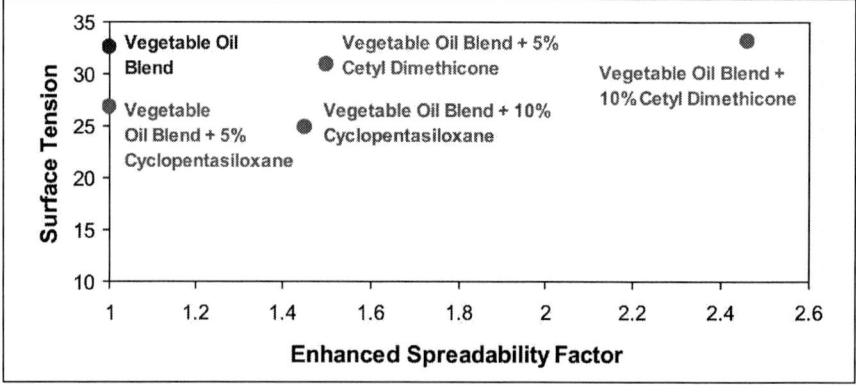

Figure 6. Relationship between surface tension and spreadability results for a vegetable oil blend

Sensory Attributes

Generally formulators are most interested in sensory enhancements that can be perceived on the skin; thus, a series of sensory panel tests was also conducted. Comparisons of pure oils and the same oils blended with silicone were tested by an experienced sensory panel of 18 Caucasian participants. The sensory evaluations were performed in a climate-controlled, with humidity at 50% ± 5%, and temperature 20°C ± 2°C. Each panelist applied 0.02g of both product samples and assigned scores for several sensory attributes during rub-in as well as after they perceived the product had been absorbed on the skin—i.e., the ratings were based on panelists perceptions, not biological skin absorption. For example, panelists found that 5% cetyl dimethicone improved a number of sensory attributes of a vegetable oil blend (see **Figures 7 and 8**). They noted less greasiness and a lighter skin feel during rub-in and after absorption, and less gloss after absorption.

Other sensory evaluations revealed that:

- 20% caprylyl dimethicone gave a lighter skin feel for borage oil during rub-in;
- 10% phenyl trimethicone reduced the tackiness of borage oil during rub-in;
- 10% cyclopentasiloxane improved the skin feel of borage oil, resulting in less greasiness during rub-in and a lighter skin feel during rub-in and after absorption; and
- 10% cyclopentasiloxane improved the feel of the vegetable oil blend, making it easier to spread and less tacky during rub-in.

Prototype **Formulas 1, 2 and 3** illustrate the use of silicones with the vegetable oil blend.

Discussion

The addition of caprylyl dimethicone resulted in a significant decrease in the surface tension and viscosity of vegetable oils and that can be translated as enhancement of spreadability on gelatin. Panelists confirmed the improved sensory properties obtained for borage oil with 20% caprylyl dimethicone. Lower addition levels were not tested by the sensory panel.

Phenyl trimethicone also decreased the surface tension and viscosity of vegetable oils. The addition of 20% phenyl trimethicone resulted in a significant improvement of the spreadability of borage oil. The panel test showed improvement of the skin feel of borage oil with the addition of 10% phenyl trimethicone.

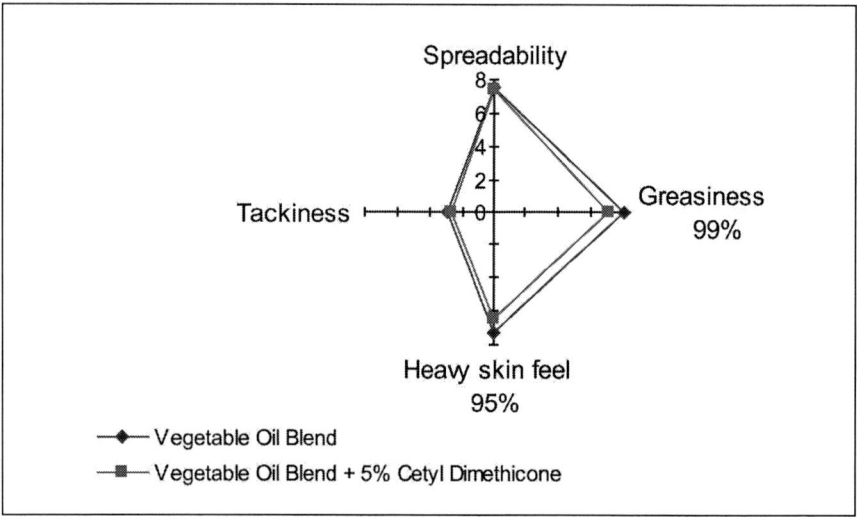

Figure 7. Sensory evaluation of a vegetable oil blend before absorption; percentages indicate level of confidence.

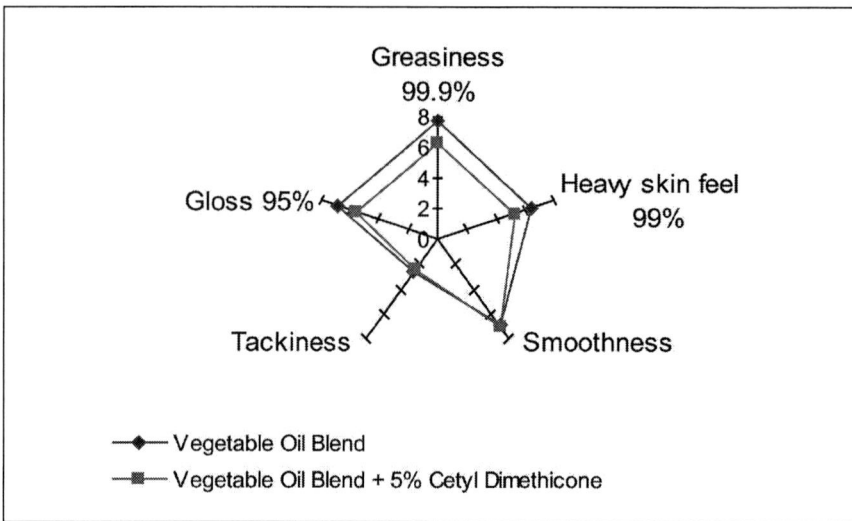

Figure 8. Sensory evaluation of a vegetable oil blend after absorption; percentages indicate level of confidence.

Cetyl dimethicone slightly decreased the surface tension of vegetable oils and slightly increased their viscosity; however, results showed an improvement in spreadability and sensory properties. Panelists were able to detect a sensory difference at 5% cetyl dimethicone in the vegetable oil blend.

The greatest reduction in surface tension was found with cyclopentasiloxane. Panelists confirmed that the addition of 10% cyclopentasiloxane in borage oil or in a vegetable oil blend improved sensory attributes.

Formula 1
Body Cream

A. *Brassica campestris* (rapeseed) seed oil (and) *Elaeis guineensis* (palm) oil (DC HY-4008 Vegetable Oil Blend, Dow Corning)	20.0% w/w
Phenyl trimethicone (DC 556 Cosmetic Grade Fluid, Dow Corning)	4.0
Sodium polyacrylate (and) dimethicone (and) cyclopentasiloxane (and) trideceth-6 (and) PEG/PPG-18/18 dimethicone (DC RM 2051 Thickening Agent, Dow Corning)	3.0
B. Water (*aqua*)	71.0
C. Fragrance (*parfum*) (Perfume Sensual 1, Givaudan)	1.0
Phenoxyethanol (and) ethylhexylglycerin (Euxyl PE 9010, schülke inc.)	1.0
	100.00

Procedure: Combine A and mix. Add B with mixing. Add C and mix until homogeneous.

Formula 2
Massage oil

Brassica campestris (rapeseed) seed oil (and) *Elaeis guineensis* (palm) oil (DC HY-4008 Vegetable Oil Blend, Dow Corning)	94.0% w/w
Cetyl dimethicone (DC 2502 Cosmetic Fluid, Dow Corning)	5.0
Essential oil	0.5
Fragrance (*parfum*)	0.5
	100.00

Procedure: Combine all and mix thoroughly.

Formula 3
Topical spray

A. *Brassica campestris* (rapeseed) seed oil (and) *Elaeis guineensis* (palm) oil (DC HY-4008 Vegetable Oil Blend, Dow Corning)	15.0% w/w
Mangifera indica (mango) seed butter (DC HY 3001 Mango Butter, Dow Corning)	4.0
B. Isopropyl myristate	18.0
Caprylyl methicone (DC Toray FZ-3196, Dow Corning)	62.5
Fragrance (*parfum*)	0.5
	100.00

Procedure: Combine A and mix with heating at 30°C until completely melted. Remove from heat and continue to mix. Add B in order and mix until homogeneous.

Summary

The present study shows that it is possible to lower the surface tension of vegetable oil and improve its spreadability with the addition of silicones such as caprylyl dimethicone, phenyl trimethicone, cetyl dimethicone or cyclopentasiloxane. In some cases, the improvements were confirmed by sensory panel testing.

Combining vegetable oils and silicone is one way for formulators to obtain improved sensory characteristics and broaden the opportunity to create innovative skin care products that expand the use of natural materials.

Published July 2008 Cosmetics and Toiletries magazine

References

1. Kline market report, Specialty Raw Materials for Cosmetics and Toiletries Volume III: Western Europe (2006)
2. M. Rieger, Cosmetic use of selected natural fats and oils, *Cosm & Toil* 109 57-68 (1994)
3. AL Girboux and M Starch, Formulation with silicone and natural lipids, *Happi* 42(12) 100 104 (Dec 2005)
4. U Zeidler, Über die taktilen eigenschaften kosmetischer öle, Upon tactile properties of cosmetic oils, *SÖFW*, 118 1001-1007 (1992)

Formulating with Surfactant Silicones

Anthony J. O'Lenick Jr. and Kevin O'Lenick
SurfaTech Corp.; Dacula, Ga., USA

KEY WORDS: *Surfactant silicones*

ABSTRACT: *The authors describe how the use of amphiphilic silicones or surfactant silicones has allowed formulators to efficiently incorporate silicone polymers into personal care products. These materials act by lowering the surface tension in the oil phase of a formulation, allowing for easier spreading on the skin and hair.*

Silicone polymers have experienced tremendous growth in the personal care market. Known since the 1860s and commercialized with the pioneering work of Rochow[1] since the 1940s they are now present in almost every personal care product category. The reason for this expansion is twofold: first, increasing classes of compounds have been developed; and second, the formulator has learned how to incorporate them efficiently into formulations. The continued development and application of silicone compounds for personal care requires the use of amphiphilic silicones—silicones with two or more groups that, in their pure form, are insoluble in one another.

These surface active or surfactant silicones move to the surface of the oil phase in which they are contained, much like sodium laureth sulfate moves to the surface of water, and lower the surface tension, allowing for easier spreading on the skin and hair. For most alkyl silicones, a concentration of 1% w/w lowers the surface tension. This makes them effective in providing a silicone-like feel to oils, most interestingly natural oils such as olive oil. If the concentration is increased to between 5-10% by weight, micelles form, providing a thixotrophic gel and change in aesthetics.

Why Silicone?

Silicones are used in formulations due to their low surface tension, which contributes to a unique feel. Silicone compounds have a surface tension of approximately 20 dynes/cm2. In contrast, oils have a surface tension in the range of 30 dynes/cm2 while water is around 72 dynes/cm2. Therefore, silicone compounds having both silicone-soluble and silicone-insoluble groups provide formulators with functional surface active agents to overcome these differences in surface tension.

The silicone-insoluble components can include oil soluble groups such as alkyl silicones as well as water soluble groups, i.e., dimethicone copolyols. This basic chemistry has been known for some time; however, new materials have been developed to impart functionality at low use levels (below 1%). These materials, referred to as *high definition polymers*, are precisely tuned to certain molecules to impart specific benefits in a formulation.

Alkyl silicones are one class of compounds that can be made into high definition polymers; other classes include dimethicone copolyols and silicone resins. The ratio of silicone to alkyl in these materials determines the degree of occlusivity of the film and the clarity of the alkyl dimethicone in natural oils. The higher the percentage of silicone in the alkyl dimethicone, the more breathable the film and the more opaque the resulting gel (see **Figure 1**). The ratio of silicone to alkyl in the alkyl dimethicone also determines the hardness it provides.

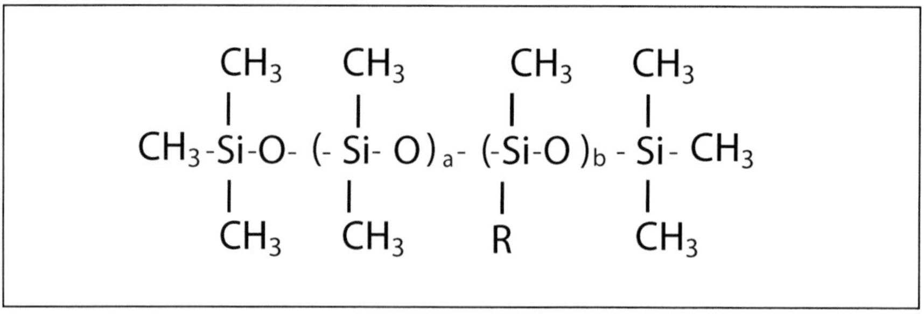

$$CH_3-\underset{\underset{CH_3}{|}}{\overset{\overset{CH_3}{|}}{Si}}-O-(-\underset{\underset{CH_3}{|}}{\overset{\overset{CH_3}{|}}{Si}}-O)_a-(-\underset{\underset{R}{|}}{\overset{\overset{CH_3}{|}}{Si}}-O)_b-\underset{\underset{CH_3}{|}}{\overset{\overset{CH_3}{|}}{Si}}-CH_3$$

Figure 1. Alkyl dimethicone structure

Structure and Function

The structure of a polymer determines its function. In **Figure 1**, R is the alkyl or oil-loving (hydrophilic) portion of the structure and the remaining portion is silicone-soluble (silliphilic). The number of a and b units and the length of the R alkyl group determine the properties of the silicone polymer. For instance, the length of the alkyl chain is the salient factor in determining its melting point of the alkyl dimethicone. In addition, waxes based on alkyl groups of 16 or less carbon atoms are liquid at room temperature, whereas those with 18 or more carbon atoms are solid; the melting point increases as the carbon length goes up (see **Table 1**).

Table 1
Melting point of alkyl dimethicone compounds

Material	State at RT	% Silicone	%Alkyl	Melting Point (°C)
Cetyl dimethicone	liquid	50.2	49.8	-
Behenyl dimethicone	solid	68.0	32.0	46
Behenyl dimethicone	soft solid	45.0	55.0	37
C26 dimethicone	solid	41.0	59.0	47
C26 dimethicone	solid	69.0	31.0	43
C26 dimethicone	solid	81.0	19.0	37
C32 dimethicone	hard solid	64.0	36.0	60

It is important to note that a material's INCI name is determined solely by its R group and does not take these a and b values into consideration. The formulation implications of this effect are that polymers having the same INCI name can function differently in a formulation—one imparting a hydrophobic feel and the other a hydrophilic feel. Generally, the lower molecular weight alkyl dimethicone compounds provide the most hydrophilic feel. Further, formulations with exactly the same label can feel different. Therefore, the INCI name often does not assist in the selection of a proper alkyl silicone polymer.

Solubility is another function related to the material's structure. Liquid alkyl dimethicone can be used as an additive to improve the solubility of polar oils in formulations. **Figure 2** depicts the addition of behenyl dimethicone to soybean oil, and **Table 2** shows the solubility of alkyl silicones in a variety of solvents.

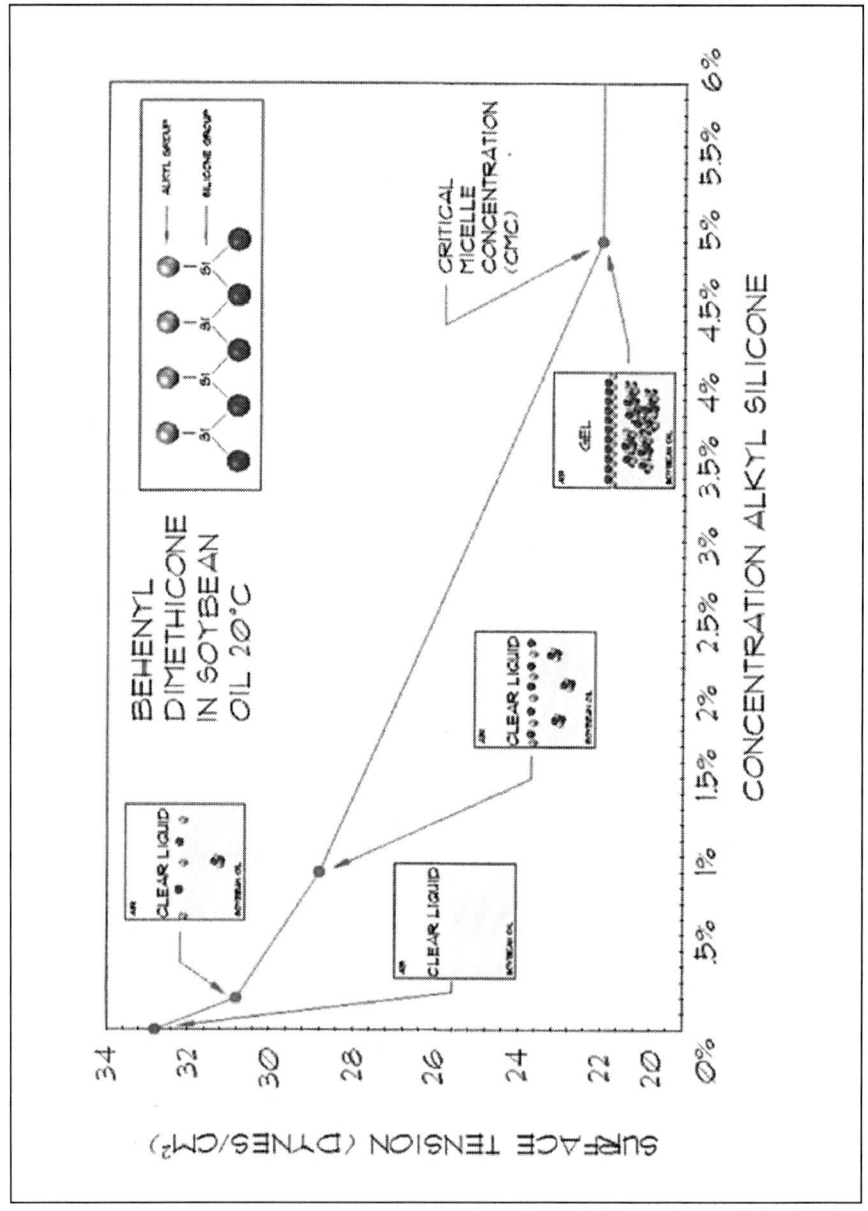

Figure 2. Addition of surfactant silicone to soybean oil

Table 2
Alkyl silicone solubility

Material	Water	Mineral oil	Mineral spirits	Propylene glycol	D5	350 visc. Dimethicone	IPA
Stearyl dimethicone	I	S	S	I	D	I	I
Behenyl dimethicone	I	S	D	I	D	D	I
C26 dimethicone	I	S	S	I	D	D	I

I = insoluble; D = dispersible; S = soluble

As noted, alkyl silicones go to the air/oil interface and act as surfactants, lowering the surface tension. The presence of both oil soluble and silicone soluble moieties in the same molecule causes this effect. This reduced surface tension makes oil feel like D5 silicone. As their concentration increases, micelles form. This property makes them amphiphilic and allows them to function at low concentrations. If an alkyl silicone with a melting point above ambient temperature is used it will form a reversible thixotrophic gel that liquefies under pressure and upon heating, and re-solidifies upon cooling. Altering the ratio of alkyl to silicone component in alkyl dimethicone the molecule will change the clarity of the gel and occlusivity of the blend (see **Figure 3**). Here, behenyl dimethicone was added to the oil with differing amounts of silicone group present.

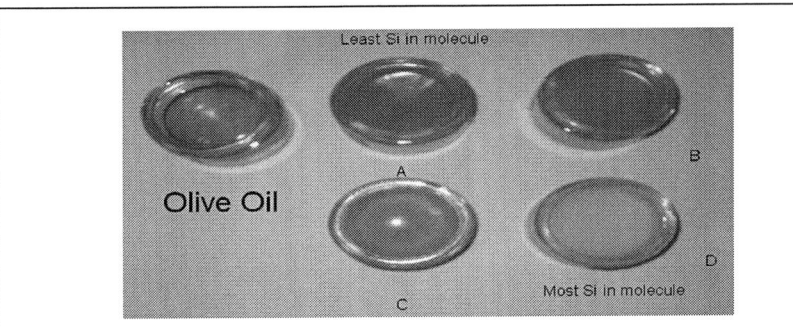

Figure 3. Behenyl dimethicone gellation of olive oil (5% additive)

Multiple Domain Silicones

The alkyl silicone surfactants discussed thus far have consisted of a single alkyl group on a silicone backbone. However, a series of patent-pending alkyl dimethicones have been developed that contain two different alkyl groups—one a liquid at ambient temperatures, and another a solid at ambient temperatures. One such polymer conforms to the structure shown in **Figure 4**.

The specific structures of the R groups in the solid and liquid domains have a profound effect on the rheology and aesthetics of a formulation and enable variations in characteristics such as cushion and playtime (see **Cushion and Playtime**). Differences in formulas containing multi-domain versus single domain silicone are clearly visible, as shown in **Figure 5**.

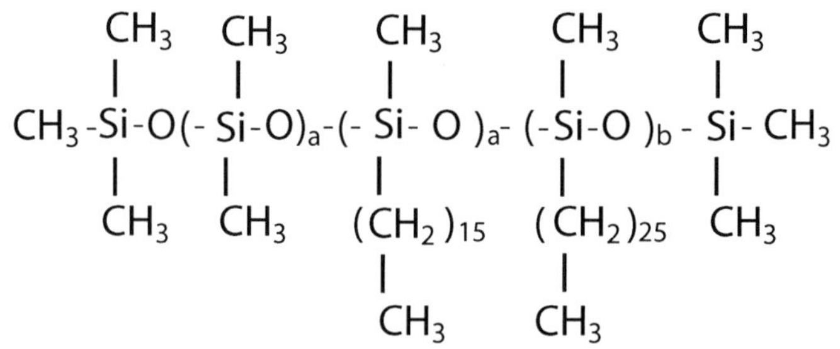

$$CH_3-Si(CH_3)_2-O-(Si(CH_3)_2-O)_a-(Si(CH_3)(C_{16}H_{33})-O)_a-(Si(CH_3)(C_{26}H_{53})-O)_b-Si(CH_3)_3$$

Figure 4. Multi-domain silicone structure

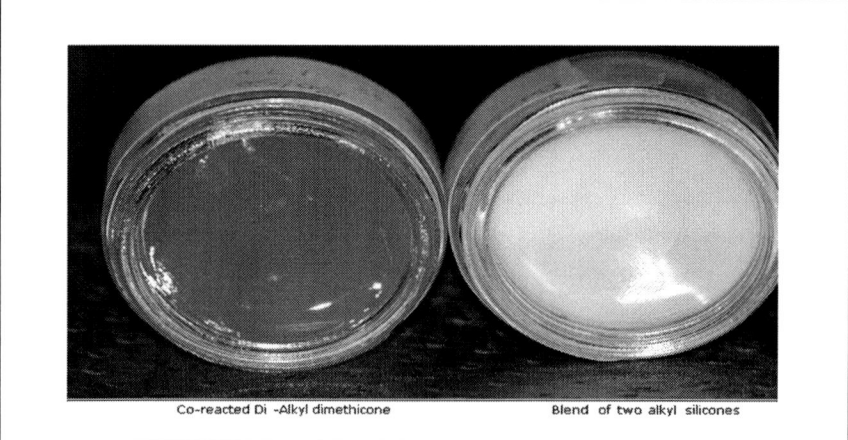

Figure 5. Multi alkyl dimethicone comparison: co-reacted di-alkyl dimethicone (left) and blend of two alkyl silicones (right)

Cushion and Playtime

The terms cushion and playtime are commonly used to describe the feel of ingredients and formulations on the skin. If one places a compound or formulation on their index finger and rubs it onto the forearm, both cushion and playtime can be evaluated. Cushion refers to the amount of compound that persists between the finger and forearm—i.e., the greater the "distance" between the finger and the forearm, the greater the cushion. Playtime refers to the length of time that cushion persists. If the cushion is felt for a long period of time, the playtime is said to be long. If the cushion collapses rapidly, the playtime is said to be short. In most compounds the cushion and playtime are directly related. Honey, for example, has both a high cushion and a high playtime. There are also materials that have good cushion but a low playtime, such as the multi-domain alkyl silicone compounds described. Many applications require a high level of cushion and a short playtime, such as lipsticks, sun products and lotions. The reason for this is to impart an initial feel that is highly desirable that quickly changes to the final desired property, i.e., a dry, non-greasy feel.

The two samples shown have exactly the same composition of C22 and C16 except one consists of a blend of two alkyl silicones that have a single alkyl group, the other has the two alkyl groups co-reacted on a single silicone backbone. The presence of the liquid portion of the molecule inhibits formulas from becoming hard solids, instead forming soft, thixotrophic gels that are translucent, that liquefy under pressure, and that have a cushion effect yet a short playtime—meaning the material rubs out rapidly.

Photomicroscopy of the two materials shows that the multi-domain silicone polymer is highly structured while the blend of the two single domain silicone polymers is random and lacks structure (see **Figure 6**). It is this structure that accounts for the different functionality between the polymers.

In this case, the INCI names also recognize the difference. The blend of the two single domain silicone molecules has the INCI name: Behenyl Dimethicone (and) Acetyl Dimethicone, while the multi-domain silicones have the INCI name: Benehyl/Cetyl Dimethicone.

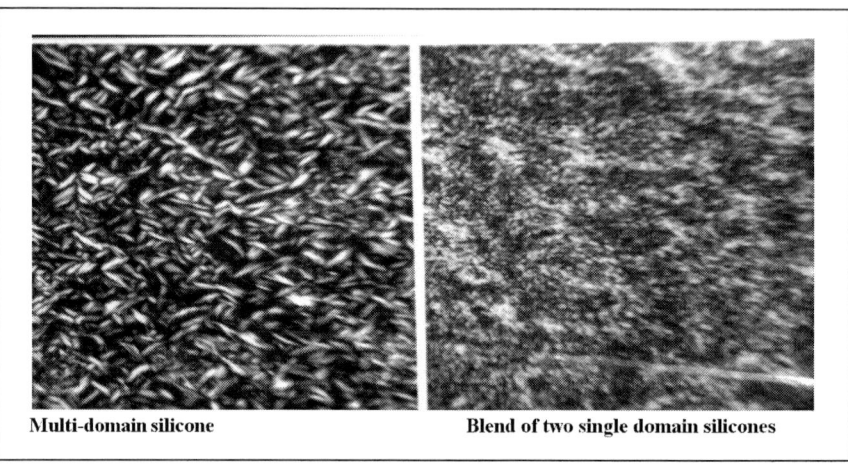

Figure 6. Photomicrograph of multi-domain silicone (left) and a blend of two single domain silicones (right)

Characterization

The two samples from **Figure 5** were compared by an independent lab[a] that characterized them as being different from one another. **Sample 1**, the multi-domain silicone, was observed as a translucent gel at room temperature. It flowed under pressure and was composed of two phases: a liquid phase at room temperature, and a solid crystalline phase whose relatively large, elongated crystals scattered light to make the product appear translucent or colorless—as if the crystals were absent. The crystalline phase melted entirely at 38°C but re-crystallized when the temperature dropped below this level.

Sample 2, the blend of two single-domain silicones, was classified as an opaque, waxy, white crystalline solid at room temperature whose color and solid phase structure were attributed to a colorless, interlocking crystal composition that melted at 56°C; this transformation was reported as reversible.

According to the studies, the crystals in **sample 1** appeared more like liquid crystals than ordinary crystals, such as those forming the waxy solid in **sample 2**. The authors note that while this has not yet been confirmed, initial observations point in this direction—the most compelling evidence being the disappearance of birefringent crystals in a thin film of **sample 1** when pressure

---

[a]Independent studies were commissioned through Microtrace LLC, Elgin, IL USA.

was applied to the coverslip, followed by their reappearance once the pressure was released.

Adjusting Formulation Parameters

The capability of changing a formula's properties using alkyl silicones was tested in sample sunscreens (see **Formulas 1a-c**). These formulas were tested for SPF on volunteers using a solar simulator lamp with a continuous light spectrum in the UVA and UVB range (290-400 nm). The spectral output of the solar simulator was calibrated according to the US Food and Drug Administration's requirements2 and the SPF test for all three formulas was performed on the same subjects.

Formula 1
Sample sunscreen formulations with and without mult-domain silicone

Ingredient	a	b	c
Water (*aqua*)	74.2% w/w	72.2% w/w	82.9% w/w
Carbomer	0.25	0.25	0.25
Disodium ethylenediaminetetraacetic acid	0.05	0.05	0.05
Triethanolamine	1.00	1.00	1.0
Octocrylene	3.00	3.00	3.00
Octisalate	3.00	3.00	3.00
Oxybenzone	2.00	2.00	2.00
Avobenzone	1.00	1.00	1.00
Stearic acid	2.00	2.00	1.00
Sorbitan isostearate	0	0	1.00
Polyglyceryl-3 distearate	0	0	1.00
Glyceryl stearate (self-emulsifying)	3.00	3.00	0
Benzyl alcohol	1.00	1.00	1.00
Dimethylpoly siloxane	0.50	0.50	0.50
VP/eicosene copolymer	0	0	2.00
Methylparaben	0	0	0.20
Propylparaben	0	0	0.10
C12-15 alkyl benzoate	8.00	8.00	0
Multi-domain silicone	0	2.00	0
Phenoxyethanol (and) isopropylparaben (and) isobutylparaben (and) n-butylparaben	1.0	1.0	0

Formula 2
Lipstick with multi-domain surfactant silicone

A. Castor oil	6.50% w/w
B. Color	5.50
Pearlescent pigment	7.00
C. Castor oil	31.00
Triisostearyl citrate	8.00
Trioctyldodecyl citrate	15.00
(Siltech CE 2000, Siltech LLC)	
Cetyl dimethicone/vinyl dimethicone crosspolymer	2.00
(Silwax CR-5016, Siltech LLC)	
Isopropyl phenyl dimethicone	2.00
(Silwax 3HMS, Siltech LLC)	
Trimethylol propane tricaprate/caprylate	2.00
(Cosmosurf ET-8, Surfatech Corp.)	
Pentaerythrityl tetra caprate/caprylate	2.00
(Cosmosurf EP-8, Surfatech Corp.)	
Cetyl/hexacosyl dimethicone	5.00
(Silwax D221M, Siltech LLC)	
Candellilla wax	3.00
Behenyl dimethicone (Silwax D222, Siltech LLC)	2.00
C32 dimethicone (Silwax J1032, Siltech LLC)	2.00
Carnauba wax	2.00
Ozokerite	2.00
Microcristalline wax	3.00
D. Preservative	qs
Antioxidant	qs

Procedure: Disperse by stirring B in A then milling. Combine C and heat with mixing to 85°C. When clear, add C to AB. Cool at 75°C, then add D.

The average SPF values for the sample formulas were: **Formula 1a**, SPF 19; **Formula 1b**, SPF 28 (very water resistant or VWR); and **Formula 1c**, SPF 29 (VWR). Based on these results, the multi-domain silicone boosted SPF in **Formula 1b**, compared with a control formula excluding a waterproofing film-former. Use of the properly selected alkyl silicone therefore resulted in a more uniform film of sunscreen on the skin and increased the SPF. Based on the results of this study, multi-domain silicones were found to be equivalent to the well-known waterproofing film-former, VP/eicosene copolymer.

Conclusions

Many interesting properties are imparted by amphiphilic surfactant silicone compounds. These materials lower surface tension, which can alter properties such as wetting, emulsification, foaming and gellation, depending on their specific structure. Since INCI names do not relate to their structure, formulators will need additional details to construct meaningful models, and since silicone polymers typically are incorporated into formulations, it is critically important for formulators to consider their interactions with the other components in a formula. The further evaluation of the effects of silicone surfactants in formulations could be an ideal topic for a computer-assisted evaluation of numerous formulations.

The ability to use this high definition polymer approach to selecting silicones for personal care products will allow formulators to optimize formulations. The amount of silicone in formulations will decrease as more efficient polymers are selected; for example, silicone fluids and cyclic silicones can be replaced with natural oils when the properly selected alkyl silicones are used. This reduction in the overall concentration of silicone in formulations will result in "greening with silicones."

Published January 2010 Cosmetics and Toiletries magazine

References

1. E Rochow, *An Introduction–Chemistry of Silicones*, John Wiley and Sons: Indianapolis (1947)
2. Spectral Output Requirements for Testing Sunscreen Drug Products for Over-the-counter Human Use, Proposed Amendment of Final Monograph, CFR Part 352.70 (b) Light Sources, Federal Register, vol 72, No. 165 (Aug 27, 2007); and the International Sun Protection Factor (SPF) Test Method (May 2006)

CHAPTER 25

Film-forming Polymers as a Strategy for Sunscreen Efficacy

Jennifer Davis and Doreen Petersen
National Starch Personal Care, Bridgewater, N.J., USA

Daniel Li
National Starch Personal Care, Shanghai, China

KEY WORDS: *Film-forming polymers, sunscreen water resistance, acrylates copolymer, acrylates/octylacrylamide copolymer, dehydroxanthan gum*

ABSTRACT: *Acrylic-based film-forming polymers lend properties of water resistance to both traditional and nontraditional sunscreen formulations. Dehydroxanthan gum is a film-forming polymer, a rheology modifier and an SPF booster in sunscreen systems containing zinc oxide. Illustrations are provided.*

Consumers are increasingly concerned about the effects of UV radiation on the skin, and with good reason. Skin cancer has become one of the leading forms of cancer in the United States, with approximately 1.2–1.5 million newly diagnosed cases per annum.[1] Demand for UV protection has made the sun care market the fastest-growing personal care sector with global sales reaching US$5.47 billion in 2005.[2]

New trends have emerged as consumers redefine what is important in their sun care products: higher Sun Protection Factor (SPF) values, broad-spectrum protection, enhanced water resistance and rub-off resistance, more aesthetically pleasing products, and perhaps most importantly, convenience. The advent of newly popular product forms such as alcohol-based aerosol and nonaerosol sprays, has created a challenge for formulators as they try to waterproof these nontraditional systems. Formulators also want to increase the efficacy of sunscreen products without increasing the levels of the sunscreen actives within the formulation.

Film-forming polymers serve as ideal technologies when formulating sunscreen products for water resistance and rub-off resistance in both traditional and newer nontraditional products. Of particular interest are combinations of film-forming polymers that show an unexpected synergy, resulting in an SPF boost. Following is a description of this synergistic formulating approach.

A Fundamental View of Film Formation

Historically, the goal of a sunscreen film has been to deliver the UV filter to the skin surface as evenly as possible.[1] In this case, the film has some hydrophobic character that retains the oil-soluble UV filters on the skin for extended periods of time. The mechanism by which a film is formed can vary depending on the formulation medium and polymer solubility. In the case of alcohol-based systems that use alcohol-soluble film-forming polymers, the quick evaporation of the solvent allows for film formation. In an emulsion system, the discrete particles pack together during the dry-down process as the water and other volatile liquids evaporate, leaving a film (**Figure 1**).[3]

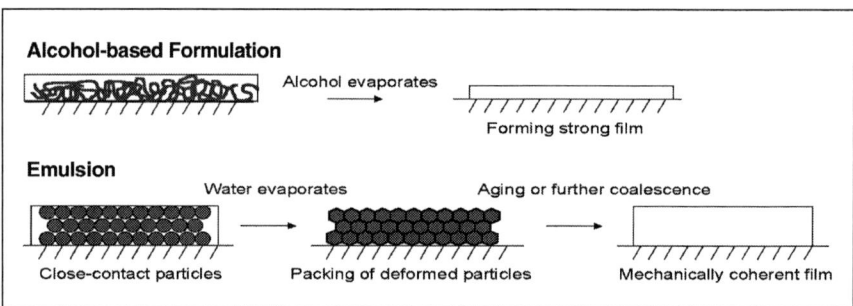

Figure 1. Mechanism of film formation

In the past, waxes such as carnauba were used in sunscreen products to promote water resistance.[1] These waxes enhanced the SPF value, not only by their hydrophobic nature, but also via their viscosity-building properties. A higher viscosity product has the advantage of forming a thicker and more uniform film on skin.[4] PVP/eicosene copolymer also protects via a very similar mechanism. Drawbacks with this type of protection mechanism include its inability to be used in a spray product form, which requires a low-viscosity product, as well as less than optimal aesthetics, such as heavy feel and drag.

More recently, silicones have been promoted to boost the SPF of products.[5,6] In addition to film formation, these classes of ingredients rely on the ability of the silicone to allow the formulation to spread more easily during application, thus creating an even film on the skin surface.[5] This mechanism, though desirable from an aesthetic-enhancing perspective, can be quite expensive and many of these silicones are not compatible in alcohol, rendering them ineffective in this solvent-based system.

Acrylic film-forming polymers also improve the SPF value and serve to enhance water resistance and rub-off resistance. These types of polymers, including acrylates copolymer and acrylates/octylacrylamide copolymer, have the advantage of forming a uniform film on the skin without an increase in product viscosity or a tacky afterfeel. The hydrophobic moieties on the polymers trap the UV filters into the film matrix upon dry-down. The hydrophobic nature of these polymers also enhances the water resistance of the films. **Figure 2** demonstrates the water resistance of acrylates/octylacrylamide copolymer in both ethanol and water solutions.

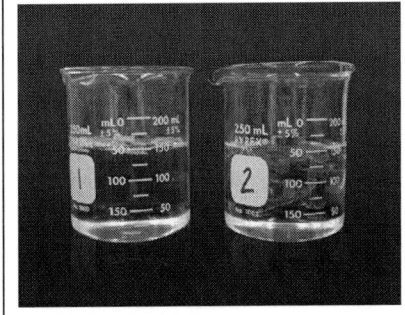
Initial

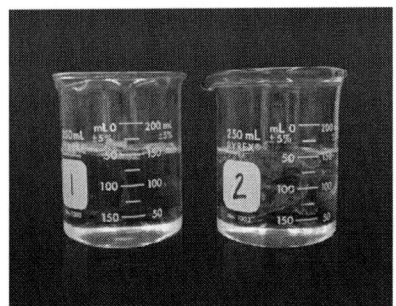
After 24 hr

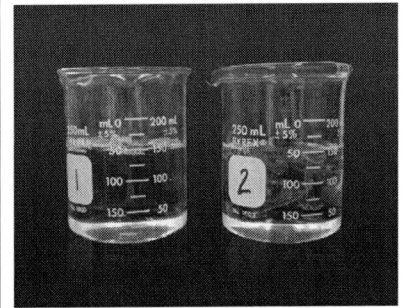
After 48 hr

Figure 2. Films of acrylates/octylacrylamide copolymer in water

Solutions of acrylates/octylacrylamide copolymer were made according to **Table 1**. These solutions then were dried in a silicone mold at 50ºC for 1 h and stored in a controlled temperature and humidity chamber (25ºC, 50% RH) overnight. The conditioned films then were placed in a beaker of water for 48 h. Photographs were taken at time zero, 24 h and 48 h. As can be seen in **Figure 2**, despite immersion in water, the films remain completely intact over the 48-h period.

Table 1
Acrylates/octylacrylamide copolymer solutions

	Ethanol solution (% w/w)	Water solution (%w/w)
Acrylates/octylacrylamide copolymer	5.00	5.00
Triethanolamine	0.00	1.61*
Ethanol	95.00	20.00
Water (aqua)	0.00	75.00
Total	100.00	100.00

* Acrylates/octylacrylamide copolymer neutralized to 90% with triethanolamine 99%

Incorporating Acrylic Polymers into Sunscreens

These types of film-forming polymers are well-suited to today's traditional and nontraditional formulations.

Acrylates copolymer: Acrylates copolymer is an emulsion-based film former that can be added to a water-based emulsion to achieve water resistance. This polymer can be incorporated at both room temperature and elevated temperatures (80ºC) during the emulsion-making process and also has the unique ability to impart water resistance to formulations as a post-added ingredient.

Acrylates copolymer has excellent compatibility with commonly used sunscreen actives, including ethylhexyl methoxycinnamate (octinoxate), ethylhexyl salicylate (octisalate), benzophenone-3 (oxybenzone), homosalate, octocrylene, avobenzone, ZnO and most coatings of TiO_2. The acrylates copolymer also is compatible with a wide range of commonly used cosmetic ingredients including carbomer, xanthan gum, acrylates/C10-30 alkyl acrylate crosspolymer, and other frequently used thickeners and emulsifiers. These compatibilities have been demonsrtated by several commercial successes in sunscreens containing this polymer.

An additional benefit is the lack of viscosity impact on formulations containing this polymer. This technology effectively lends water resistance properties to formulations without the need to thicken the system. All of these benefits combine to allow the formulator to deliver a variety of product forms and SPF values.

Acrylates/octylacrylamide copolymer: Acrylates/octylacrylamide copolymer is a distinctive film-forming technology because the powder is completely soluble in alcohol, as demonstrated by its long history of use in many alcohol-based sunscreen products. It also is compatible with many UV actives and has a negligible impact on viscosity, making this polymer a good choice for alcohol-based sunscreen spray applications. As with acrylates copolymer, unpublished safety data is available to support the use of acrylates/octylacrylamide copolymer in spray applications, which is vitally important to many formulators.

This polymer also can be used in hydro-alcoholic systems, upon neutralization with a base. Incorporation of the polymer into these clear systems is accomplished first by the dissolution of the acrylates/octylacrylamide copolymer into the alcohol, in a polymer-to-alcohol ratio of 1:4, followed by the neutralizer and finally water, UV filters and other ingredients. The ability to impart water resistance and rub-off resistance in these types of systems is quite unusual and lends itself to new spray product concepts.

Acrylic Film-forming Polymers to Enhance SPF Water Resistance

Water-resistance and SPF were enhanced by using acrylates copolymer and acrylates/octylacrylamide copolymer in a variety of formulations, as demonstrated here using both in vitro and in vivo testing methodologies.

In vitro testing: The in vitro SPF testing was performed by a third-party facility[a] using its proprietary substrate[b] following a Very Water Resistant SPF test protocol. In this protocol, the SPF

---

[a]IMS Inc., Milford, Conn., USA
[b]VITRO-SKIN N-19 is a product of IMS Inc. VITRO-SKIN is a registered trademark of IMS Inc.

measurements were made both prior to and following sample immersion in water with stirring for 80 min, a time frame utilized in the in vivo protocol for very water-resistant sunscreens published by the US Food and Drug Administration (FDA). An ultraviolet transmittance analyzer[c] was used to determine UV absorption for each formulation within the wavelength range of 290–400 nm. For each sunscreen formulation (**Tables 2 and 3**), three samples of the substrate were evaluated with 10 measurement sites on each substrate sample. The individual SPF values for each sample were calculated based on the average of all runs for each product.

Table 2 In vitro-tested emulsions (Formulas 1 and 2)

	1 Blank Control (% w/w)	2 With Film Former (% w/w)
A. Water (*aqua*)	5.00	5.00
Disodium EDTA	0.04	0.04
Acrylates/C10-30 alkyl acrylate crosspolymer	0.20	0.20
Glycerin	3.00	3.00
Phenoxyethanol (and) methylparaben (and) ethylparaben (and) butylparaben (and) propylparaben (and) isobutylparaben	1.00	1.00
Acrylates copolymer	0.00	4.40
B. Ethylhexyl methoxycinnamate	7.50	7.50
Ethylhexyl salicylate	5.00	5.00
Homosalate	10.00	10.00
Butyl methoxydibenzoylmethane	2.00	2.00
Cetearyl alcohol	0.30	0.30
Sorbitan oleate	0.45	0.45
C. Vitamin E acetate	0.50	0.50
Triethanolamine	qs to pH 6.5	qs to pH 6.5
Total	100.00	100.00
In vitro static SPF	25	31
In vitro SPF after 80-min immersion	20	32
% SPF retained	80	103

[c]UV 1000S Ultraviolet Transmittance Analyzer is a product of Labsphere, Inc., North Sutton, New Hampshire, USA.

Table 3 In vitro-tested alcohol-based formulations (Formulas 3 and 4)

	3 Blank Control (% w/w)	4 With Film Former (% w/w)
A. Ethanol	48.00	46.00
Acrylates/octylacrylamide copolymer	0.00	2.00
Ethylhexyl salicylate	5.00	5.00
Homosalate	10.00	10.00
Butyl methoxydibenzoylmethane	3.00	3.00
Benzophenone-3	6.00	6.00
Diethylhexyl 2,6-napthalate	4.00	4.00
B. Isobutane	24.00	24.00
Total	100.00	100.00
In vitro static SPF	50	61
In vitro SPF after 80-min immersion	31	43
% SPF retained	62	70

Four sunscreen formulations (**Tables 2 and 3**) were tested:

- An emulsion containing no film-forming polymer (**Formula 1**)
- An emulsion containing acrylates copolymer (**Formula 2**)
- An alcohol-based system containing no film-forming polymer (**Formula 3**)
- An alcohol-based system containing acrylates/octylacrylamide copolymer (**Formula 4**).

In each case, the system that contained the film-forming polymer (**Formulas 2 and 4**) achieved higher SPF values and an increase in the percentage of SPF retained after 80 min of water immersion.

In vivo **testing:** In vivo Very Water Resistant SPF testing was used to compare the water-resistance property of formulations with and without acrylates copolymer (**Formulas 6 and 5**, respectively, in **Table 4**). The in vivo SPF testing was conducted by a third-party facility[d] according to the FDA's final monograph[7] for very water-resistant sunscreens. SPF testing was performed

---

[d]Consumer Products Testing Co., Fairfield, N.J., USA

using five human panelists. Readings were taken before and after an 80-min immersion in water. The results demonstrate that the formulation containing acrylates copolymer (**Formula 6**) offers 97% SPF retention.

Visual imaging: Retention of film structure after submersion in water is an indication of water resistance and can also be visualized in the images of **Figure 3**, where **Formulas 1 and 2** were compared to an identical formulation containing PVP/eicosene copolymer instead of acrylates copolymer as the film former.

Table 4
In vitro-tested emulsions (Formulas 5 and 6)

	5 Blank Control (% w/w)	6 With Film Former (% w/w)
A. Water (*aqua*)	48.90	44.50
Glycerin	5.00	5.00
Carbomer	10.00	10.00
Acrylates/C10-30 alkyl acrylate crosspolymer	0.20	0.20
Phenoxyethanol (and) methylparaben (and) butylparaben (and) ethylparaben (and) propylparaben	1.00	1.00
Triethanolamine	0.40	0.40
Acrylates copolymer	0.00	4.40
B. Ethylhexyl methoxycinnamate	7.50	7.50
Benzophenone-3	6.00	6.00
Ethylhexyl salicylate	4.00	4.00
Octocrylene	9.00	9.00
Glyceryl stearate	2.50	2.50
Stearic acid	2.50	2.50
Isostearyl alcohol	1.00	1.00
DEA-cetyl phosphate	2.00	2.00
Total	100.00	100.00
In vivo static SPF	32	32
In vivo SPF after 80-min immersion	<21	31
% SPF retained	<66	97

A yellow dye was added to the formulations to enhance the visual differences and 0.1 g of the formulations then were applied to a synthetic skin substrate[e]. The sunscreens were allowed to dry for 10 min at ambient conditions before the substrate was placed in a warm water bath at approximately 35°C. After 30 min, the substrate was removed and rinsed with warm water for 5 min. This cycle was repeated two more times, the second and third soakings for 30 min and 60 min, respectively, until a total of 2 h had elapsed.

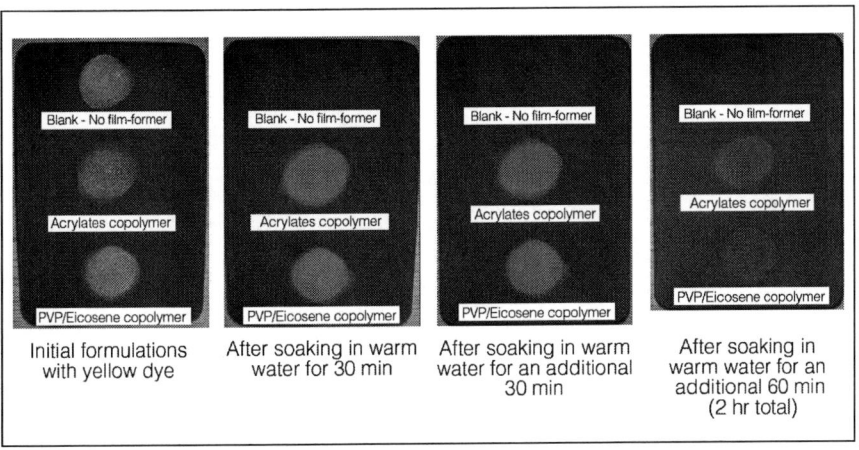

Figure 3. Images of water resistance on a substrate

The photographs in **Figure 3** depict the film's appearance on the synthetic skin at each time point: initial application and after soaking of 30 min, 60 min and 120 min. The visual performance of **Formula 2**, containing acrylates copolymer in this study, correlates well with what is seen in the in vitro and in vivo studies of this polymer in various formulations (see SPF results in **Formulas 1–4**).

Enhanced SPF via Combinations of Dehydroxanthan Gum and Acrylic-based Film-forming Polymers

Dehydroxanthan gum is a heat-treated variant of xanthan gum that gives very different performance properties from its xanthan gum parent.[8] Unlike traditional xanthan gum, this polymer is both a film-former and a rheology modifier. It has been used previously

---

[e]Bioskin, a product of Beaulax Co., Ltd., Tokyo, Japan. Bioskin is a registered trademark of Beaulax Co., Ltd.

in hair styling formulations.[8] As reported here for the first time, the use of dehydroxanthan gum in conjunction with acrylic-based film-forming polymers has been shown to enhance SPF. This is especially useful because in sunscreen systems containing zinc oxide there are few choices for rheology modifiers due to compatibility issues. Dehydroxanthan gum acts to boost the SPF enhancement of acrylic-based film-forming polymers such as acrylates copolymer, an effect not seen with the xanthan gum that is commonly used in these formulations.

The four emulsion formulations (**Table 5**) were tested in vitro utilizing the same methodology previously described:

- **Formula 7** containing only dehydroxanthan gum.
- **Formula 8** containing both dehydroxanthan gum and acrylates copolymer.
- **Formula 9** containing both traditional xanthan gum and acrylates copolymer.
- **Formula 10** containing traditional xanthan gum and PVP/eicosene copolymer.

The resulting data in **Table 5** indicates that an SPF boost exists between dehydroxanthan gum and acrylates copolymer. As can be seen, **Formula 7** containing only dehydroxanthan gum does not have any SPF retention; however, **Formula 8** containing both dehydroxanthan gum and acrylates copolymer has an SPF value of 34 after immersion for 80 min. **Formulas 9 and 10** containing traditional xanthan gum do not provide much SPF retention, although **Formula 9** containing acrylates copolymer performed better than **Formula 10** containing PVP/eicosene copolymer.

A possible mechanism for this SPF enhancement is thought by these authors to be a combination of the individual polymer benefits. The hydrophobic nature of the acrylates copolymer increases the water resistance of the UV filters. Dehydroxanthan gum both thickens the sunscreen film and suspends the inorganic particulate sunscreens to increase optical path length and subsequently the SPF value. Traditional xanthan gum does not have this effect, as indicated by its lack of SPF retention.

Table 5
In vitro-tested emulsions (Formulas 7, 8, 9, 10) with varying amounts of dehydroxanthan gum (DG), acrylates copolymer (AC), xanthan gum (XG) and PVP/eicosene (PE)

	7 DG only (% w/w)	8 DG and AC (% w/w)	9 XG and AC (% w/w)	10 XG and PE (% w/w)
A. Isohexadecane	1.50	1.50	1.50	1.50
C12-15 alkyl benzoate	5.00	5.00	3.00	3.00
Cyclopentasiloxane	2.25	2.25	2.25	2.25
Sorbitan stearate	1.00	1.00	1.00	1.00
Glyceryl stearate (and) PEG-100 stearate	2.00	2.00	2.00	2.00
Octocrylene	2.00	2.00	2.00	2.00
Ethylhexyl methoxycinnamate	7.50	7.50	7.50	7.50
Benzophenone-3	3.00	3.00	3.00	3.00
Zinc oxide (and) C12-15 alkyl benzoate (and) polyhydro-xystearic acid	6.00	6.00	6.00	6.00
PVP/eicosene copolymer	0.00	0.00	0.00	2.00
B. Water (*aqua*)	58.65	54.25	54.25	56.65
Dehydroxanthan gum	0.50	0.50	0.00	0.00
Xanthan gum	0.00	0.00	0.50	0.50
Acrylates copolymer	0.00	4.40	4.40	0.00
Glycerin	3.00	3.00	3.00	3.00
Titanium dioxide (and) alumina (and) silica (and) sodium polyacrylate	7.00	7.00	7.00	7.00
C. Cornstarch modified	2.00	2.00	2.00	2.00
DMDM hydantoin (and) iodopropynyl butylcarbamate	0.60	0.60	0.60	0.60
Citric acid	qs to pH 7	qs to pH 7	qs to pH 7	qs to pH 7
Total	100.00	100.00	100.00	100.00
In vivo static SPF	34	50	50	54
In vivo SPF after 80-min immersion	9	34	21	13
% SPF retained	26	68	42	13

Conclusion

Acrylic-based film-forming polymers lend water-resistance properties to both traditional and nontraditional sunscreen formulations. The effects delivered from the water-resistance technology are further enhanced by the unexpected SPF boost produced from select combinations of dehydroxanthan gum and acrylates copolymer in formulations containing inorganic particulate sunscreens. This finding on SPF enhancement and dehydroxanthan gum's known properties as a rheology modifier offer formulators another choice for thickening zinc oxide-containing formulations and boosting their SPF.

As the sun care market continues to grow at an accelerated rate, these polymers provide versatile, effective tools to deliver the performance characteristics that the consumers want today and will want in the future.

Published May 2007 Cosmetics and Toiletries magazine

References

1. G Langer, The evolution of sun care, *Functional Foods & Nutraceuticals,* 38–45 (Sep 2006)
2. C Wang, Sun care, *Spray Technology & Marketing* 16(5) 10–13 and 24–26 (2006)
3. S Muroi and I Morino, Chapter 1, *Polymer Latex* (Dec 1998) (In Japanese)
4. A Hunter and M Trevino, Film-formers enhance water resistance and SPF in sun care products, *Cosmet Toil* 119(7) 51–56 (2004)
5. I Van Reeth, S Postiaux and H Van Dort, Silicones bring multifunctional performance to sun care, *Cosmet Toil* 121(10) 41–54 (2006)
6. N Shaath, Sunscreens: regulations, technical and commercial development, *Household and Personal Care Today* 18–23 (Spring 2005)
7. Sunscreen drug products for over-the-counter human drugs, Rule, 21 CFR Part 352, Subpart D, *Federal Register* 64(98) (May 21, 1999) Proposed Amendment; Docket number 78N-0038/CP12 (Jun 21, 1999)
8. H Cao, K Maurer and MJ Vitale, Dehydroxanthan gum, *Happi* 41(5) 82–86 (2004)

CHAPTER 26

Silicones Bring Multi-functional Performance to Sun Care

Isabelle Van Reeth
Dow Corning Co., Ltd., Shanghai, China
Stéphanie Postiaux
Dow Corning S.A., Seneffe, Belgium
Heidi Van Dort
Dow Corning Corp., Midland, Mich., USA

KEY WORDS: *Silicone acrylate copolymer, silicone carbinol, silicone elastomer, silicone, SPF, sun care, sunscreen, UV, wash-off resistance*

ABSTRACT: *Silicones give formulators choices for a variety of high-performance sun care products and delivery systems. Silicones can boost SPF, add wash-off resistance and help prevent sand from sticking to the skin.*

Amidst heightened awareness over the effects of the sun on skin, the world sun care market, the fastest-growing personal care sector, rose 43% in retail value between 2000 and 2005. Sales reached US$5.47 billion in 2005, with Western Europe and North America contributing US$2.3 billion and US$1.2 billion respectively. The compound annual growth rate over this period was about 7.4%.[1]

This increase reflects consumers' concern about skin cancer, premature aging and an interest in a broader variety of sun care product forms. Demand is increasing for protective sun products as well as those developed for self-tanning and after-sun, and focus has turned to specialty formulations developed for children or those that provide extra benefits such as antiaging ingredients, vitamins, scents, quick-drying characteristics, insect repellency and even sheen or glittery effects on the skin.

In the hair care segment, an increasing number of sun care products include sunscreens that aid color retention by protecting hair from UV radiation. But no matter how novel sun care products become, consumers know what they want in terms of the fundamentals: UVB and UVA protection, high SPF, photostability, safe and nonirritating products, water-resistance and good aesthetics—all at a reasonable cost.

An Expanded Role for Silicones

Despite growing sales, sun care products still retain a stigma in the minds of some consumers, who perceive many as unpleasantly sticky, greasy or difficult to apply. Silicones are known for their positive effect on the sensory profiles of both sun care formulations, where silicones impart a light, nongreasy and silky feel,[2] and skin care products in general. Use of silicones in sun care products continues to increase, and as silicone technology evolves, greater interest is focused on their multifunctional properties. In the newest sun care products and product forms, silicones also can be used to provide substantivity, sebum control, resistance to wash-off and to boost SPF. In part, this broader use is reflected in the number of sun care products containing at least one silicone. In the United States, 63% of 102 sun care products introduced in 2004 contained silicones;[3] of 66 sun care products launched in France that year, 92% contained silicones.[4]

Sunscreen actives are compatible with a variety of silicone materials, including selected silicone polyethers, low-viscosity dimethicones and cyclomethicones. In addition, several classes of silicone materials, including silicone acrylate copolymers, elastomers, resins, alkylmethylsiloxanes and high molecular weight emulsions, offer formulating advantages.

Silicone Acrylate Copolymers

Among the newest materials are silicone acrylate copolymers that provide enhanced durability on the skin and easy formulation. Composed of blends of acrylates/polytrimethyl-siloxymethacrylate in organic or silicone solvent (see **Figure 1**), these waterlike silicone and organic hybrids form nonocclusive films that resist wash-off. Their acrylate backbone grafted with demidentritic silicone functionalities results in a unique structure where the acrylate portion is responsible for the film formation on the skin, and the silicone functionalities increase the film suppleness as well as decrease the tackiness. Silicone acrylates are compatible with a range of common cosmetic ingredients including organic sunscreens, pigments and triglycerides. They can be incorporated into creams and lotions to provide sebum resistance or reduction, and they also offer good film-forming properties.

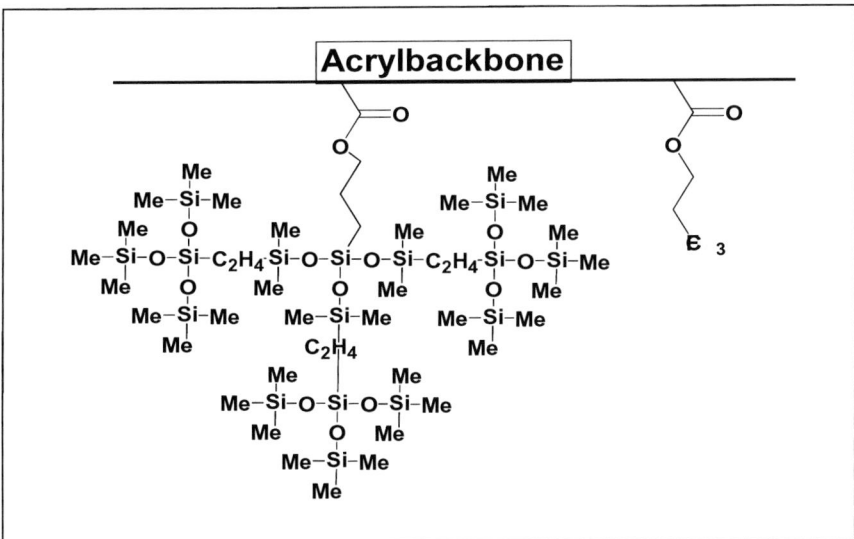

Figure 1. Schematic of the silicone acrylate copolymer

Individual applications may require silicone acrylate copolymers with an isododecane or cyclopentasiloxane solvent. These organic solvents evaporate quickly, leaving a high molecular weight silicone acrylate polymer film on the skin. For slower evaporation or other formulation requirements, the silicone solvent may be more appropriate (see **Figure 2**).

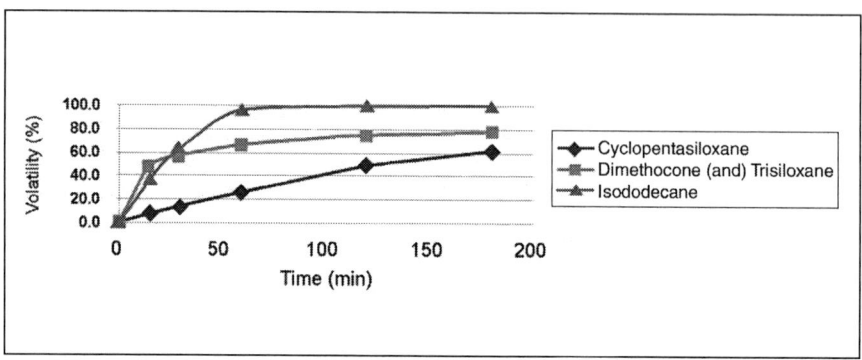

Figure 2. Evaporation profiles of three solvents at 25°C: isododecane, cyclopentasiloxane, and dimethicone (and) trisiloxane

Silicone Carbinol Fluid

Mono-oxyalkylene-functional silicone that contains a carbinol (or C-OH functional) group, has applications in sun care products as well as color cosmetics, and in skin care, underarm and hair care products. Although it offers both polar and silicone functionality, its behavior is considerably different from existing polar silicone materials such as silicone polyethers and silanol fluids. Also referred to as silicone carbinol fluid, mono-oxyalkylene-functional silicone can provide a solution for aesthetic, compatibility and delivery limitations associated with organic oils and some silicone oils.

This clear, low-viscosity, hydrolytically stable fluid can easily be incorporated into personal care formulations, where it imparts hydrophilic and wetting characteristics. It does not appreciably contribute to the odor of finished formulations. In addition, compared to many polar organic materials, it is nonirritating.[5] The presence of hydroxyethoxypropyl functionalities at both ends of the molecules increases its polarity as well as improves its compatibility with organic materials

Silicone carbinol fluid has been shown in vitro to enhance the SPF of formulations containing sunscreen actives. A Meyer rod was used to apply 2 mg/cm^2 samples of the lotion shown in **Formula 1** to a quartz substrate to provide an even coating with minimal variation. Operator variance was reduced from >15% to 5%. Test revealed a 35% boost in SPF when the silicone carbinol fluid was used in place of dimethicone, 5 cSt.[6]

Formula 1
Sunscreen Lotion

A. Cetyl dimethicone (DC 2502 Cosmetic Fluid, Dow Corning)	3.00% w/w
B. bis-Hydroxyethoxypropyl dimethicone (DC 5562 Carbinol Fluid, Dow Corning)	7.00
Lauryl PEG/PPG-18/18 methicone (DC 5200 Formulation Aid, Dow Corning)	6.00
Cyclopentasiloxane (DC 245 Fluid, Dow Corning)	6.00
Ethylhexyl methoxycinnamate (Uvinul MC80, BASF Corp.)	7.50
C. Sodium chloride	2.00
Water (*aqua*)	65.10
Glycerin	3.00
Propylene glycol (and) diazolidinyl urea (and) methylparaben (and) propylparaben (Germaben II, Sutton Laboratories)	0.40
	100.00

Procedure: Warm A slightly before using. Combine A and B. In a separate container, combine C. Slowly add C to AB while mixing A at 800–1300 rpm.

Alkylmethylsiloxanes

Ingredients from the alkylmethylsiloxane (AMS) family are silicone-organic hybrids that offer the best qualities of both materials—molecules based on a silicone backbone on which alkyl chains of different lengths have been grafted. They are compatible with a wide range of organic materials and offer the soft and nongreasy feel of silicones.[7] AMS materials were found to enhance the effectiveness of sunscreen ingredients and increase resistance to wash-off.[8] In addition, they can be used to help build viscosity and add body,[9] reduce moisture loss from the skin via their occlusivity and provide moisturization.[10]

AMS impacts the SPF of a formulation by optimizing its rheology, making it spread easily on the skin during application. This permits an even distribution of the sunscreen, followed by a "rebuild" in viscosity to maintain a homogeneous film of the sunscreen active.[11] In these organo-modified materials, methyl groups are partially replaced by long-chain alkyl groups. Varying the chain length of the silicone backbone and the alkyl group, as well as the degree of substitution, makes it possible to produce three classes of AMSs with a range of melting points (25–70°C): volatile fluids, nonvolatile fluids and waxes.[7]

Cetyl dimethicone is a translucent, white, nonvolatile AMS fluid that imparts substantivity and occlusivity on the skin, retains the soft, nontacky aesthetics of silicones and their emolliency, and provides controlled moisturization. It also demonstrates the key property of increasing the effectiveness of sunscreens—in particular, physical sunscreens. The increased effectiveness in physical sunscreens may be due to an improvement of the dispersion of TiO_2 in the final formulation, reducing the aggregation phenomenon. Cetyl dimethicone is compatible with a broad range of organic cosmetic ingredients and is easy to incorporate into the oil phase of a formula. In most formulations, the fluid can be used to partially or completely replace mineral oil or petrolatum.[8]

Formula 2 illustrates the use of cetyl dimethicone in an o/w sun cream containing physical sunscreens. Addition of the silicone increases the in vitro SPF from 9.1 to 22.4.[7]

Stearyl dimethicone is a soft AMS wax that melts on contact with skin, spreads easily to a thin film and provides moisturizing benefits. Like cetyl dimethicone, it is substantive on the skin for extended protection. While cetyl dimethicone provides the best SPF improvement in physical sunscreens, stearyl dimethicone works best with organic sunscreens as it has the highest impact on the formulation thixotropy, which correlates with an increase of the in vitro SPF.[11] In the case of organic sunscreens such as ethylhexyl methoxycinnamate and butyl methoxydibenzolylmethane, especially with stearyl dimethicone, it has been demonstrated that the silicone forms an intimate blend with the UV absorbers, also helping to form a homogenous film on the skin.[11]

Formula 3 incorporates stearyl dimethicone in an o/w sun lotion, resulting in an in vivo SPF of 49.7.[11] This SPF is reached with 11% UVB absorbers, or an SPF-to-percent UVB ratio of 4.5, thus demonstrating high efficiency. The in vitro SPF value for the same formulation was respectively 43 and 49, measured using an SPF analyzer on a substrate using two different formulation batches.[8] When replacing the stearyl dimethicone with cetyl dimethicone, the in vivo SPF value dropped to 29.4. The in vitro SPF also was measured, resulting in a value of 28. These results show an acceptable correlation between in vivo and in vitro SPF for this specific formulation.[11]

Based on **Formula 3**, additional studies evaluated the impact of stearyl dimethicone on the in vitro SPF of creams containing decreasing levels of organic sunscreen actives (see **Figure 3**).[8]

Formula 2
O/W Sunscreen cream with SPF enhancement
(In vitro SPF 22.4)

A. Cetyl dimethicone (DC 2502 Cosmetic Fluid, Dow Corning)	2.00%w/w
Cyclopentasiloxane (DC 245 Fluid, Dow Corning)	5.00
Paraffinum liquidum (mineral) oil	6.00
Myristyl lactate (Crodamol ML, Croda Inc.)	2.00
Cetyl alcohol	2.00
Glyceryl stearate SE (Cithrol GMS S/E, Croda Inc.)	1.20
Ceteareth-20 (Procol CS-20, Protameen Chemicals Inc.)	0.40
Stearic acid	1.00
Propylparaben	0.05
B. Water (*aqua*)	qs to 100.00
Glycerin	1.00
Triethanolamine	1.00
Aloe vera gel	0.50
Methylparaben	0.15
Titanium dioxide (and) water (aqua) (Tioveil AQ-N, Uniqema)	18.75
C. Fragrance (*parfum*)	qs
D. Imidazolidinyl urea (Sepicide CI, Seppic S.A.)	0.30
	100.00

Procedure: Combine A and heat to 70–75°C. In a separate container, combine B and heat to 70–75°C. Add A to B with gentle mixing. Homogenize using a high shear mixer. Cool to 50°C with mixing. Add C to AB. Continue to cool to 35°C. Add D to batch with stirring.

Formula 3
High protection sun cream (In vivo SPF 49)

A. Carbomer, 1% (Carbopol 980, BF Goodrich Chemical S.A.)	10.00% w/w
Propylene glycol	2.50
B. Potassium hydroxide, 1%	qs
C. Disodium EDTA (Titriplex III Solution, Merck KGaA)	0.10
Water (*aqua*)	qs to 100.00
Ethylhexyl methoxycinnamate	
(Parsol MCX, DSM Nutritional Products)	6.00
Butyl methoxydibenzoylmethane (Parsol 1789,	
DSM Nutritional Products)	3.00
4-Methylbenzylidene camphor (Uvinul MBC 95, BASF)	3.00
Phenyl trimethicone (Dow Corning 556 Cosmetic Grade Fluid)	3.00
Stearyl dimethicone (Dow Corning 2503 Cosmetic Wax)	2.00
Glyceryl stearate (Cithrol GMS N/E, Croda Inc.)	3.00
C12-15 alkyl benzoate (Crodamol AB, Croda Inc.)	4.00
Cetyl alcohol	0.25
Preservative	qs
D. Potassium cetyl phosphate (Amphisol K, DSM Nutritional Products)	2.00
E. Cyclopentasiloxane (Dow Corning 245 Fluid, Dow Corning)	4.00
Tocopheryl acetate (Vitamin E Acetate, Roche Vitamins)	0.50
F. Phenylbenzimidazole sulfonic acid (Parsol HS,	
DSM Nutritional Products)	2.00
Water (*aqua*)	20.00
Potassium hydroxide, 10%	qs
G. bis-PEG-18 methyl ether dimethyl silane (Dow Corning 2501	
Cosmetic Wax, Dow Corning)	<u>2.00</u>
	100.00

Procedure: Mix A. Adjust A to pH 7 with B. Heat AB to 75°C. Mix C and heat to 85°C. Add D to C with gentle mixing. Add AB to CD with strong agitation. Continue mixing while cooling to 45°C. Mix E and add to ABCD with strong agitation. Mix F and adjust to pH 7 with additional B; add to batch. Heat to 30°C and add G to batch. Check pH of final formulation. If necessary, adjust to 7 with additional B. Add water to compensate for water loss during heating.

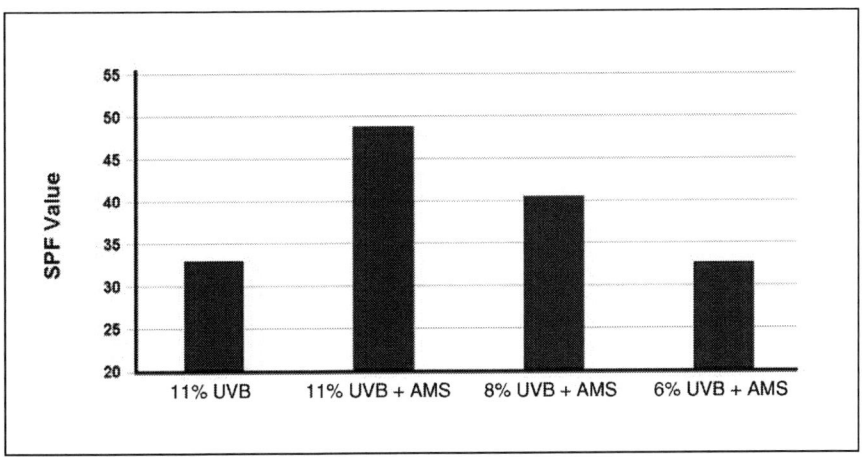

Figure 3. Effect of stearyl dimethicone on in vitro SPF based on decreasing levels of organic sunscreen

Results indicated that the addition of stearyl dimethicone allowed a reduction in the quantity of UVB sunscreen used—from 11% to 6%—to achieve the same SPF value. Both cetyl dimethicone and stearyl dimethicone (samples 2502 and 2503, respectively) demonstrated greater resistance to wash-off compared to other silicone materials (see **Figure 4**).

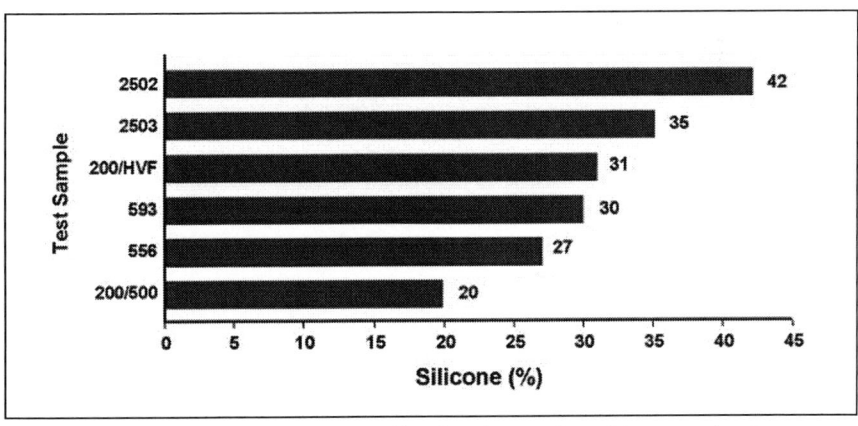

Figure 4. Percent of silicone remaining on skin after three washes with soap and water

Another alkylmethylsiloxane, C30-45 alkyl methicone (and) C30-45 olefin, is a high melt-point wax (70–158°F) whose structural matrix-building properties combine with the rich, smooth and silky sensory aesthetics of silicone. It provides shape and structural integrity for stick-form applications and is used to build viscosity and add body to emulsions. The wax acts as a moisturizing agent and provides occlusivity to help reduce moisture loss. It too can be used to enhance SPF in combination with physical sunscreens, especially in w/o systems, where its structuring ability is the strongest.

Like related AMS materials, the silicone wax is compatible with a variety of organic ingredients, including other waxes, esters, sunscreens, vegetable oils and hydrocarbons. It can be combined with or replace conventional natural and synthetic waxes to minimize the greasy, oily feel. Resulting emulsions also were perceived by a sensory panel as being thicker, with greater "cushion" and body. Depending on the desired characteristics for a formulation, the wax is effective at concentrations from 1–2%.

Formula 4 compares the viscosities of a w/o system containing physical sunscreens with and without the AMS wax. When a 2% addition of the silicone wax replaced an equal portion of mineral oil, the viscosity of the final formulation nearly doubled[8] and the in vitro SPF increased from 9.7 to 17.1.

An internal Dow Corning test method[8] also demonstrated a w/o system containing 2% of this wax improved resistance to wash-off of organic sunscreens; in this case, ethylhexyl methoxycinnamate and avobenzone. Without the wax, 40% of the sunscreens were washed away, compared to less than 5% with the wax.

Phenyl Trimethicone

Phenyl trimethicone, often recognized for its ability to add shine in hair and skin care products, also can contribute to a broad range of sun care products. Phenyl trimethicone spreads easily to form a nonoily, nontacky film that can aid wash-off resistance. The presence of phenyl groups makes it compatible with commonly used organic sunscreens and other ingredients used in sun care formulations. Phenyl trimethicone, like other silicones, can boost SPF. This likely is because of its good spreadability and its compatibility with organic sunscreens. In vitro SPF measurements showed that the addition of 5% phenyl trimethicone to a prototype sunscreen formulation increased in vitro SPF nearly five-fold, from 5.87 to 27.5.[6]

Formula 4
W/O sunscreen with high melt point silicone wax

	% w/w	
	A	B
A. Laurylmethicone copolyol (DC 5200 Formulation Aid, Dow Corning)	3.0	3.0
Ethylhexyl palmitate (and) titanium dioxide (and) alumina (and) polyhydroxystearic acid (and) silica (Tioveil OP, Uniqema)	12.5	12.5
Paraffinum liquidum (mineral) oil (Klearol, Witco)	5.0	7.0
C12-15 alkyl benzoate (Crodamol AB, Croda)	3.0	3.0
Isopropyl myristate	2.0	2.0
C30-45 alkyl methicone (and) C30-45 olefin (DC AMS-C30 Wax, Dow Corning)	2.0	----
Preservative	q.s.	q.s.
B. Water (*aqua*)	qs to 100.0	
C. Sodium chloride	1.0	1.0
Glycerin	4.0	4.0
	100.0	100.0

Procedure: Combine A. Mix until uniform using a dual blade and turbulent style mixing action. Heat to 70–80°C. Combine B. Mix until uniform and heat to 80°C. Increase mixing speed of A to a tip velocity of 900 ft/min (2-in blade = 1376 rpm).
Add B to A very slowly. Addition time should take at least 10 min. Continue mixing for 20 min after B addition is completed. Cool to 45–50°C. Add C to batch and mix well. Cool to RT. Viscosity (cP): (A) 22,400 and (B) 7,500; in vitro SPF: (A) 17.1 and (B) 9.7.

An unusual advantage of phenyl trimethicone is its sand-proofing effect. With its lack of tackiness and greasiness, the ingredient forms a film on the skin that reduces the adherence of sand, as compared to other formulas. Seven formulas, each in its original form and then in a variation incorporating 5% phenyl trimethicone, were applied on the forearms of three panelists for a total of 14 sample formulations per test subject. After application, the forearms were covered with fine sand, which causes poor aesthetics and discomfort because it adheres to skin. Researchers visually observed that less sand was present on the forearms treated with formulations containing phenyl trimethicone.

Ultra HMW Silicone Emulsion

An ultra high molecular weight (HMW) silicone emulsion[a] was developed to design formulas with a high degree of water resistance. The emulsion was applied to two novel formulation concepts—sprayable sun formulas and sun protection wipes for children. **Formula 5** shows an example of the lotion incorporating the HMW silicone emulsion.

Formula 5
Sun care sprayable lotion

A. Sucrose palmitate (and) glyceryl stearate (and) glyceryl stearate citrate (and) sucrose (and) mannan (and) xanthan gum (Arlatone V-175, Uniqema)	1.0% w/w
B. Water (*aqua*)	62.5
C. Glycerin	5.0
Preservative	qs
Disodium EDTA	0.1
D. Ethylhexyl methoxycinnamate (Neo Heliopan AV, Haarman & Reimer)	7.0
Butyl methoxydibenzoylmethane (Neo Heliopan 357, Haarman & Reimer)	2.0
4-methylbenzilidene camphor (Neo Heliopan MBC, Haarman & Reimer)	3.0
Cyclomethicone (DC 345 Fluid, Dow Corning)	3.0
C12-15 alkyl benzoate (Crodamol AB, Croda)	5.0
C15-19 alkane (Gemseal 40, Totalfinaelf)	3.0
E. Divinyldimethicone/dimethicone copolymer (and) C12-13 pareth-3 (and) C12-13 pareth-23 (DC HMW2220 Nonionic Emulsion, Dow Corning)	<u>5.0</u>
	100.0

Procedure: Slowly add A to B. With strong agitation speed, mix for 10 min. Combine C in order with AB, mixing until uniform. Heat to 80°C. In a separate vessel, blend D and heat to 80 °C. Add D to ABC while mixing. Homogenize. Cool to RT. Add E to batch and mix until uniform.

---

[a]HMW 2220 Non-ionic Emulsion (INCI: Divinyldimethicone/dimethicone copolymer (and) C12-13 pareth-23 (and) C12-13 pareth-3) is a product of Dow Corning.

Silicone Elastomers

Silicone elastomer technology offers new formulation options. One versatile material, cyclopentasiloxane (and) dimethicone crosspolymer, is based on a silicone elastomer that forms a gel in a solvent of cyclopentasiloxane. This material was developed to thicken w/o and w/s formulations, as well as volatile cyclic silicones and other silicone fluids, essentially converting these fluids to gels. The elastomer particles entrap the fluid to be thickened, forming a gel matrix structure. The elastomer blend allows cold processing and can be diluted with nonpolar oils or solvents to reduce its viscosity.

The ability of the silicone elastomer blend to enhance SPF in o/w sunscreen formulations containing organic sunscreens has been evaluated through in vivo tests. Two prototype formulations were used; one with a combination of organic sunscreens and the silicone elastomer, the other with the same sunscreen active ingredients but without the silicone elastomer blend. Although the mechanism behind this effect is not completely understood, it likely results from the impact of the silicone elastomer on the formulation rheology.[12]

The addition of 4% silicone elastomer blend to a sun care formulation containing organic sunscreens increased the in vivo SPF from 5.7 to 18 (**Figure 5**). This SPF enhancing property of the silicone elastomer allows formulators to maximize the effectiveness of sunscreen agents in a formulation while reducing the amount needed to achieve the desired SPF. Other important characteristics afforded by the silicone elastomer are the unique sensory properties of silkiness, powdery feel and reduced glossiness.

Formula 6 illustrates the use of silicone elastomer in the highly efficient sunscreen of **Figure 5**.

Using an internal test method,[8] researchers screened a variety of silicones in o/w and w/o formulations and compared them with a common organic resin benchmark. A formulation containing phenyl trimethicone was mixed with the organic resin to reduce the tackiness associated with the material and to make it aesthetically more comparable to the same formulation substituted with a silicone elastomer blend that ultimately imparts a smooth feel to the final formulation.

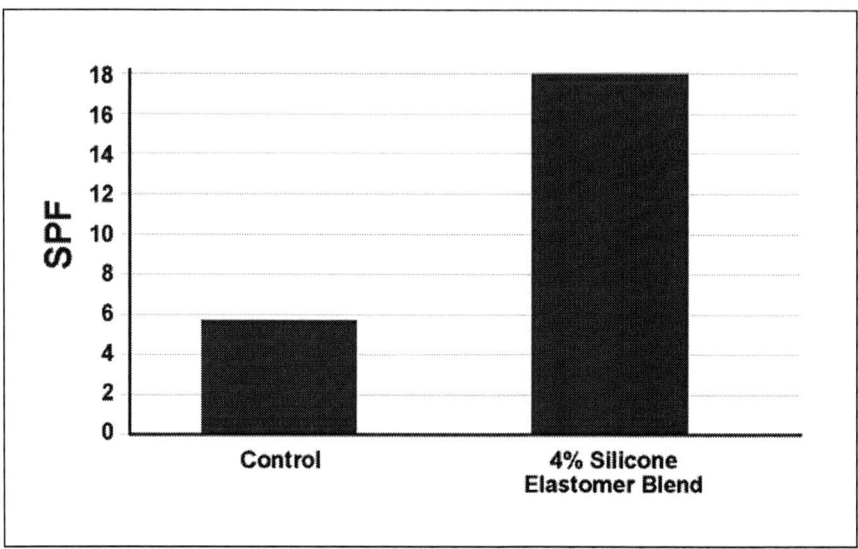

Figure 5. Silicone elastomer blend as an SPF enhancer

Table 1
Screening of materials with wash-off simulator

Test Material Screened	% Ethylhexyl Methoxycinnamate Washed Away	% Butyl Methoxydibenzoylmethane Washed Away
Oil-in-Water Systems		
Control	31	30
PVP/eicosene copolymer/ phenyl trimethicone (3%/3%)	20	17
Cyclopentasiloxane (and) dimethicone cross-polymer (and) cyclohexasiloxane (4%)	19	16
Water-in-Oil Systems		
Control	39	38
PVP/eicosene copolymer/phenyl trimethicone (3%/3%)	24	24
Cyclopentasiloxane (and) dimethicone cross-polymer (and) cyclohexasiloxane (4%)	14	11

Table 1 summarizes the results of the screening studies. Initial tests were conducted for two organic sunscreens—ethylhexyl methoxycinnamate and butyl methoxydibenzoylmethane. In o/w systems, performance equal to the organic resin was obtained in the formulation using 4% silicone elastomer blend. This formulation also showed superior sensory characteristics due to the presence of the silicone elastomer. The internal SPF screening results indicated a loss of 19% and 17%, respectively.

Formula 6
O/W sunscreen (in vivo SPF 18)

A. Ethylhexyl methoxycinnamate (Parsol MCX, DSM Nutritional Products)	4.0% w/w
Butyl methoxydibenzoylmethane (Parsol 1789, DSM Nutritional Products)	1.5
Stearyl dimethicone (DC 2503 Cosmetic Wax, Dow Corning)	2.0
Glyceryl stearate (Cithrol GMS N/E, Croda)	3.0
Caprylic/capric triglyceride (Crodamol GTCC, Croda)	3.0
Phenoxyethanol (and) methylparaben (and) ethylparaben (and) propylparaben (and) butylparaben (Sepicide HB, Seppic)	0.5
B. Potassium cetyl phosphate (Amphisol K, DSM Nutritional Products)	2.0
C. Water (*aqua*)	to 100.0
D. Carbomer (Carbopol 980, BF Goodrich)	0.1
E. Propylene glycol	3.5
Disodium EDTA (Titriplex III, Merck KGaA)	0.1
F. Potassium hydroxide, 10% (Potassium Hydroxide, Merck KGaA)	qs
G. Cyclopentasiloxane (DC 245 Fluid, Dow Corning)	4.0
Cyclopentasiloxane (and) dimethicone crosspolymer (DC 9040 Silicone Elastomer Blend, Dow Corning)	<u>4.0</u>
	100.00

Procedure: Combine A. Using a water bath, heat A to 85°C and mix until uniform. Add B to A and mix while keeping the temperature at 85°C. In a separate container, heat C to 75°C and disperse D in C until homogeneous. Add E to CD and neutralize with F until pH 7. Ensure temperature is kept at 75°C. Add AB to CDEF with strong agitation. Continue mixing while cooling to 40°C. Blend G in a separate container and add to batch with strong agitation. Cool to RT while mixing. Check the pH and adjust with additional F (10%) if necessary. Add water to compensate for water loss during the heating phase. Incorporate the formulation in aerosol cans (two-chamber spraying system from MEGATEC GmbH, Germany).

As a comparison, an in vivo wash off resistance test was conducted according to FDA guidelines on **Formula 6** incorporating 4% ethylhexylmethoxycinnamate and 1.5% avobenzone. For an initial value of 18 prior to immersion, the SPF value after immersion was 10. The internal test method also measured a loss of 19% and 17%, indicating a reasonable correlation between the test methods.

In w/o, the silicone elastomer blend showed good wash-off resistance, whereas the organic resin did not perform as well.[13] This data indicates that in final in vivo tests, one could expect improvement in wash-off resistance when using the silicone elastomer blend.

In skin care applications, the ability of silicone elastomers to absorb various oils and sebum is also important when considering the formulation of specialty sun care products.[14] Among the newest of these materials is a silicone elastomer cosmetic powder, dimethicone/vinyl dimethicone crosspolymer (and) silica.

Sun Care for Hair

Global hair care market trend reports indicate that consumer use of hair colorants has significantly increased. Because hair colorants damage the hair cuticle and leave the hair brittle, dull and dry, consumers with colored hair seek specialized treatments to maintain healthy hair. Washing is the main parameter affecting fading and significant color loss can be observed after one shampooing. Rinse-off conditioner applications also contribute to hair discoloration. However, because the effects of UV exposure can intensify these effects, formulators are challenged to develop hair care products that help reduce discoloration from both sources.

Although silicones do not directly protect against UV rays as organic sunscreens do, studies have demonstrated that the use of rinse-off conditioners containing silicones help to protect hair treated with permanent dyes against discoloration caused by UV radiation. A study was conducted to evaluate different silicones.

To replicate normal conditions of wear and shampooing over time, a protocol was developed to include up to six wash cycles, coupled with UV exposure cycles.[15] Hair was first colored with a leading commercial permanent color-ant, then washed with a commercial shampoo without silicones, followed by treatment with a rinse-off conditioner containing silicones to be evaluated and exposure to UV light for 7 h. The hair was washed for 1 min and rinsed with water at 37°C. A variety of silicone types including amine-functional silicones, silicone elastomers, a silicone polyether and a high molecular weight silicone emulsion were formulated into a prototype rinse-off conditioner for evaluation. Color measurements were taken with a colorimeter/spectrophotometer after 7 h of exposure in a UV chamber, and hair was evaluated by a Dow Corning internal panel for its sensory attributes.

The study helped to identify silicone families that preserved the color of hair exposed to UV radiation and washing, and also that provided conditioning benefits such as shine, improved drying time, moisturization and a smooth, light feel without negatively impacting body and volume. Results of rinse-off conditioner evaluations indicated that silicones showed excellent potential for their ability to aid in color-lock. Although one silicone type did not stand out for overall best performance in color retention, all of the silicones tested proved good in color retention in general.[12]

In addition to amodimethicone and amodimethicone (and) C12-14 sec-pareth-7 (and) C12-14 sec-pareth-5, other silicone materials showed promise for use in these applications, including silicone polyether and the ultra high molecular weight dimethicone and silicone elastomer emulsion, giving formulators broader latitude in selecting the type of silicone most suitable for benefits beyond color protection.

Conclusions

Silicones provide formulators with choices for a variety of sun care product forms and delivery systems—from creams to lotions, sprays to sticks, and mousses to gels—and benefits such as protection of hair. Advanced silicone technology offers silicones that are substantive on the skin to help prevent wash-off so that sun care products are optimized and last longer.

Combined with organic or inorganic sunscreens, silicones also can boost the SPF of sun care formulations, making it possible to develop products with greater protection and enhanced claims without added cost. Additionally, in products designed for children or individuals with sensitive skin, silicones may lower the levels needed of potentially irritating sunscreen actives while maintaining the degree of protection.

Because of their proven impact on SPF, silicones also are very good candidates for skin care, color cosmetic and self-tanning products where sun protection also is needed. With their differing sets of properties, silicone materials offer combinations of performance characteristics or compatibilities for individual formulations. By considering a range of silicone options, formulators can capitalize on the characteristics of these versatile ingredients.

Published October 2006 Cosmetics and Toiletries magazine

References

1. Sun Care, *The world market for cosmetics and toiletries*, Euromonitor 15 (2005)
2. DiSapio, Silicones as adjuvants in sun products, *Cosm & Toil*, 102 3 102–106 (1987)
3. Cosmetic Research/USA News (2002–2004)
4. Cosmetic Research/Fiches France (2002–2004)
5. HM van Dort, A Urrutia, G Brissette, P Pretzer, R Haller, I van Reeth and V Caprasse, Silicone Carbinol Fluid, *Household and Personal Care Product Industry*, 41 8 77–80 (2004)
6. M Starch, H Van Dort, M Pretzer, A new in vitro approach for screening SPF values in sun care product development, poster at *Florida Sunscreen Symposium* (Sept 2005)
7. G LeGrow, A Wilson and A Harashima, Alkylmethylsiloxanes: A novel family of silicone-organic hybrid polymers for the cosmetic industry, presented at the *17th IFSCC International Congress*, Yokohama, Japan (Oct 13–16, 1992)
8. I Van Reeth and J Blakely, Use of current and new test methods to demonstrate the benefits of alkylmethylsiloxanes in sun care products, presented at the *European UV Sunfilter Conference*, Paris, France (Nov 3–4, 1999)
9. I van Reeth and A Wilson, Understanding factors which influence permeability of silicones and their derivatives, *Cosm & Toil*, 109 7 87–92 (1994)
10. I van Reeth and M Starch, Novel silicone thickening technologies: Delivering the appropriate rheology profile to optimize formulation performance, *J of Appl Cosmet* 213 97–107 (2003)
11. I Van Reeth, F Dahman and J Hannington, Alkylmethylsiloxanes as SPF enhancers: Relationship between effects and physico-chemical properties, presented at the *19th IFSCC Congress*, Sydney, Australia (Oct 22–25, 1996)
12. Silicone Elastomer Blends as Ingredients to Increase the Sun Protection Factor (SPF) of Personal Care Formulations, research disclosure, 442 252–253 (2001)
13. I Van Reeth, New method for the evaluation of wash-off resistance of organic sunscreen, Dow Corning internal report (2001)
14. G Gacic-Vukovljak, I Li and A Vagts, Next-generation applications for silicone elastomers: Beyond superior feel in skin care, presented at *Personal Care Ingredients Asia*, Shanghai, China (Mar 19–21, 2002)
15. B Moss, V Ungvary and S Marchioretto, Silicones as color-lock aid in rinse-off hair care products, *Dow Corning internal publication* (2003), www.dowcorning.com/content/publishedlit/27-1152-01.pdf. (Accessed on Jan 19, 2006)

CHAPTER 27

Thermoplastic Silicone Elastomers Improve Nail Polish Performance

Dr. Arndt Schlosser and Lois Hassenzahl
Wacker Chemical Corporation, Adrian, Mich., USA

KEY WORDS: *elastomer, scratch resistance, chip-off, tear strength, energy absorption properties, nail polish*

ABSTRACT: *A new thermoplastic silicone elastomer (TPSE) is shown here to improve scratch resistance, chip-off, feel, smoothness, gloss, and color in a nail polish formulation when compared with a formulation without TPSE. The new ingredient proves to be an interesting technology for optimizing nail polishes.*

Editor's Note: The use of this substance has been banned from the European Union (EU). In the US, it was added to the California list of teratogens in November 2006 and all major producers began eliminating it from nail polishes in the Fall of 2006.

Nail polishes are one of the traditional applications in color cosmetics and have been well developed over the years. Yet consumers are still looking for nail polishes with attributes such as more scratch resistance and less sensitivity to chipping. Such products would enable consumers to reduce the reapplication of nail polish by minimizing the damage occurring from daily life. We tested the ability of thermoplastic silicone elastomers[a] (TPSE) to improve the film-forming and elastomeric properties of nail polish formulations.

---

[a]The Geniomer line of TPSEs is a product of the Wacker Chemical Corporation

Technology

Silicone polyurea copolymers are TPSEs.[1] The basic technology behind these products is the copolymerization of α-ω aminosilicone fluids with diisocyanates.[2-4] As shown in **Figure 1**, the resulting silicone polyurea copolymer has alternating silicone soft blocks and so-called organic hard blocks.

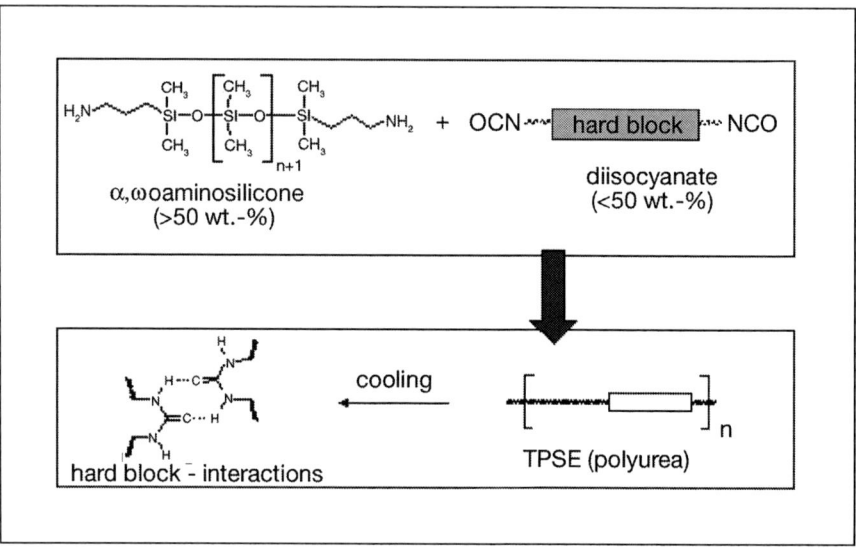

Figure 1. Mechanism for the copolymerization to a TPSE

The thermoplastic properties of TPSEs are based on intermolecular interactions. Hydrogen bridge bonds make them elastomers at low temperatures. An increase in temperature loosens these bonds, causing the products to soften and finally to become liquid. Lowering the temperature reverses this process and reverts the product back to its elastomeric state. The temperature at which softening begins can be adjusted by ratio and type of soft and hard blocks used in the reaction. This reversible property of TPSEs makes formulating easier.

Properties

TPSEs have several other interesting properties:[5,6]

- They have good tear strength.
- They absorb energy and "fill-in" scratches or marks.

- They are transparent and the first kind of silicone elastomers that can be easily colored (see sidebar)
- They provide a smooth feeling to the surface.

The combination of these properties should allow the formulation of a one-step, colored nail polish that improves scratch resistance, nail feel and chip-off. We tested TPSEs in nail polishes for increasing scratch resistance and chip-off.

Formulation

A nail polish without TPSE was our standard; its composition is shown in **Table 1**. We then modified this standard formulation by adding 25% of a 20% active ethanol TPSE solution, resulting in a 5% TPSE nail polish formulation. The TPSE was predissolved in ethanol to make incorporation into the formulation easier. This solution was added to phase A as shown in **Table 1**.

Table 1
Nail polish formulas used in this study (a) without TPSE and (b) with TPSE

	a	b
A. Cellulose nitrate	13.3	10.0
TPSE (20% active in ethanol)	----	25.0
Ethyl acetate	26.7	20.0
Butyl acetate	16.7	12.5
Dibutyl phthalate*	9.3	7.0
Toluene	34.0	25.5
B. Fragrance (parfum)	qs	qs
Preservative	qs	qs
Color	qs	qs

*See Editor's note regarding the regulatory status of dibutyl phthalate

Test Methods

One complete coat of each nail formulation was applied with a commercially available brush to artificial resin nails purchased from a local nail salon. The nails were allowed to dry for 24 hours under standard test conditions (approx. 70ºC, standard humidity). The coated nails were then evaluated for scratch resistance, chip-off, feel, smoothness, color, and shine.

Scratch resistance: Scratch resistance was evaluated by placing nails painted with the standard formulation and those treated with the TPSE-containing formulation into a standard lab rotator partially filled with round metal beads (4.5 mm diameter). Both nails were placed in the rotator and tumbled. Every 5 minutes, up to 30 minutes, the rotator was stopped and the nails were evaluated.

Chip-off: To study chip-off, the different nail polishes were applied in squares (approx. 5 cm X 5 cm) to aluminum panels (15 cm long X 7.5 cm wide X 0.5 mm thick). These panels were placed with the color side down onto a block with a hole in the center. A weight of 2 pounds was dropped from defined heights through a tube centered over the hole in the base block. The starting height was 5 in., and we increased it in 5-in. increments up to 35 in. For this test we examined not only the standard sample formulation and the TPSE-containing formulation (see **Table 1**) but also a commercially available nail polish.

In a second series of tests, the aluminum sheet was placed onto the block with the colored side up so the weight hit directly on the nail polish. For the color check, we used a colorimeter[b] (via the L*a*b color system) to measure the influence of the TPSE on the color of the nail polish.

Sensory evaluation: Feel, smoothness, and shine were evaluated by 22 test panelists. During the panel test, the artificial nail coated with the standard formula was compared with the formula containing TPSE. The test was set up as a blind evaluation so panelists did not know which samples were which.

Results

Scratch resistance: During the rotator scratch-resistance test, the TPSE-containing formulation showed no change in appearance or color after the total 30 minutes. No scratches/

---

[b]968 colorimeter is a product of X-Rite.

marks or discoloration were observed. The nail treated with the standard formula showed the first visible changes after 15 minutes. After 30 minutes, several marks and areas with color loss were observed and the nail was split at one end. **Figure 2** shows both nails tested with the different formulations, before and after the test.

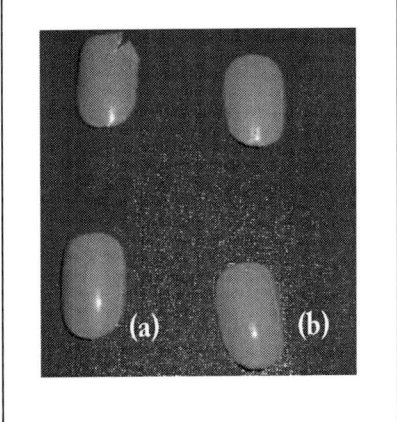

Figure 2. Scratch resistance test: (a) the standard formulation vs. (b) the TPSE-containing formulation. The bottom nails are before the experiment, the top are after the experiment.

Chip-off: The nail polish containing TPSE did not show any color peel-off or chip-off up to a maximum height of 30 inches. No differences were observed before or after the treatment. The first minor damage was seen at 35 inches and it made no difference whether the aluminum sheet was faced with its colored side up or down on the block, so even a direct hit from the weight did not cause visible damage. The commercially available nail polish showed color chip-off beginning at five inches and the standard formulation at ten inches. A comparison of these results is shown in **Figure 3**.

The height where first damage is visible was compared for the three different nail polishes. The addition of 5% TPSE improved the performance by 3.5 times, compared to the standard formulation.

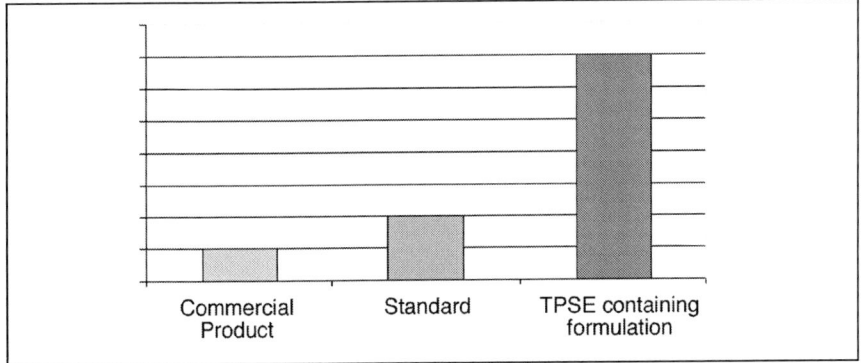

Figure 3. Comparison of height first damage in chip-off tests

Color: The addition of the TPSE to the formulation did not change the color when examined via the L*a*b method. Both samples have a C value of 73.3 ± 0.5. C is defined as $C = (a^2 + b^2)^{1/2}$. Lightness (L) is 49.7 ± 0.8 for both.

Panel test: During the panel test, the TPSE formula was rated by 92 % of the panelists as the sample with better feel and by 90 % of panelists as having better smoothness. In the evaluation of shine, the panelists group was split; 53 % said the standard showed more gloss and 47 % rated the TPSE formula higher. Detailed results are shown in **Figure 4**.

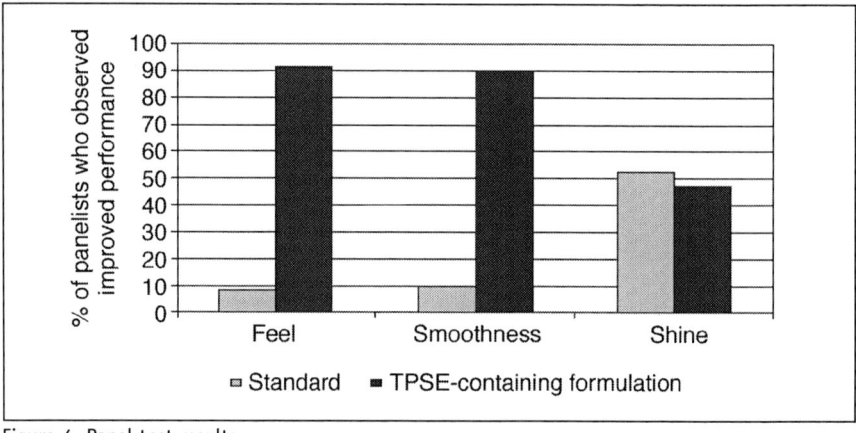

Figure 4. Panel test results

Discussion

The given results show that the addition of 5 % TPSE to a standard nail polish improved the properties of scratch resistance, chip-off, feel and smoothness but does not affect the color or shine of the nail polish. The improvement of scratch resistance can be explained by the tear strength and energy absorption properties of the TPSE. Because of the tear resistance, the nail polish film does not crack. The energy absorption and flexibility of the ingredient help to protect the nail polish from marks. The better performance in the chip-off test can also be explained by the high flexibility of the film build of TPSE.

One formulation benefit of TPSE is that it can be used in existing colorant compositions without the need to reformulate them, since it does not affect color. This property is caused by the transparency of the ingredient and its compatibility with colors. It also makes it one of the first paintable silicone-based polymers (see sidebar).

> **Paintable Silicone-Based Polymers**
>
> All silicone elastomers are not paintable. If you take a silicone elastomer, you can color it by incorporating pigments into it, but you cannot paint over it because of the hydrophilicity of the silicone. TPSEs are silicone-based elastomers that can be painted over because of their combination of silicone and organic components in one material.
>
> -Arndt Schlosser

The panel test results can be explained by typical silicone elastomer properties. Silicones are known for providing a smooth and very pleasant feel. Because of the transparent film, we did not expect a major change in shine. This expectation was proven by the panel test results showing no preference in shine for either the standard or TPSE-containing formulations.

Conclusion

The results of our studies show that the new technology can be used to optimize a nail polish according to scratch resistance, chip-off and feel. It demonstrated a significant improvement against a standard formulation and outperformed a commercially available nail polish in the chip-off test. These improvements came along with a smoother feel of the applied nail polish.

At the same time for the nail polish important properties as color and shine stayed unchanged, so a reformulation of existing products can be easily done without the need of adjusting the color composition.

Published July 2005 Cosmetics and Toiletries magazine

References

1. O Schaefer, J Weis, S Delica, F Csellich and A Kneissl, Thermoplastic Silicone Elastomers, poster presentation, 2nd European Silicone Days, Munich (2003)
2. DE 10137855, Organo-polysiloxane/polyurea/polyurethane block copolymers, Schafer et al, assigned to Wacker (October 21, 2004)

3. WO 03014194, Organo-polysiloxane/polyurea/polyurethane block copolymers, Pachaly et al, assigned to Wacker (October 21, 2004)
4. DE10141235, Moisture crosslinking elastic composition, Schindler et al, assigned to Wacker (December 23, 2004)
5. Technical Data Sheets, Geniomer 60, 80, 100, 140, 200; Wacker Chemie GmbH, www.geniomer.com (2004)
6. Geniomer product brochure; Wacker Chemie GmbH (2004)

CHAPTER 28

Silicone Compounds– New Formulation Possibilities

Anthony J. O'Lenick Jr.
Siltech LLC, Dacula, Georgia USA

Thomas G. O'Lenick
Department of Chemistry, Georgia Southern University, Statesboro, Georgia USA

KEY WORDS: *Silicone compounds, water solubility, wetting, alkyl dimethicones, silicone waxes*

ABSTRACT: *Tapping into little understood products selected from a class of well known compounds can provide formulation advantages. PEG/PPG dimethicone compounds, alkyl dimethicone compounds and alkyl PEG/PPG dimethicone compounds are three classes of compounds that offer far more utility in personal care products than is generally appreciated by formulators.*

Silicone compounds have been known since the 1860s, but have seen explosive growth in their utilization since the late 1980s. In the early days, silicone fluids were essentially the only type of silicone polymer used. They are still widely used in many personal care applications, for example conditioning in hair care products and in pigmented products. There are however a large number of formulations in which silicone fluids cannot be used, due in large part to their inherent insolubility in oil and water. There are many silicone polymers that offer functional attributes in aqueous and oil-based systems that remain largely unappreciated. The classes of compounds are known but the selection of the lesser-known products can provide benefits not offered by the better-understood products.

Silicones with Increased Water Solubility

PEG/PPG dimethicone compounds: PEG/PPG dimethicone compounds are a very versatile class of compounds that, in addition to offering increased water solubility over silicone fluids, can be altered to provide properties like wetting, emulsification and conditioning. The products of this class have been known by a variety of names over the years. Our industry is most comfortable calling them dimethicone copolyols, notwithstanding the switch to the term PEG/PPG dimethicone. In other industries, these products are referred to as silicone glycols, silicone super wetting agents, and silicone surfactants. Regardless of what they are called, they are a class of compounds that offer many formulation benefits. They conform to the structure shown in **Figure 1**.

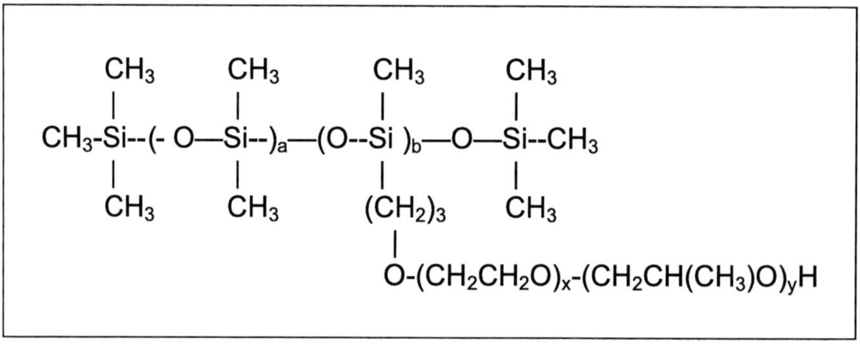

$$\begin{array}{cccc} CH_3 & CH_3 & CH_3 & CH_3 \\ | & | & | & | \\ CH_3-Si-(-O-Si-)_a-(O-Si\;)_b-O-Si-CH_3 \\ | & | & | & | \\ CH_3 & CH_3 & (CH_2)_3 & CH_3 \\ & & | & \\ & & O\text{-}(CH_2CH_2O)_x\text{-}(CH_2CH(CH_3)O)_yH \end{array}$$

Figure 1. Structure of dimethicone copolyol compounds

Depending on the exact structure and molecular weight, the compounds of this class can be what are called super wetters, traditional wetting agents, conditioners or emulsifiers.

Creating formulations requires the ability to pick ingredients for a variety of formulation functions. For example, a number of functions need to be incorporated into a hair conditioner. First, there needs to be a cationic agent that provides antistatic properties and conditioning. Second, there needs to be a wetting agent that allows for thorough and efficient spreading of the conditioning agent over the hair to avoid "gunkiness." Third, there needs to be an agent that reduces the fiber-to-fiber friction, resulting in better wet comb. And lastly, it is advisable to add ingredients that improve gloss.

These attributes come not from one but a number of compounds. Some need to be low molecular weight compounds, others high molecular weight, some branched polymers and others linear - and polymers need to have an increased refractive index.

Silicones are currently used for each and every application, but one silicone cannot provide all properties. The obligation for this selection falls upon the formulator, who not only must answer all these technical questions but at the same time provide a product to marketing that meets the perceived needs of the consumer, is cost effective and is free of infringing the plethora of patents covering such products. It is no wonder product development has become a more difficult, time-consuming activity than it was 20 years ago.

The variability of relatively well known silicones to provide differing functionalities is a good reason why these materials continue to experience growth in the personal care market. Knowledge of the structure/function attributes of these materials is key to efficient formulation. To demonstrate this, we have chosen a homologous series of compounds each having 8 moles of polyoxyethylene present. Although the total molecular weight increases over the series, the equivalent molecular weight changes little. What we are essentially doing is putting more and more groups on the molecule, knitting them together. This results not only in the modification of molecular weight but in very different performance properties. **Table 1** shows the differences in properties of the tested series of compounds as a function of molecular weight.

Wetting: Wetting is a very important phenomenon that is key to the formulation of cost efficient products. However, the term has been confused in different ways. The term "super wetting" is one term. We prefer "super spreader," because we believe it is more technically correct. The term relates to the ability of a 1% solution of the test surfactant to spread spontaneously on paraffin without mechanical means. This attribute is very important to the formulation and use of agricultural products, because they are often sprayed on waxy plants and left to spread without any additional touching of the leaf.

Table 1
The differences in properties of the tested series of PEG/PPG dimethicone compounds as a function of molecular weight

Product	Molecular Weight	Wetting 0.1% Sol	CMC mg/L @ CMC	Surface Tension 1 day/7day	Eye Irritation	Super Wetting
A-008	633	7 sec	20	20	28 / 4	56
A-208	855	8 sec	20	20	13 / 2	5
B-208	1398	10 sec	20	20	5 / 2	2
C-208	2105	18 sec	23	22	4 / 0	2
D-208	2706	257 sec	23	22	2 / 0	2
J-208	6334	-	23	23	0 / 0	-

The trisiloxane[a] is the only product in the series that demonstrates these properties. However, it also is the material with the most limited hydrolytic stability and is the highest eye and skin irritant. Blending this material with another silicone glycol has been done, but neither overcomes the hydrolytic instability of the trisiloxane, nor does it improve the wetting of the non-trisiloxane component.

While super wetting is very structure specific, thankfully, Draves Wetting – the ability to sink a cotton skein in a surfactant solution – is far less restrictive in terms of structure than super spreading. This type of wetting is of much more interest in our industry, since we always use application techniques that are more complicated than simple spraying, and the substrate is always more complex than paraffin.

We have observed that there is a gradual increase in wetting time as a function of increased molecular weight. Eye irritation of the surfactant drops off as molecular weight increases. This means there are a relatively large number of compounds that have outstanding Draves Wetting, and at the same time low irritation.

Wetting turns out to be a critical factor in almost every application for silicone surfactants. Silicone surfactants used for conditioning are high molecular weight materials. They are

---
[a]Silsurf A-008 is a product of Siltech, LLC.

also poor wetting agents. Therefore these high molecular weight surfactants have difficulty spreading uniformly on substrates, resulting in non-uniform films. It is recommended that a lower molecular weight silicone surfactant be added to wet out the higher molecular weight silicone surfactant. This is true for textile fabrics, plastics and hair. Since wetting occurs at or below the critical micelle concentration (CMC), one should add enough to have the product present at that concentration available after the formulation has been cut to use concentration.

Table 1 describes the molecular weight of several of the products and describes the wetting time for those same compounds. As can be easily seen, these products show quite a variation in the speed of wetting. The formulator can choose any one of these products for the specific properties it delivers.

The proper selection of silicone polyether for a given application will most likely include a lower molecular weight product for wetting and a higher molecular weight component for slip and feel modification as well as a silicone quaternary compound for conditioning.

Silicone Compounds with Increased Oil Solubility

Alkyl dimethicones: Alkyl dimethicones are another class of compounds of which many cosmetic chemists know a great deal about a very narrow subsection. This is because the commercial offering of most suppliers is highly limited. If one takes the time to explore the structure/function relationship between the alkyl chain length and the length of the silicone portion, the products offer a far wider range of formulation possibilities. Alkyl dimethicone compounds conform to the structure shown in **Figure 2**.

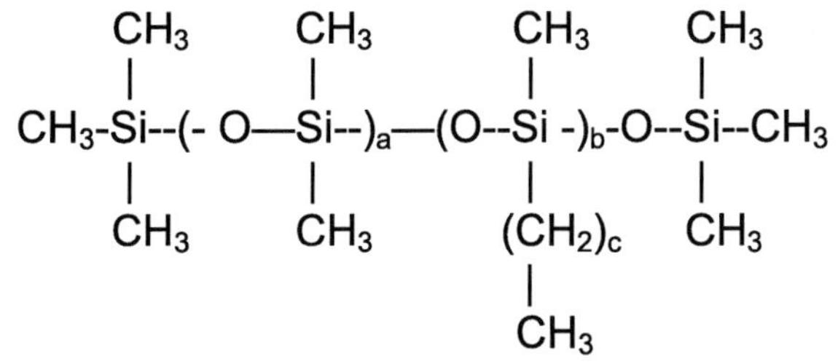

$$CH_3-\underset{\underset{CH_3}{|}}{\overset{\overset{CH_3}{|}}{Si}}--(-O—\underset{\underset{CH_3}{|}}{\overset{\overset{CH_3}{|}}{Si}}--)_a—(O--\underset{\underset{(CH_2)_c-CH_3}{|}}{\overset{\overset{CH_3}{|}}{Si}}-)_b-O--\underset{\underset{CH_3}{|}}{\overset{\overset{CH_3}{|}}{Si}}--CH_3$$

Figure 2. Structure of alkyl dimethicone compounds

The inclusion of a very small amount of alkyl group into the molecule results in a product that is soluble in mineral oil (**Table 2**). This solubility offers the ability to use these materials in a variety of clear systems based upon many oils, where the use of silicone fluids in these systems is not possible.

Table 2
Solubility (10% Weight) of alkyl dimethicones

Product	Water oil	Mineral spirits	Mineral	PG	D-5	Sil fluid 350 visc	Iso-propanol	Aromatic hydrocarbon
Cerotyl dimethicone (Silwax D-026, Siltech)	I	S	D	I	D	D	I	D
Cerotyl dimethicone (Silwax J-226, Siltech)	I	S	S	I	D	D	I	S
Stearyl dimethicone (Silwax H-418, Siltech)	I	S	S	I	D	I	I	S
Stearyl dimethicone (Silwax L-118, Siltech)	I	S	S	I	I	I	I	S

Note: I = insoluble D = dispersible S = soluble

Physical Properties of Silicone Waxes

There are several important trends that become apparent when one looks at the structure/property relationships in **Tables 3** and **4**. These trends include:

- The length of the alkyl chain has a dramatic effect upon the melt point of the wax. Waxes based upon alkyl groups having between 12 and 16 carbon units are liquids at room temperature. At carbon lengths of 18 and above, products become solid and the melt point increases as the carbon length goes up.
- The amount of silicone in the molecule for a given alkyl length has a minimal impact on melting point.
- The amount of silicone in the molecule for a given alkyl length

has a minimal effect on wax hardness. As the amount of alkyl group in a wax is increased in a wax having over 18 carbon atoms in the alkyl group, the wax becomes harder.

Table 3
Structure/Property relationships of silicone waxes having differing amounts of alkyl group on same silicone backbone

Wax	Alkyl Group	State RT	% Silicone	% Alkyl	MP (oC)
Lauryl dimethicone	Lauryl	Liquid	82.0	18.0	Liquid(thin)
Cetyl dimethicone	Cetyl	Liquid	77.0	23.0	Liquid (thin)
Stearyl dimethicone	Stearyl	Liquid	75.0	25.0	Liquid (viscous)
Behenyl dimethicone	Behenyl	Soft solid	72.0	28.0	20.0
Cerotyl dimethicone	Cerotyl	Solid	68.0	32.0	46.0
Lacceroic dimethicone	Lacceroic	Hard solid	64.0	36.0	60.5

Table 4
Structure/Property relationships of silicone waxes having differing amounts of silicone using the same alkyl group

Wax	Alkyl Group	State RT	% Silicone	% Alkyl	MP (oC)
Cerotyl dimethicone (Silwax D1026, Siltech)	Cerotyl	Solid	69.0	31.0	42.0
Cerotyl dimethicone (Silwax D2026, Siltech)	Cerotyl	Solid	81.0	19.0	37.0
Cerotyl dimethicone (Silwax D3026, Siltech)	Cerotyl	Solid	86.0	14.0	36.0
Stearyl dimethicone (Silwax H-418, Siltech)	Stearyl	Liquid	61.0	39.0	Liquid (Thin)
Stearyl dimethicone (Silwax P-418, Siltech)	Stearyl	Soft Solid	58.0	42.0	Liquid (Viscous)
Steryl dimeyhicone (Silwax L-118, Siltech)	Stearyl	Soft Solid	38.0	62.0	30.0

Understanding these trends allows for the selection of a wax for the specific application chosen. All silicone waxes offer improved oil solubility over silicone fluids. Waxes added to oil phases offer an ability to alter the viscosity and skin feel of a formulation. Mineral oil can be gelled by addition of the proper wax. Petrolatum can be thinned out and made less grainy by adding liquid waxes. The play time at a given melt point can be altered by selecting the specific alkyl chain (melt point) and adding differing amounts of silicone to the molecule (hardness).

In addition, silicone waxes are great at minimizing syneresis in pigmented products. The alteration of the amount of alkyl group relative to silicone group determines which wax is best at lowering syneresis in a given formula.

Modification of the physical properties of esters: Silicone waxes can be added not only to mineral oil-based products to modify melt point, hardness, play time, viscosity, syneresis and the like, they can be added to esters and other more polar products to alter the very same properties.

The addition of two different products, both having the same INCI name, can provide very different properties when blended into common cosmetic esters at 10% by weight. The differences are both in physical form and in properties.

Silicone Compounds as Emulsifiers

Alkyl dimethicone copolyol compounds: Alkyl dimethicone copolyol compounds are a series of surface active materials that contain both alkyl- and water-soluble groups on the same polymer. These very versatile emulsifiers conform to the structure shown in **Figure 3**. **Formula 1** shows the functionality of these emulsifiers.

A series of products has been designed with different solubilities in a variety of solvents. These molecules are described in terms of the percentage by weight of the water-soluble groups present as well as by the percentage of hydrocarbon group present. This is because the introduction of three mutually insoluble groups into a molecule results in the need for more descriptive information than is needed with standard surfactants that have only hydrocarbon-soluble groups and oil-soluble groups.

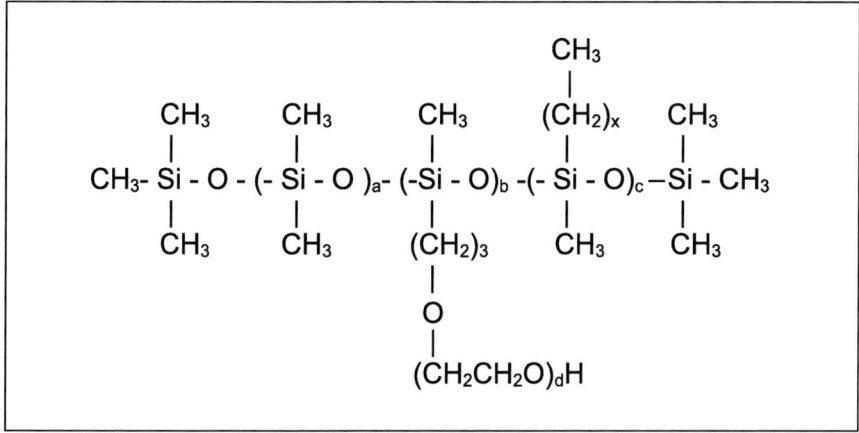

Figure 3. Structure of alkyl dimethicone copolyol compounds

Formula 1
W/O emulsion

A. Lauryl dimethicone copolyol (Silsurf J-208-812, Siltech)	5.0% wt/wt
D-5 Cyclomethicone	35.0
B. Water (*aqua*)	59.0
NaCl	1.0
	100.0

Procedure: Mix A and B separately. Add B to A and mix until uniform.

Silicone surfactants result in a less sticky, more cosmetically elegant emulsions than do the standard fatty surfactants; this is particularly in invert emulsions, the so called water-in-oil emulsions.

Solubility: The polymers from this class of materials become more water-soluble as the percentage of water-soluble group increases. As the percentage of water-soluble group decreases the polymers go from water-dispersible to water-insoluble. The interesting fact is that all products are soluble in isopropanol, regardless of their solubility in water.

Other properties: The inclusion of alkyl groups having 16 or more carbon atoms in the alkyl group results in a product that offers improved wet comb when compared to PEG dimethicone compounds.

Conclusion

Fatty esters can be modified for skin feel, viscosity, and other aesthetic properties by the addition of alkyl dimethicones. The modifications can result in clear gels. This ability to modify the properties is an important attribute of alkyl silicones making them cost effective additives of many formulations.

Published April 2005 Cosmetics and Toiletries magazine

CHAPTER 29

Equilibration Reaction of Silicone Fluids

Anthony J. O'Lenick Jr.
Siltech LLC, Dacula, Georgia USA

Kirk N. Wiegel
Department of Chemistry, University of Wisconsin, Eau Claire, Wisconsin USA

Thomas G. O'Lenick
Department of Chemistry, Georgia Southern University, Statesboro, Georgia USA

KEY WORDS: *Silicone compounds, water solubility, wetting, alkyl dimethicones, silicone waxes*

ABSTRACT: *Tapping into little understood products selected from a class of well known compounds can provide formulation advantages. PEG/PPG dimethicone compounds, alkyl dimethicone compounds and alkyl PEG/PPG dimethicone compounds are three classes of compounds that offer far more utility in personal care products than is generally appreciated by formulators.*

Silicone fluids are used in many cosmetics and personal care products. This chapter looks at the synthesis of silicone fluids and evaluates whether that process can be viewed as an equilibrium reaction.

Silicone Fluids

Silicone fluids are a class of compounds that have become known by a variety of names including silicone oils, dimethyl fluids, dimethyl polysiloxane, and polydimethyl siloxane. Silicone fluids have become an important class of materials over the years. These materials are unique in terms of chemistry when compared to hydrocarbon-based materials. While much has been learned about these compounds since they were developed in the 1940s, the available published data remains somewhat limited related to certain aspects of the chemistry.

Silicone fluids are sold by their viscosity. Commercial products range in viscosity from 0.65 centistokes to 1,000,000 centistokes. If the product is not made by blending two different viscosity fluids, the viscosity is related to molecular weight. Silicone fluids conform to the structure shown in **Figure 1**. The viscosity allows for an approximate calculation of the value of "n" as shown in **Table 1**.

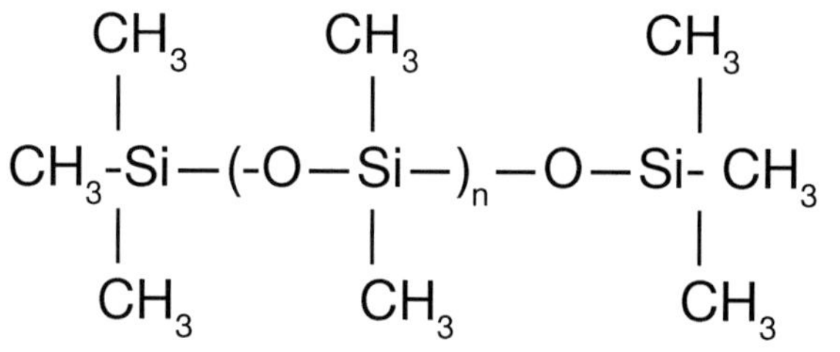

$$CH_3-Si(CH_3)_2-(-O-Si(CH_3)_2-)_n-O-Si(CH_3)_2-CH_3$$

Figure 1. General structure of silicone fluids

Table 1
The "n" value for selected silicone fluids

Approximate Viscosity at 25°C (Centistokes)	Approximate molecular weight	"n" Value
5	800	9
50	3,780	53
100	6,000	85
200	9,430	127
350	13,650	182
500	17,350	230
1,000	28,000	376
10,000	67,700	910
60,000	116,500	1,570
100,000	139,050	1,875

These materials have found a home in many cosmetic products as outlined in **Table 2**.

Table 2
Cosmetic usage of silicone fluids[1]

Product Type	Desired effect	Use level
Skin Lotion	Desoaping	0.1%
	Rub-out	0.1 - 0.5%
	Protection	1 - 30%
	Feel	0.5 - 2%
Skin Cleaner	Lubricity	0.1 - 0.5%
	Wetting	0.1%
Antiperspirant	Anti-whitening	0.5 - 2%
	Detackification	0.5 - 2%
Preshave Lotion	Lubricity	0.5 - 2%
Aftershave Lotion	Feel	0.5 - 2%
Makeup	Water Resistance	1 - 5%
Shaving Cream	Reduce Razor Drag	0.5 - 2%

Synthesis

Silicone fluids are synthesized by the equilibration reaction of MM (Author: Please spell out MM.) and cyclomethicone. Typical of the synthesis of fluids is the reaction in which one MM is reacted with one D-4 (Author: Please spell out D-4.) compound to make MD4M, a simple silicone fluid.

The reaction may be run with either an acid or base catalyst. In one method, the reaction is conducted at room temperature for 12 hours, with sulfuric acid as a catalyst resulting in a mixture of about free cyclic product (Author: Is something missing in the yellow?) and linear fluid. If the catalyst is neutralized and the cyclic is stripped off, a stable fluid results. If the catalyst is not neutralized during stripping, the fluid will degrade.[2,3]

The equilibration process is critical not only to the production of stable silicone fluids, but also as a means of introducing functional groups into the polymer. This is done using a process called hydrosilylation, a process used to make organofunctional silicone compounds.

It is also quite interesting to note that a "finished silicone fluid" may be placed in contact with D-4 and catalyst and re-equilibrated to make a higher viscosity fluid. Conversely, a "finished silicone fluid" may be re-equilibrated with MM and catalyst to make a lower viscosity fluid. Finally, silicone rubber may be decomposed into MM, and D-4 via stripping of the product in the presence of catalyst. This property of silicone polymers makes them decidedly different from organic compounds.[4]

Equilibration

It is thought that silicone polymers form in equilibrium with their reactants and could be pushed back towards the reactant side of the equation under the correct circumstances. The reactants are $Si(CH_3)_3$-O-Si$(CH_3)_3$ (MM) and $-(Si(CH_3)_2-O)_4$ or D-4. Since D-4 is a six-member ring, having alternate silicon and oxygen atoms, its reaction with MM gives linear polymers in the presence of MM and catalyst. To be a true equilibrium reaction when MM is added to an already existing linear polymer one might expect to get the equilibrium mixture of D-4 and a smaller linear molecule. If an excess of MM is combined with a linear polymer chain one might expect to get a different polymer consuming the MM. Little is published on the nature of the reversibility of the reaction known as equilibration.

In order to evaluate the nature of the equilibrium, a study was undertaken which included:

- Reacting MM and D-4 and building it up to a viscosity of 350 centistokes, and also to 1,000 centistokes;
- Adding MM to break down the 1,000 centistoke fluid made in step 1 and also to break down a commercially obtained 1,000 centistoke fluid;
- Neutralization of the catalyst, followed by;
- Analysis via Gel Permeation Chromatography of the products to determine the linear polymer concentration and the concentration of D-4 found in each.

One objective is to determine if the composition of product made by build up is the same as the composition made by the break down process. Specifically, the concentration of D-4 will be of major interest. One possibility is that there will be a comparable amount of D-4 present regardless if the process is build up or break down. Another possibility is that since commercial 1,000 centistoke product is stripped of D-4 after processing, the break down product may be very low in D-4.

The build up reaction is shown in **Figure 2**. The break down reaction is shown in **Figure 3**.

What is not clear from the literature is if the equilibrium mixture made by the build up process is the same as that of the break down product. If the reaction is a true equilibrium, it should not matter which path the reaction takes, but should be only determined by the ratio of reactants introduced. On the other hand it is possible when one breaks down a pre-existing silicone polymer, the silicone polymer might be the same but no D-4 would form. This would mean the reaction is not a true equilibrium.

The average structures of the two silicone fluids used in this study are shown in **Figure 4**.

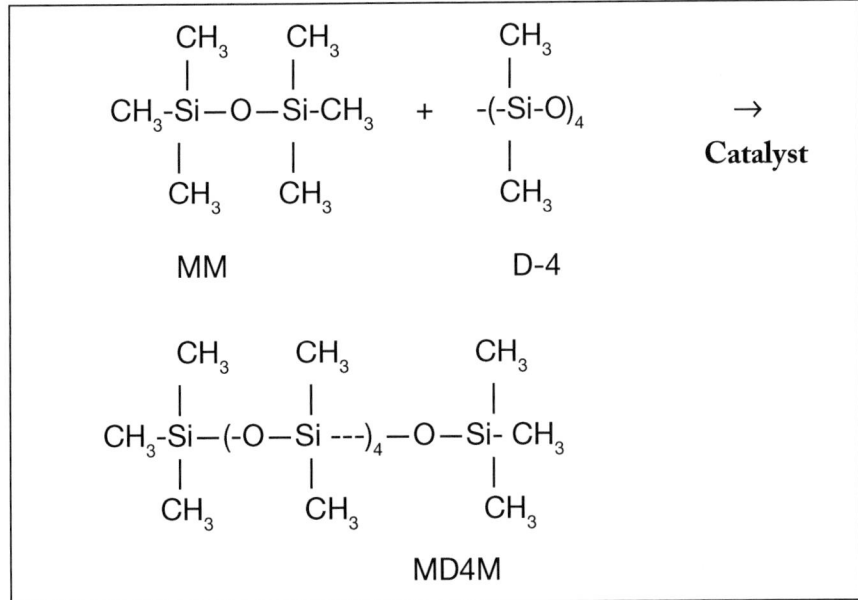

Figure 2. The build up reaction

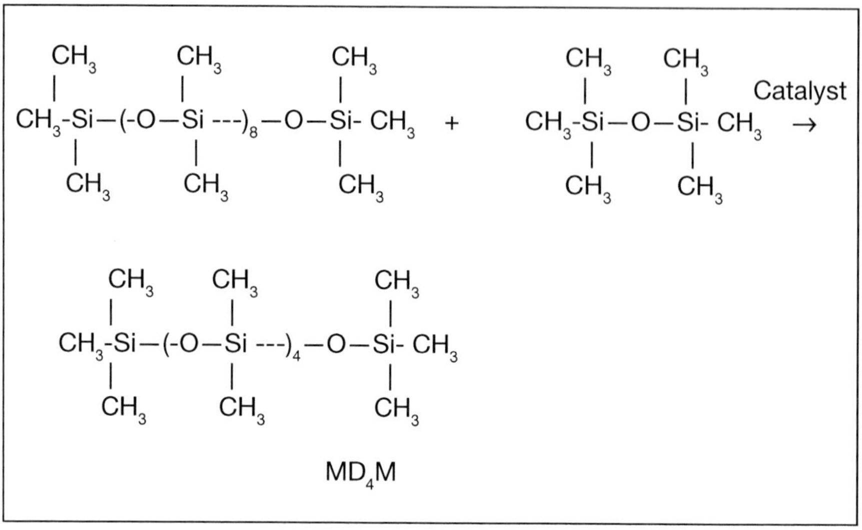

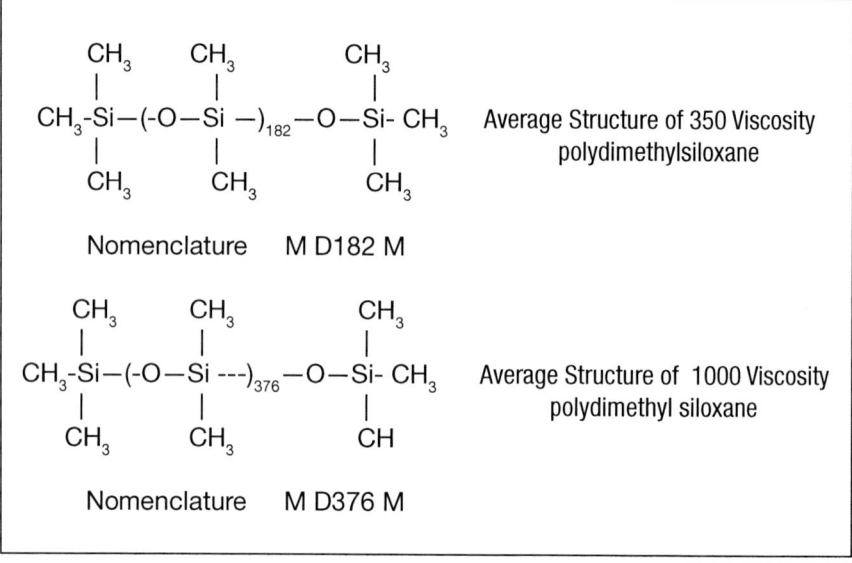

Figure 3. The break down reaction

Figure 4. The average structures of the silicone fluids used in this study

If the silicone polymer made by the break down process results in no D-4, a cyclic free product might be possible by breaking down higher molecular weight polymers with MM. This is very important to the cosmetic industry because cyclic silicones are not desirable in cosmetic products. Many companies go through different synthesis to minimize the concentration of cyclic in their final product.

Methods and Materials

In our study we used the five samples described in **Table 3**.

The equipment used for gel permeation chromatography analysis included an HPLC pump[a], a differential refractometer detector[b] and a column heater module[c]. The columns were Styagel HR 3, 1 and 0.5 in series with a flow rate of 1.0 mL/min, a mobile phase THF, a column temperature of 55°C and a detector temperature of 45°C.

Results

The results of the gel permeation chromatography analysis are presented in **Table 4**. The time shown in the table is the time needed to exit the column. The shorter the time te higher the molecular weight.

Discussion

Both the build up mechanism and the break down mechanism had a comparable quantity of cyclic products present. The break down from 1,000 to 350 had 5.29% cyclic silicones present before distillation, while the build up product had 4.65%. The commercial 350 viscosity product had less cyclic silicones present in it, at 1.58%. This is related to the degree of strip used after the catalyst is neutralized. It is surprising to see that a product that was built up, neutralized but not stripped, followed by a break down had twice as much cyclic silicone as the direct build up. The build up to 350 had 4.65% and the build up and break down had 10.39%. It appears that in the case of this sample there were in fact two different mechanisms occurring simultaneously, a build up and a break down, giving different equilibration concentrations of product. One of the other products had MM, D-4, and linear silicone present at the same time, representing a different reaction sequence.

---

[a]Waters HPLC Pump Model 515, manufactured by Waters and Associates, Milford, Massachusetts, USA
[b]Waters Differential Refractometer Detector Model 410, manufactured by Waters and Associates
[c]Waters Column Heater Module, manufactured by Waters and Associates

Table 3
Materials used in the study, showing composition in parts

A = 1000 cst (Build Up Process)
B = 350 cst (Break Down Process) from commercial 1000 cst silicone fluid
C = 1000 cst (Build Up Process) broken down to 350 cst
D = 350 cst (Build Up Process)
E = Commercial 350 cst product

Ingredient	A	B	C	D	E
Cyclomethicone	99.4		99.4	98.8	
Hexamethyl disiloxane	0.6	0.6	0.6	1.2	
Sulfuric acid	5.0	5.0	5.0	5.0	
Sodium bicarbonate	15.0	15.0	15.0	15.0	
Commercial 1,000 cst fluid		99.4			
Commercial 350 cst fluid					100.0

Procedures for samples A, C, D: Combine the amounts of hexamethyl disiloxane and cyclomethicone in a 400 mL flask. Stir well. Add sulfuric acid. Mix for 24 hours (under good agitation for sample A). Slowly add sodium bicarbonate. Foam will be encountered requiring venting of carbon dioxide. Filter.

Procedures for sample B: Combine the amounts of hexamethyl disiloxane and commercial 1,000 cst fluid in a 400 mL flask. Stir well. Add sulfuric acid. Mix for 24 hours. Slowly add sodium bicarbonate. Foam will be encountered requiring venting of carbon dioxide. Filter.

Table 4
Results of the gel permeation chromatography analysis, showing composition in % wt and time in minutes

A = 1000 cst (Build Up Process)
B = 350 cst (Break Down Process) from commercial 1000 cst silicone fluid
C = 1000 cst (Build Up Process) broken down to 350 cst
D = 350 cst (Build Up Process)
E = Commercial 350 cst product

Sample	Component	% Wt	Time
A	D-4	3.05	23.97
	Fluid	96.95	15.29
	Total	100.00	
B	D-4	5.29	23.38
	Fluid	94.71	15.57
	Total	100.00	
C	D-4	10.39	23.34
	Fluid	89.61	15.66
	Total	100.00	
D	D-4	4.65	23.45
	Fluid	95.35	15.64
	Total	100.00	
E	D-4	1.58	24.10
	Fluid	98.42	15.76
	Total	100.00	

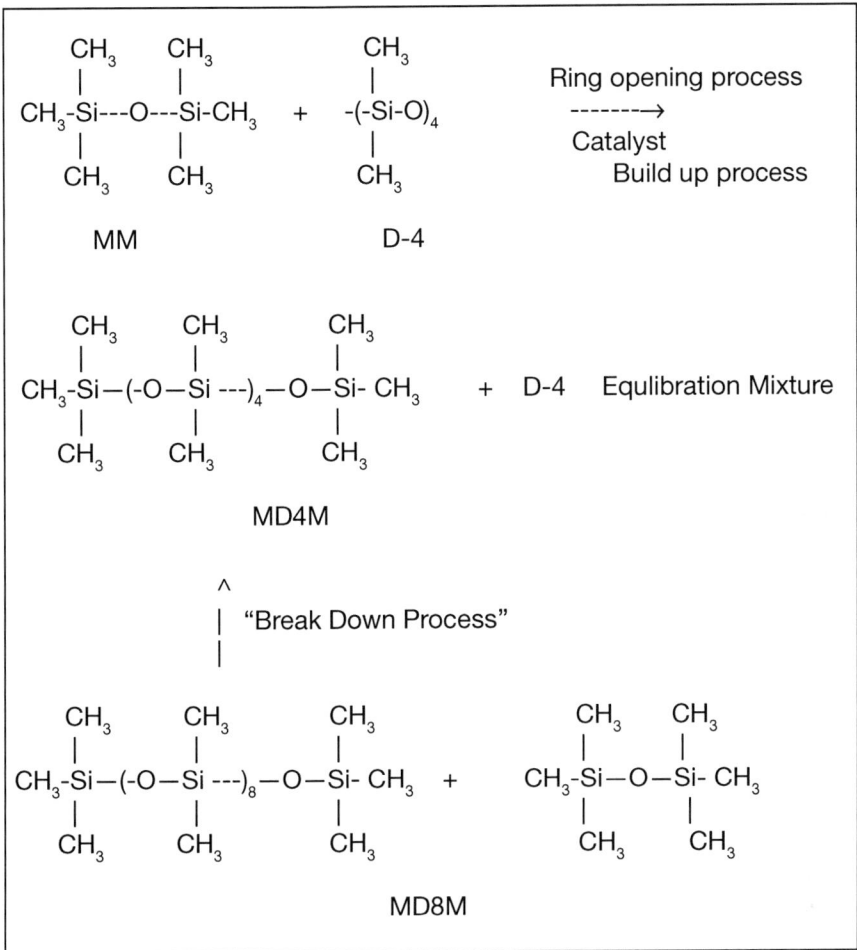

Figure 5. Silicone equilibration reaction scheme

Conclusions

Reference to the results in **Table 4** suggests several interesting conclusions.

- There are two different ways to make a 350 viscosity dimethyl polysiloxane – by build up (Sample D) or break down (Sample B). They result in the same mixture of D-4 to polymer. **Figure 5** shows the two reactions and the common product mixture.
- Commercial 350 viscosity silicone is stripped to reduce the % D-4 to under 2% (Sample E), from the original level of around 5% (Samples B and D).

- The equilibrium mixture of dimethyl polysiloxane having a viscosity of 1,000 (Sample A) has a lower concentration of D-4 in the equilibrium mixture than the 350 viscosity product (Sample D).
- The surprising result is Sample C, the product in which a 350 viscosity dimethyl polysiloxame was built up to 1000 viscosity and then broken down to 350 viscosity. That sample had a very high level of D-4 – twice the expected amount based on Samples B and D.

Published May 2004 Cosmetics and Toiletries magazine

References

1. A O'Lenick, Silicones of Personal Care, Carol Stream, Illinois: Allured Publishing (2003) p 22
2. US Pat 2,384,384 issued in 1945 to McGregor
3. US Pat 2,443,353 issued in 1947 to Hyde

CHAPTER 30

Stimuli-responsive Polymer Systems: A Review of Thermo-associative Thickening

Robert Y. Lochhead
The University of Southern Mississippi, Hattiesburg, Miss., USA

KEY WORDS: *stimuli-responsive, thermal gelling, thermo-thickening, lower critical solution temperature, hydrophobically modified hydrophilic polymers*

ABSTRACT: *This chapter reviews recent trends in thermally initiated stimuli-responsive materials and provides some insight into the physicochemical mechanisms that underpin this behavior.*

Water-soluble polymers and thickeners continue to grow in market volume and diversity. Today there is a noticeable trend toward cosmetic applications that depend upon stimuli-responsive behavior that results in thermo-associative thickening at desired temperatures. This chapter reviews recent trends in thermally initiated stimuli-responsive materials and provides some insight into the physicochemical mechanisms that underpin this fascinating behavior.

The Flory-Huggins Theory of Polymer Solutions

The thermodynamics of polymer solubility are classically described by the Flory-Huggins equation shown in **Figure 1**. The first two terms on the right-hand side describe the combinatorial entropy of mixing, and this always will be favorable to molecular mixing of the

> $\Delta G_{mix}/RT = x_{solvent} \ln\Phi_{solvent} + x_{polymer} \ln\Phi_{polymer} + \chi\, x_{solvent} \Phi_{polymer}$
>
> where:
> ΔG_{mix} is the free energy of mixing of the polymer and solvent.
> $x_{solvent}$ is the mole fraction of solvent in the solution.
> $x_{polymer}$ is the mole fraction of polymer in the solution.
> $\Phi_{solvent}$ is the volume fraction of solvent in the solution.
> $\Phi_{polymer}$ is the volume fraction of polymer in the solution.
> χ is the Flory-Huggins interaction parameter for polymer-solvent interaction.

Figure 1. The Flory-Huggins equation

polymer and the solvent. In the original conceptual thinking of the Flory-Huggins theory, the third term arises only from the enthalpy of mixing; the polymer and solvent are completely miscible over the entire composition range if the following statement is true:[1-4]

$$\chi < \tfrac{1}{2}\left(1 + (V_{polymer}/V_{solvent})^{-1/2}\right)^2$$

where:
$V_{solvent}$ is the solvent's molar volume.
$V_{polymer}$ is the polymer's molar volume.

This equation predicts that the solubility of a polymer should decrease with an increase in the polymer's molar volume and hence its molecular weight. Also, a polymer and solvent should be completely miscible if the value of the Flory-Huggins interaction parameter, χ, is less than 0.5.

The simple Flory-Huggins theory has several drawbacks that limit its applicability to real systems:[4]

- is not a constant; it varies with polymer concentration and temperature.
- cannot be easily found experimentally.
- is characteristic of only a polymer-solvent pair and it is not easily extended to multicomponent formulations.
- is not a simple term; it has to be modified to include terms for molecular orientation and specific binding such as hydrogen bonding.

- If the system becomes more ordered when a solution is formed, χ can have anomalous large positive values.
- Finally, classical Flory-Huggins theory cannot explain the fact that polymer solutions can separate into two phases upon heating or cooling beyond certain critical temperatures.[3,5,6] This is especially pertinent to the subject of thermo-associative polymers.

Polymer Solution Phase Behavior

A generalized phase diagram for a polymer solution is shown in **Figure 2**. At intermediate temperatures, this polymer is in solution at all concentrations as indicated by the "one-phase" region on the diagram. As the temperature of the system is lowered or raised, it eventually will cross over into a two-phase region and phase separation will occur as indicated on the diagram. The upper critical solution temperature (UCST) is the highest temperature of the bottom two-phase region and the lower critical solution temperature (LCST) is the lowest temperature of the top two-phase region.

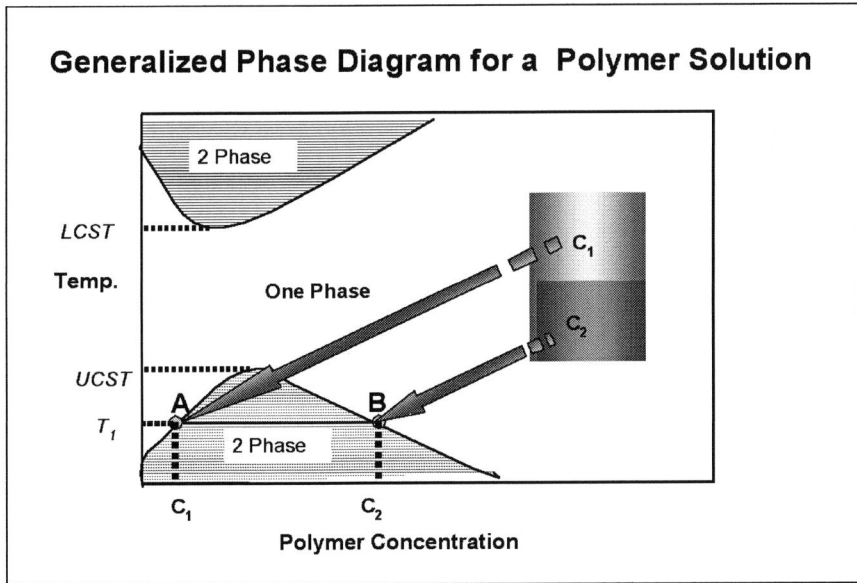

Figure 2. A generalized phase diagram for polymer solution as a function of temperature and polymer concentration. The miscible polymer solution separates into two phases upon cooling below the UCST or heating above the LCST. The compositions of the separated phases can be determined by the intersection points of the tie lines on the two-phase envelope.

The composition of each phase is indicated by the envelopes surrounding the two-phase regions. The horizontal lines inside these envelopes are called *tie-lines*; they connect the polymer concentrations of the separated phases. For example, at temperature T_1 this system separates into a solvent-rich phase, A, and a polymer-rich phase, B. Phase A is a solution that has a polymer concentration C_1, and phase B is a solution that has a polymer concentration C_2.

A system reaches chemical equilibrium, and this includes phase equilibria, when the free energy of the system reaches a minimum. The change in Gibbs free energy (ΔG) is related to the changes in enthalpy (ΔH) and entropy (ΔS) of a process at temperature, T, by the familiar equation:

$$\Delta G = \Delta H - T\Delta S$$

Phase separation below the UCST requires a significant negative enthalpy of mixing, and phase separation above the LCST requires both a negative enthalpy and entropy of mixing.

Polymer solution behavior is better understood by considering the relative values of the excess Gibbs free energy of mixing ($\Delta^{excess}G_{mix}$) as a function of polymer composition (**Figure 3**).[4] In **Figure 3(a)** it can be seen that the excess free energy of mixing is lower than the ideal free energy for all polymer concentrations. **Figure 3(a)** is indicative of a system that is miscible in all proportions. For the two-phase system in **Figure 3b**, however, there are two free energy minima and a free energy maximum. Thermodynamics predicts that for compositions between points A and B, the system will be driven to the two energy minima and this will cause the system to separate into two phases of

$$\left(\frac{\partial \mu_{polym}}{\partial C_{polym}}\right)_{T,P} = \left(\frac{\partial^2 \Delta^{excess}G_{mix}}{\partial C_{polym}^2}\right)_{T,P}$$

composition C_1 and C_2.

The chemical potential is the normalized change in excess free energy with concentration:

$$\mu_{polym} = \left(\frac{1}{C_{polym}}\right)\left(\frac{\partial \Delta^{excess}G_{mix}}{\partial C_{polym}}\right)_{T,P}$$

Stimuli-responsive Polymer Systems: A Review of Thermo-associative Thickening

Solutes dissolve spontaneously when their chemical potential is negative; that is, when $(\partial \Delta^{excess} G_{mix}/\partial C_{polym})$ is negative. The chemical potential is merely the slope of the lines in **Figure 3**. First, note that the slope of the line at point p in **Figure 3(b)** is positive. Therefore, for a composition of polymer concentration x, the polymer has to overcome a positive chemical potential in order to get "over the hump" and reach the free energy minimum at C_2.

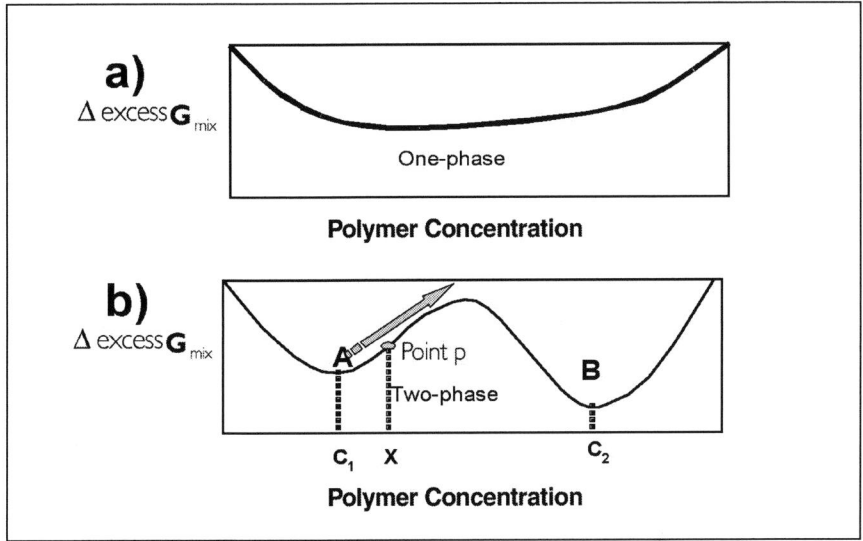

Figure 3. The excess free energy as a function of polymer concentration for a) a miscible solution and b) a phase-separated system

For thermo-associative thickening, phase separation at equilibrium is not a sufficient condition; the process by which the system diffuses toward phase separation is also important. According to Fick's Second Law, the diffusion of a polymer into solution is described by:

$$D_{polym} = C_{polym} M_{polym} (\partial \mu_{polym}/\partial C_{polym})_{T,P}$$

where
D_{polym} is the polymer's diffusion coefficient.
C_{polym} is the polymer concentration.
M_{polym} is the polymer mobility.
μ_{polym} is the polymer's chemical potential.

Fick's Second Law states that the diffusion coefficient is proportional to $\partial\mu_{polym}/\partial C_{polym}$. This is the slope of the line just considered; that is:

For a curve such as this there must be points of inflection between the minima and the maximum turning points and at these turning points $(\partial\mu_{polym}/\partial C_{polym})$ is equal to zero. This means that at these inflection points, from Fick's Second Law, $D_{polymer} = 0$. (See exploded view in **Figure 4**.) Below the inflection point, spontaneous diffusional concentration of the polymer solution is thermodynamically disfavored. Above the inflection point, diffusion of the polymer to the more concentrated phase is thermodynamically favored. The curve through these inflection points is known as the *chemical spinodal* (**Figure 5**).

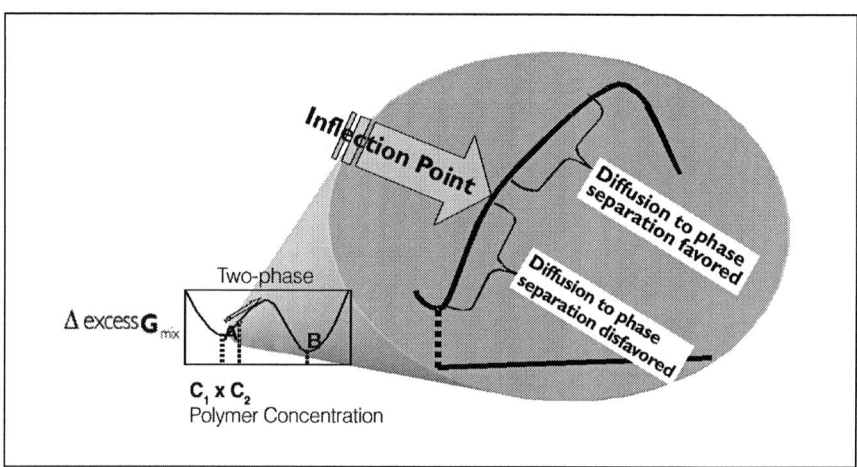

Figure 4. Exploded view of a segment of the free energy curve in Figure 3b showing the inflection point

Diffusion-driven phase separation is favored in regions within the locus of points defined by the chemical spinodal and spontaneous separation into two phases usually occurs. In regions between the free energy minima and the chemical spinodal (i.e., the point of inflection in the excess free energy curve, which often is called the miscibility gap), the molecules have to diffuse uphill against the chemical potential. Large compositional fluctuations are required before phase separation can occur. This process is known as *spinodal decomposition*. If the compositional fluctuations are sufficiently large, phase separated nuclei are generated and they serve as initiation points upon which growth of the separated phase can occur. Nucleation and growth occur within the spinodal and for this stage the chemical potential favors diffusion to the separate phase.

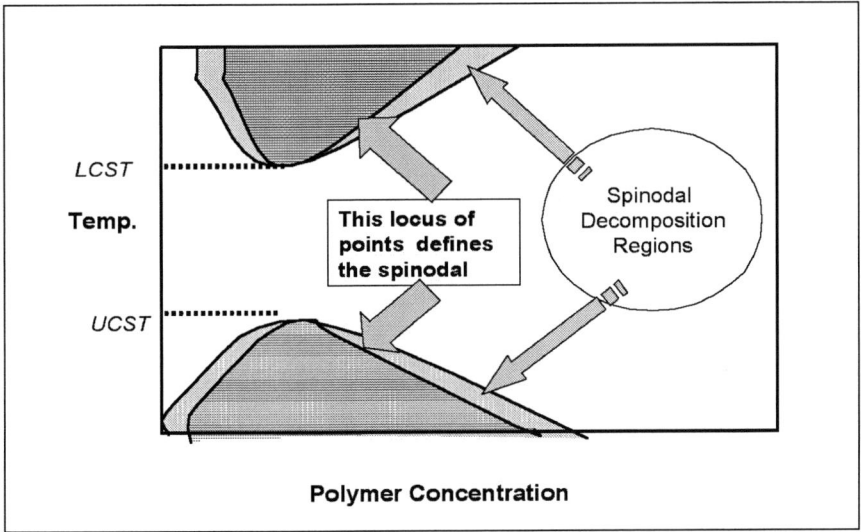

Figure 5. A schematic representation of a generalized phase diagram showing the location of the chemical spinodal and the miscibility gap in which spinodal decomposition would occur

The Lower Critical Solution Temperature

Thermal-responsive performance in polymer solutions is based upon the phase behavior of the system as a function of temperature. It generally is accepted that the incorporation of hydrophobic groups into hydrophilic polymer molecules will lead to a decrease in the Lower Critical Solution Temperature (LCST).[7] However, the effect of polymer structure on LCST is only qualitatively understood.[8]

For example, according to the Flory-Huggins theory, the effect of polymer molecular weight on the LCST is predicted by the ratio $(V_{polymer}/V_{solvent})^{-1/2}$. That ratio will decrease as polymer molecular weight decreases and this indicates that χ will increase concomitantly. This theory, therefore, predicts that the LCST would increase with decrease in the polymer molecular weight. However, the LCST of poly (N-isopropylacrylamide) (PNIPAM) has been reported to increase,[9] decrease[8,10,11] or remain unchanged[12] with increase in polymer molecular weight. Polymer end-groups can influence the LCST, but this effect has been observed only for low-molecular-weight polymers.[8]

The LCSTs of polymers are conventionally measured by methods such as light-scattering, UV-visible absorption, differential scanning calorimetry or infrared spectroscopy. Unfortunately, there are numerous subtle solvent and polymer structure effects that influence the LCST phenomenon, especially in the region of spinodal decomposition, and the low-throughput of conventional methods limits the ability to generate sufficient data to elucidate the details of the underlying molecular mechanism(s) involved.

Professor Bergbreiter of Texas A&M has developed a high throughput method to meet this challenge.[13] The apparatus is a microfluidics device with an imposed linear temperature gradient. The LCST is detected by the position on the temperature gradient at which the solution becomes cloudy. This apparatus allowed Bergbreiter to investigate the effect of salts on the LCST of PNIPAM. Anions lowered the LCST in accordance with the Hofmeister series ($I^- < Br^- < Cl^- < F^-$) and cations lowered it in the order observed for salting out of proteins ($Li^+ < Cs^+ < Rb^+ < K^+ < Na^+$). The Hofmeister series was introduced originally as a classification of the ability of common ions to precipitate soluble proteins from aqueous solution:[14]

$$CO_3^{2-} > SO_4^{2-} > S_2O_3^{2-} > H_2PO_4^- > F^- > Cl^- > Br^- > F^- \sim NO_3^- > I^- > ClO_4^- > SCN^-$$

The ions at the CO_3 end are called *kosmotropes* or *water-structure makers* and those at the SCN end are called *chaotropes* or *water-structure breakers*. Recently proposed hypotheses cast doubt on Hofmeister water-structure theories and have attributed the effect to related polarizabilities and specific ion binding, but there was a paucity of data to support the new hypothesis.[15–16] Use of a method employing a high throughput temperature gradient enabled Bergbreiter et al. to investigate the effect of dissolved ions on the LCST of PNIPAM solutions.[17] From measured turbidities they observed that the LCST showed two distinct steps in the presence of kosmotropes. They deduced that the effect of kosmotropes on PNIPAM solvation could be explained on the basis of three distinct interactions:

- The anions can polarize water molecules that are positioned to hydrogen-bond with the polymer's amide groups.
- The anions interfere with the hydrophobic hydration and reduce the interfacial tension of the cavity surrounding the polymer backbone and the isopropyl group.
- The anions bind directly to the polyamide.

The first two interactions would lead to salting-out of the polymer and the last interaction would cause salting-in. The effect of salts on the LCST can be modeled by the equation:

$$T = T_0 + c[M] + \frac{B_{max} K_A[M]}{1 + K_A[M]}$$

T0 is the LCST of PNIPAM in the absence of salt. The constant, c, in the second term is directly proportional to the ion's hydration entropy for kosmotropes and is proportional to the surface tension decrement due to the ion for chaotropes. Ion-binding to the polymer chain is considered by the third term, in which KA is the binding constant of the ion to the polymer and Bmax is the increase in LCST due to ion-binding at saturation.

Thermo-associative Thickening

Some polymers, such as PNIPAM and poly(ethylene oxide), display LCST in the range of human body temperature. This property makes these polymers useful as copolymer units to confer temperature-triggered stimuli-response properties.

One such property is thermo-thickening of these polymer solutions as the temperature is raised. This is observed, for example, for polysaccharides having grafts of PNIPAM and poloxamers in aqueous solution. For example, polymers having a backbone of carboxymethylcellulose (CMC) and side-chains of PNIPAM are soft critical gels below the threshold association temperature (T'_{assoc}) and stiff critical gels above that temperature.[18] The gel is a *physical* gel in which the polysaccharide chains are linked by junction zones formed by hydrophobic interaction between the PNIPAM grafts. This behavior corresponds to weak segregation of PNIPAM below T'_{assoc} and strong segregation of PNIPAM above T'_{assoc}. This phenomenon has been widely reported for polymers with hydrophilic backbones and hydrophobic side-chains.

Thermo-associative thickening in aqueous solutions depends upon the formation of molecular networks in which the water-soluble chains remain in solution and the LCST moieties attached to the chain phase-segregate into junction zones. This type of phase-segregation is hindered in the miscibility gap where spinodal decomposition is relied upon to produce the network. In addition, once the gel begins to form, the mobility of the polymer in the medium will be reduced greatly and Fick's Second Law would predict that the diffusion constant would decrease. Moreover, once the first chains segregate, the reptation of additional LCST moieties to the junction zone will be limited by the molecular relaxation processes of the participating polymers. For these reasons, the preparation of reproducible thermo-gelling systems is far from a trivial pursuit. Fortunately, this has not discouraged research in this field and a number of researchers have claimed success.

An example of LCST polymers is provided by ethoxylated poly(organophosphazenes) that are soluble in water below their LCST and they precipitate above that temperature. However, when these molecules are substituted with hydrophobic grafts of L-isoleucine ethyl ester, they exhibit thermo-thickening to a clear gel.[19] As the temperature is raised above T'_{assoc}, the gel shrinks and at higher temperatures it becomes a precipitate. The underlying mechanism was probed using ^{31}P NMR, and it was found that the phosphorus resonance peak broadened as the gel formed at body temperatures, but then sharpened as the temperature was raised further to 60°C and the polymer precipitated. The NMR indicates that the chains are restricted in the gel region but when the gel breaks and a precipitate forms, the polymer molecules move freely in solution. This was interpreted as a segregative separation into two phases; one a precipitate and the other a solution. The sharpening peak was attributed to the solution phase. So the gel appears to be an intermediate phase in which the molecules are trapped between a solution and a precipitated state.

Thermo-thickening can be achieved from water-soluble polymers with attached blocks or grafts of LCST polymers.[20] These polymers can be synthesized by various methods:

- Grafting LCST polymer chains onto water-soluble macromolecular backbones to produce comb-type structures.[21] This is difficult to scale to a commercial process.[20]
- Copolymerization of an LCST macromonomer with a water-soluble monomer.[22] Water-soluble thickeners cannot be synthesized in water in commercially viable solid concentrations. They are, therefore, preferably made by precipitation polymerization[23] or by inverse emulsion polymerization.[22] Graft copolymers of N-acryloyl taurate with commercially available macromonomers can be clear thickening emulsifiers[23,24] or thermo-thickeners[23] or both. This class of polymers is useful for thickening acid solutions. In this context, low-pH formulations have presented a challenge to conventional thickeners, because polysaccharides are hydrolyzed at these pH values and polyelectrolyte thickeners undergo polyion collapse at low pHs. However, 2-acrylamido-2-methylpropanesulphonic acid copolymers can thicken low-pH solutions[25] and high molecular weight versions can confer desired Ellis rheology with a yield stress and shear-thinning characteristics. Thus, acryloyl taurate/vinyl pyrrolidone copolymer can thicken and stabilize emulsions that contain alpha and beta hydroxy acids.[26]
- Preparation of amphipathic block copolymers. For example, one type is prepared by end-capping poloxamers with poly(acrylic acid).[27] These polymers enable the facile preparation of multiple emulsions.[28]
- Free-radical polymerization of water-soluble monomers with monomers bearing oxyalkylated derivatives. For example, thermo-thickening also has been observed for polymers having a poly(acrylic acid) or a copoly(acrylic acid/PVP) backbone[29,30] and side chains of poly(ethylene oxide) or poly(propylene oxide). Thermo-thickening of foams is one possible useful application of graft copoly-mers of this general

structure.[31] Flash-foaming occurs best with low viscosity liquids but these foams can break and run on application and give poor aesthetics. The stimuli-responsive polymers allow the composition to be foamed at room temperature and to thicken at body temperature to confer the desired attributes throughout the foaming and subsequent application steps. It is interesting, in this context, that poly(acrylic acid) has been hydrophobically modified with renewable resources such as cashew nutshell liquid.[32] There is one drawback of these acrylic acid polymers and that is their precipitation by divalent metal salts.[33]

Surfactants influence the temperature of thermo-gelation. Anionic surfactants dramatically increase the gelation temperature of PNIPAM and nonionic surfactants have little or no effect. Adsorption isotherms constructed by Moran and Tsujii of Kao Corp. and the late Professor Tanaka of Massachusetts Institute of Technology revealed three possible locations of surfactant in these gels. As illustrated in **Figure 6**, these locations are direct adsorption on the polymer chain, entrapment within the gel matrix or presence in the bulk aqueous solution outside the gel.[34]

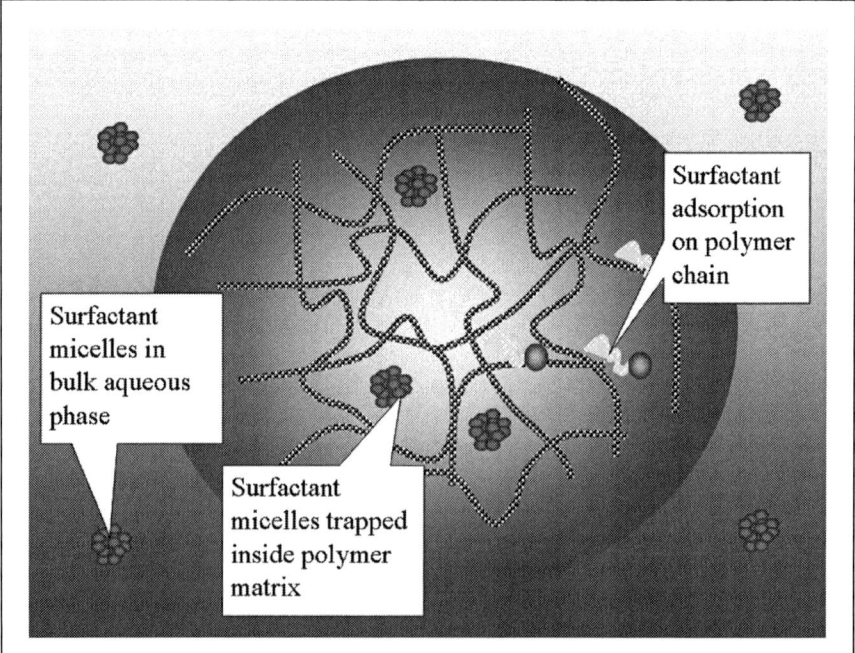

Figure 6. The possible location of nonionic surfactants in poly(N- isopropylacrylamide) gels according to Murase et al[34]

Sodium lauryl sulfate adsorbs on the polymer chain and increases the polymer solubility and concomitantly increases the temperature of gelation. The driving force for this adsorption is hydrophobic interaction and this conclusion is reinforced by the fact that there is no such surfactant adsorption on hydrophilic polymer chains such as polyacrylamide. The concentration of surfactant entrapped within the polymer matrix is less than that in the bulk water and this is explained by mutual repulsion between the polymer matrix and the surfactant micelles. A nonionic surfactant resides principally in the bulk water phase. That is, the nonionic surfactant is neither bound nor entrapped within the PNIPAM matrix. Nonionic surfactant micelles are large and they might be unable to fit into the mesh of the polymer net. Another explanation is that the large nonionic micelles phase-segregate from the polymer microgel because the mixing of polymers and large micelles would produce only a small increase in entropy.

This behavior contrasts with that exhibited by hydrophobically modified water-soluble polymers (**Figure 7**).[35] For example copolymers of acrylic acid and N-octadecylacrylamide show dramatic increases in viscosity in the presence of certain nonionic surfactants when the surfactant concentration is close to the critical micelle concentration (CMC);[36] the viscosity decreases again above the CMC (**Figures 7a and 7b**). The viscosity increase is attributed to comicellization between the polymer hydrophobes and the surfactant leading to physical cross-linking of the polymer chains. Comicellization still occurs at higher surfactant concentrations but the stoichiometry of the hydrophobes disfavors cross-linking, the network is lost and the viscosity decreases with increase in surfactant concentration (**Figure 7c**). The viscosity decrease can be prevented if the micelles are large, worm-like surfactant aggregates (**Figure 7d**).[37] Systems comprising hydrophobically modified hydrophilic polymers and nonionic surfactants also can display thermo-thickening and this has been correlated with the transition of micelle structure from regular micelles to lamellar vesicles (**Figure 7e**).[38]

Amphiphilic block copolymers self-associate in aqueous solution to form large micelle-like structures.[39–40] For example, the block copolymer of caprolactone and PEG 550 spontaneously forms micelles of size 15–125 nm.[41] Block copolymer micelles can be tailored to confer specific rheologies on solutions.[42] It now has been found that amphipathic block copolymers interact synergistically with associative thickeners and the rheologies of the resulting composites can be tailored for optimization.[43]

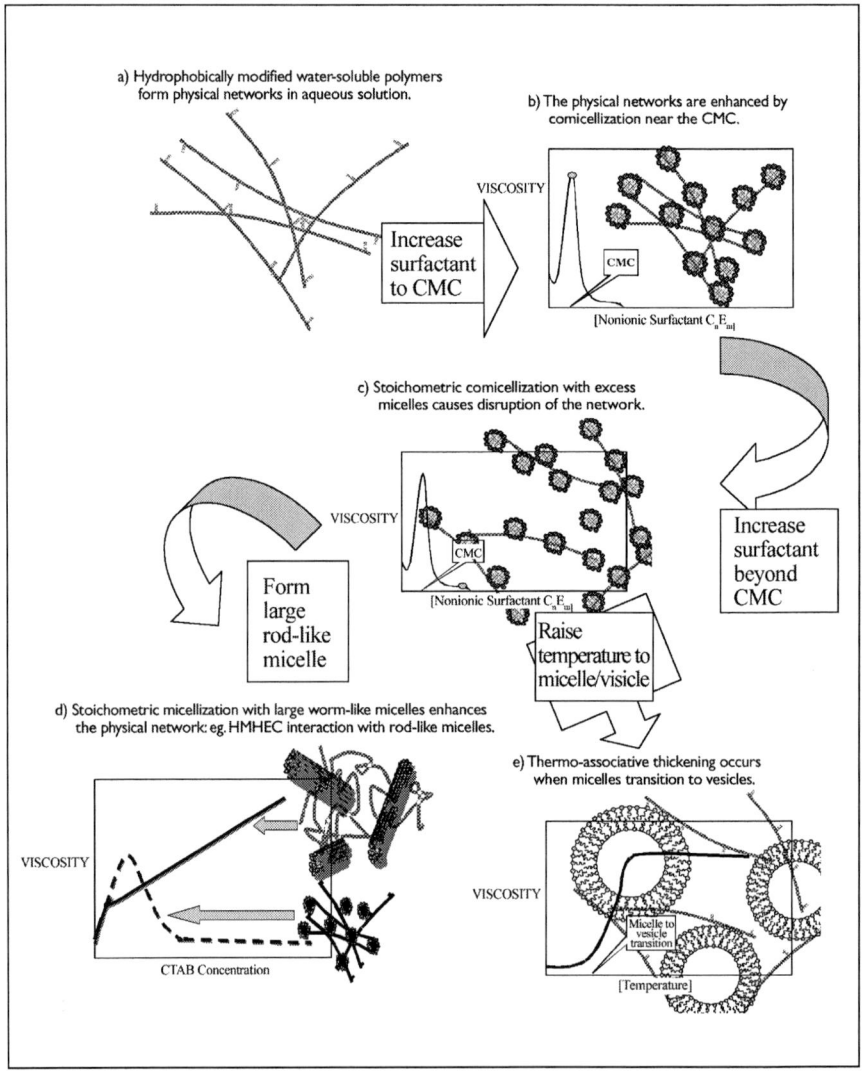

Figure 7. Hydrophobically modified hydrophilic polymers form physical networks in aqueous solution. The networks can be enhanced by addition of surfactant close to the CMC, but for small micelles the network is disrupted by excess micellar concentration. The viscosity is maintained in the presence of large rod-like or worm-like micelles and the thermally induced micelle-to-vesicle transition can be utilized to thermo-thicken these systems. (From Reference 37)

Summary

In personal care, the development of thermo-responsive systems is emerging as a notable trend as judged by the increasing numbers of patent applications being filed within this area. Thermo-associative gelation is a significant thrust area within this trend. This chapter discussed important factors in this trend and considered the underlying mechanisms.

Existing polymer solution theories such as Flory-Huggins theory need to be rethought or updated to accurately explain thermo-gelation. The Hofmeister series is inadequate to accurately define the role of dissolved salts in thermo-gelation and new, more-detailed theories are being developed. Thermo-gelation arises from microphase separation in polymer solutions in which phase-separation is thermodynamically favored but frustrated by chemical potential gradients that disfavor diffusion of the system towards a polymer-rich phase and a polymer-poor phase. Discrete microdomain junction zones within soluble polymer networks are further favored by restricted diffusion in the viscous polymer regions and the resulting retardation of polymer reptation processes.

There is a need for more detailed mechanistic understanding and we can be assured that as this trend continues to gain commercial significance, the detailed mechanisms will be unraveled and, as current theories are remodeled, predictive structure-property relations will be revealed.

Published October 2006 Cosmetics and Toiletries magazine

References

1. PJ Flory, Thermodynamics of high polymer solutions, *J Chem Phys* 10 51 (1942)
2. PJ Flory, *Principles of Polymer Chemistry*, Ithaca, New York: Cornell University Press (1953)
3. D Patterson, *Macromolecules* 2 672 (1969)
4. AFM Barton, *Handbook of Solubility Parameters and Other Cohesion Parameters,* Boca Raton, Florida: CRC Press (1983)
5. D Patterson, Thermodynamics of non-dilute polymer solutions, *Rubber Chem Technol* 40 1 (1967)
6. D Patterson, G Delmas and T Somcynsky, A Comparison of lower critical solution temperatures of some polymer solutions, *Polymer* 8 503 (1967)
7. LD Taylor and LD Cerkowski, *J Polymer Sci, Polymer Chem Ed* 13 2551 (1975)
8. S Furyk, Y Zhang, D Ortis-Acosta, PS Cremer and DE Bergbreiter, Effects of end-group polarity and molecular-weight on the lower critical solution temperature of poly (N-isopropylacrylamide), *J Polymer Sci Part A* 44 1492 (2006)

9. Z Tong, F Zeng, X Zheng and T Sato, *Macromolecules* 32 4488 (1999)
10. T Baltes, F Garret-Flaudy and R Freitag, *J Polymer Sci Part A: Polymer Chem* 37 2977 (1999)
11. HG Schild and DA Tirrel, *J Phys Chem* 94 4352 (1990)
12. El Tiktopulo, VN Uversky, VB Lushchick, SL Klenin, VE Bychkova and OB Ptytsin, *Macromolecules* 28 7519 (1995)
13. H Mao, C Li, S Furyk, PS Cremer and DE Bergbreiter, High throughput studies of the effects of polymer structure and solution components on the phase separation of thermo responsive polymers, *Macromolecules* 37 1031 (2004)
14. F Hofmeister, *Arch Exp Pathol Phamakol* 24 247 (1888)
15. M Bostrom, DRM Williams and BW Ninham, *Biophys J* 85 686 (2003)
16. M Bostrom, DRM Williams and BW Ninham, *Phys Rev Lett* 87 168103 (2001)
17. Y Zhang, S Furyk, DE Bergbreiter and PS Cremer, Specific ion effects on the water solubility of macromolecules, *J Amer Chem Soc* 127 14505 (2005)
18. T Aubry, F Bossard, G Staikos and G Bokias, Rheological study of semidilute aqueous solutions of a thermoassociative copolymer, *J Rheology* 47(2) 577–587 (2003)
19. BH Lee, YM Lee, YS Sohn and S-C Song, A thermosensitive poly(organophosphazene) gel, *Macromolecules* 35 3876 (2002)
20. US Pat 6,689,856, Water-soluble polymers with a water-soluble backbone and side units with a lower critical solution temperature, process for preparing them, aqueous compositions containing them and cosmetic use thereof, F L'Alloret, assigned to L'Oréal (Feb 10, 2004)
21. D Hourdet, F L'Alloret and R Audebert, *Polymer* 38 2535 (1997)
22. US Pat 6,838,514, Polymers which exhibit thermothickening properties and process making same, D Yeung, DW Kwing, LZ Liu, BRC Langlois, D Charmot and P Corpart, assigned to Rhodia (Jan 4, 2005)
23. US Pat 6,964,995, Grafted comb polymers based on acryloyldimethyltaurine acid, R Morschhauser, M Löffler and I Maier, assigned to Clariant (Nov 15, 2005)
24. US Pat 6,891,011, Comb-shaped copolymers based on acryloyldimethyltaurine acid, R Morschhäuser, J Glauder, M Löffler, C Kayser and A Tardi, assigned to Clariant (May 10, 2005)
25. US Pat Applic 20060046949, Water-soluble thickener and liquid acidic detergent, K Ito and Y Mori (Mar 2, 2006)
26. US Pat 6,986,895, Thickened cosmetic compositions, AJ Suares and JH Zhang, assigned to Unilever Home & Personal Care USA division of Conopco (Jan 17, 2006)
27. US Pat 6,316,011, End modified thermal responsive hydrogels, ES Ron, L Bromberg and M Temchenko, assigned to Madash LLC (Nov 13, 2001)
28. US Pat 6,995,209, Thermally reversible water in oil in water emulsions, L Olivieri and ES Ron, assigned to Madash LLC (Feb 7, 2006)
29. US Pat Applic 20040214913, Polymer comprising water-soluble units and lcst units, and aqueous composition comprising same, F L'Alloret (Oct 28, 2004)
30. US Pat Applic 20060111518, Polymer comprising water-soluble units and LCST units, and aqueous composition comprising it, F L'Alloret (May 25, 2006)
31. US Pat 6,878,754, Heat-induced gelling foaming composition and foam obtained, F L'Alloret, assigned to L'Oréal (Apr 12, 2005)
32. US Pat Applic 20060142501, Hydrophobically modified poly(acrylic acid) [PAA] and process of preparation thereof, MV Badiger, PP Wadgaonkar, AK Lele, A Subhash, D Hourdet, P Perrin and C Chassenieux, assigned to Council of Scientific and Industrial Research (Jun 29, 2006)
33. US Pat 6,645,476, Water-soluble polymers and their use in cosmetic and pharmaceutical compositions, R Morschhauser and M Loffler, assigned to Clariant GmbH (Nov 11, 2003)
34. Y Murase, K Tsujii and T Tanaka, Aggregation behavior of surfactants in polymer gel networks, *Langmuir* 16 6385 (2000)

35. US Pat Applic 20040109838, Compositions containing copolymers based on acryloyldimethyl aminoethylsulfonic acid and synergistic additives, R Morschhuser, C Kayser, M Loffler, KH Heier, A Tardi, M Schade and G Botthof, (Jun 10, 2004)
36. A Sarrazin-Cartalas, I Iliopoulos, R Audebert and U Olsson, Association and thermal gelation in mixtures of hydrophobically modified polyelectrolytes and nonionic surfactants, *Langmuir* 10 1421 (1994)
37. S Panai, RK Prud'homme and DG Peiffer, *Colloids & Surfaces* 147 3 (1999)
38. K Loyen, I Iliopoulos, R Audebert and U Olsson, Reversible thermal gelation in polymer/surfactant system, *Langmuir* 11 1053 (1995)
39. RL Xu, MA Winnik, FR Hallett, G Riess and MD Croucher, Light scattering study of the association behavior of styrene-ethylene oxide block copolymers in aqueous solution, *Macromolecules* 24 87–93 (1991)
40. M Wilhelm, CL Zhao, Y Wang, RL Xu, MA Winnik, JL Mura, G Riess and MD Croucher, Ooly(styrene-ethylene oxide) block copolymer micelle formation in water: A fluorescence probe study, *Macromolecules* 24 1033–1044 (1991)
41. US Pat Applic 20060034797, Polymeric micromulsions, AME Arien, ME Brewster, A Nathan, J Rosenblatt, LM Ould-Ouali and V Preat (Feb 16, 2006)
42. ANS Cameron, MK Corbierre and A Eisenberg, Symmetric amphiphilic block copolymers in solution: A morphological wonderland, *Can J Chem* 77 1311–1326 (1999)
43. US Pat Applic 20060140898, Use of a combination of at least one associated polymer and at least one amphiphilic diblock copolymer for thickening cosmetic compositions, C Dubief, LN Morgantini, A-L Bernard and F Simonet (Jun 29, 2006)

CHAPTER 31

Citrate Polyesters

Kevin O'Lenick and Andrew O'Lenick
SurfaTech Corporation

Over the last decade, our industry has undergone a dramatic metamorphosis. This change has been a result of consumer demand, government regulation and a realization that we are stewards of our environment.

The introduction of new materials for use in the personal care market has been complicated by several factors. The successful products will:

1. be based upon sustainable raw materials;
2. be polymers (meeting the requirements of REACH);
3. be free of vinyl monomers which are considered toxic (that is, they will be made from raw materials that are friendly both to the consumer and the environment);
4. offer the formulator advantages that cannot be found in other materials meeting the other three requirements.

A new series of Citrate Esters that meet all of the requirements listed above have been developed.

Sustainable Raw Materials

The raw materials used in the preparation of citrate esters are derived from natural, sustainable renewable raw materials. The raw materials are as follows:

Stearyl Alcohol. Stearyl alcohol is:

$$CH_3(CH_2)_{17}\text{-}OH.$$

It is derived from coconuts.

Octyldodecanol. Octyldodecanol is:

$$\begin{array}{c} (CH_2)_7CH_3 \\ | \\ CH_3\text{-}(CH_2)_9\text{-}CH\text{-}CH_2\text{-}OH \end{array}$$

It is derived from coconuts.

1, 3 Propanediol. **1,3 Propanediol is HO-(CH2)3-OH.** Zemea® propanediol is a colorless and highly purified glycol derived from a sustainable and renewable corn sugar fermentation process. Approved by Ecocert™ and certified by the Natural Products Association (NPA), Zemea® is a 100% natural ingredient. Zemea® propanediol is the perfect glycol compound for formulations where non-petroleum based ingredients are desired. The benefits of Zemea® propanediol include purity, lack of irritation and sensitization, and environmental sustainability

Citric Acid. Citric acid is:

$$\begin{array}{c} H_2C\text{-}C(O)OH \\ | \\ HO\text{-}C\text{-}C(O)OH \\ | \\ H_2\text{-}C\text{-}C(O)OH \end{array}$$

Citric acid is a product of the fermentation of glucose.

Polymer Molecular Design

The citrate polymers of interest are made by the polymerization of mono citrate esters and di citrate esters polymerized using 1,3 propane diol.

There are several classes of materials that are related to the polymer preparation. The first class is the triester. For example tri-octyldocecyl citrate is a known material.

Molecules with no Reactive Carboxyl Groups

Tri-substituted citrate esters

$$\begin{array}{c} H_2C\text{-}C(O)OR \\ | \\ HO\text{-}C\text{-}C(O)OR \\ | \\ H_2C\text{-}C(O)OR \end{array}$$

R is a mixture of

$$-(CH_2)_{17}\text{-}CH_3 \quad (50\%)$$

and

$$\begin{array}{c} (CH_2)_7CH_3 \\ | \quad\quad (50\%) \\ CH_3\text{-}(CH_2)_9\text{-}CH\text{-}CH_2\text{-} \end{array}$$

The product is a slushy liquid when the alkyl group is 50% octlydodecyl and 50% stearyl.

This is in contrast to when the R group is pure:

$$\begin{array}{c} (CH_2)_7CH_3 \\ | \\ CH_3\text{-}(CH_2)_9\text{-}CH\text{-}CH_2\text{-} \end{array}$$

When the R group is pure octyldodecyl, the compound is called tri-octyldodecyl citrate1. It is a liquid C66 ester. It is not a polymer under REACH. And since all three acid groups are esterified, it cannot be incorporated into a polymer (although some may argue that the OH could be reacted into a polymer, but with difficulty).

High Definition Polymers®

High Definition Polymers® are a series of products offered by SurfaTech that are the product of molecular modeling, allowing the chemist to focus in on every detail of the molecule in order to dial in the desired aesthetics. In order to develop a wide range of products, three different types of alcohols are incorporated in order to provide different properties to these products. They are a liquid C_{20} octyldodecanol, a saturated low melting C_{18} alcohol (stearyl alcohol) and a higher melting C_{22} alcohol (behenyl alcohol).

The inclusion of the octyldodecyl group into the polymer results in a liquid product that provides cushion, spread on the skin and a very light, dry feel on the skin.

The inclusion of a C_{18} (stearyl alcohol) results in a solid polymer that leaves a soft barrier on the skin and provides structure. A polymer with predominantly C_{18} as the alkyl group has a melting point close to body temperature allowing it to liquefy when applied to the skin.

The inclusion of a C_{22} (benenyl alcohol) results in a hard, solid polymer with a melting point of about 45ºC and is used in lipsticks.

Chain Terminators

Chain terminators have one group that is reactive. For simplicity, we are showing the carboxyl group on the third carbon as the reactive species, but from an esterification point of view it would be equally reactive on each of the three positions.

$$H_2C\text{-}C(O)OR$$
$$|$$
$$HO\text{-}C\text{-}C(O)OR$$
$$|$$
$$H_2C\text{-}C(O)OH$$

Chain Extenders

Chain extenders have two groups that are reactive. For simplicity, we are showing the second and third carbon as the reactive ones, but from an esterification point of view all three are equally reactive.

$$\begin{array}{c} H_2C\text{-}C(O)OR \\ | \\ HO\text{-}C\text{-}C(O)OH \\ | \\ H_2C\text{-}C(O)OH \end{array}$$

Chain Branching

Chain branching groups have all three groups available for reaction.

$$\begin{array}{c} H_2\text{-}C\text{-}C(O)OH \\ | \\ HO\text{-}C\text{-}C(O)OH \\ | \\ H_2C\text{-}C(O)OH \end{array}$$

Crosslinked Groups

The reactive carboxyl groups are linked to each other using a 1,3 propanediol derived from corn.

$$HO\text{-}(CH_2)_3\text{-}OH$$

It is only when all of these components (di substituted, mono substituted and crosslinked) are combined in the proper ratio that the products giving specific cosmetic properties are obtained. The reaction forms a polyester, includes no vinyl reactive groups and no undesirable monomers.

When the mono and di substituted esters and crosslinked are simply combined with each other as individual components in the same ratio used to make a polymer, the mixture is a non-uniform mixture of all components (see **Figures 1** and **2** later in the chapter).

When reacted with the same ratio of components and then crosslinked with 1,3 propanediol, a polymer is formed that no longer is simply a mixture, but is a condensation polymer with a very specific structure and very specific properties.

The simplest representation of the polymers is one in which all the reactive positions are as shown here.

Chain Terminator   **Chain Extender**   **Chain Terminator**

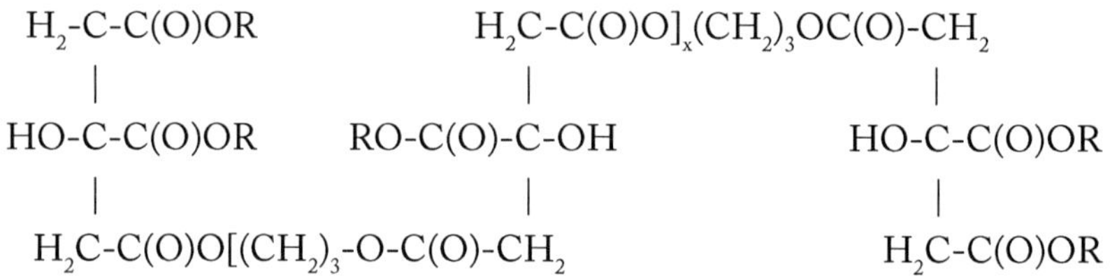

H_2-C-C(O)OR H_2C-C(O)O]$_x$(CH$_2$)$_3$OC(O)-CH$_2$
| | |
HO-C-C(O)OR   RO-C(O)-C-OH   HO-C-C(O)OR
| | |
H_2C-C(O)O[(CH$_2$)$_3$-O-C(O)-CH$_2$ H_2C-C(O)OR

Photomicrographs

The following samples were submitted for photomicrographic evaluation:

Non-crosslinked. Citrate ester with no crosslinking having:

- 50% by weight C18 (stearyl) and
- 50% C20 branched (octyldodecanol)

Crosslinked. Citrate ester having:

- 50% by weight C18 (stearyl) and
- 50% C20 branched (octyldodecanol), crosslinked with 1,3 propane diol

Non-crosslinked Photomicrograph

All four components are clearly seen in **Figure 1**.

The non-crosslinked material is a viscous liquid containing three types of anisotropic crystals suspended in an isotropic liquid phase. The crystals have a bimodal particle size distribution.

The large blocky crystals melt over the range of 39°–42.2°C.

The small needle-like crystals melt over the range of 44°–55.8°C. Melting is appreciably complete by 50°C with only a few crystals melting at 55.8°C. The crystals disappear into the liquid phase as they melt.

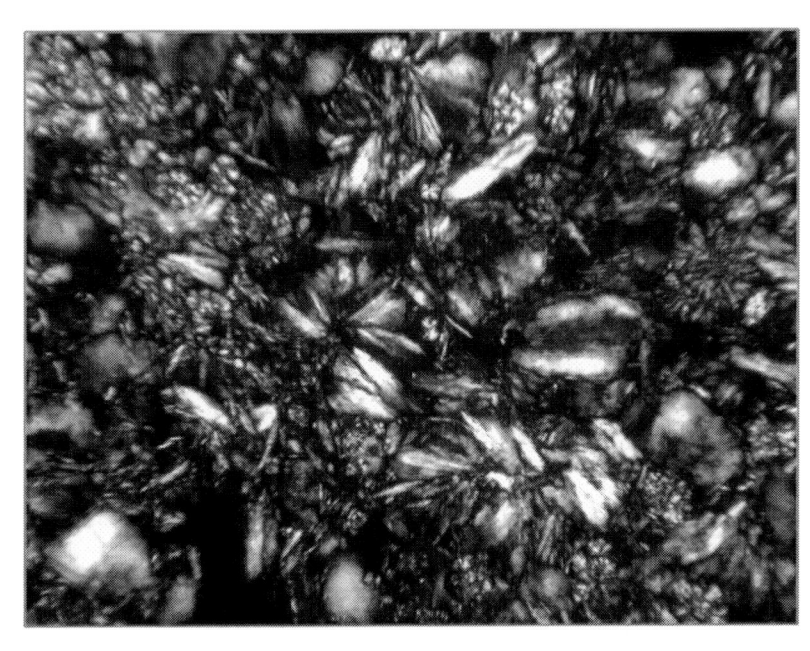

Figure 1 Non-crosslinked Photomicrograph

The onset of melting is approximate since it is difficult to see individual crystals melting when there are many of them in the field.

Crosslinked Photomicrographs

The introduction of crosslinking makes the product a polymer, rather than a collection of non-polymeric materials (see **Figure 2**).

The crosslinked polymer consists of uniformly-sized acicular-to-narrow lath shaped crystals. Melting of the crystals occurs over a wide temperature range. The onset of melting is difficult to recognize (approximately 42°C) and approximately one half of the crystals have melted by 45°C. The last of the crystals melts by 48.4°C. Black regions are the liquid crystal phase.

The crosslinked product is a thick paste consisting of a single anisotropic crystalline phase.

The crystalline phase melts over the range of 42°C to 48.4°C. By 45°C most of the crystals have melted and disappeared into the liquid phase.

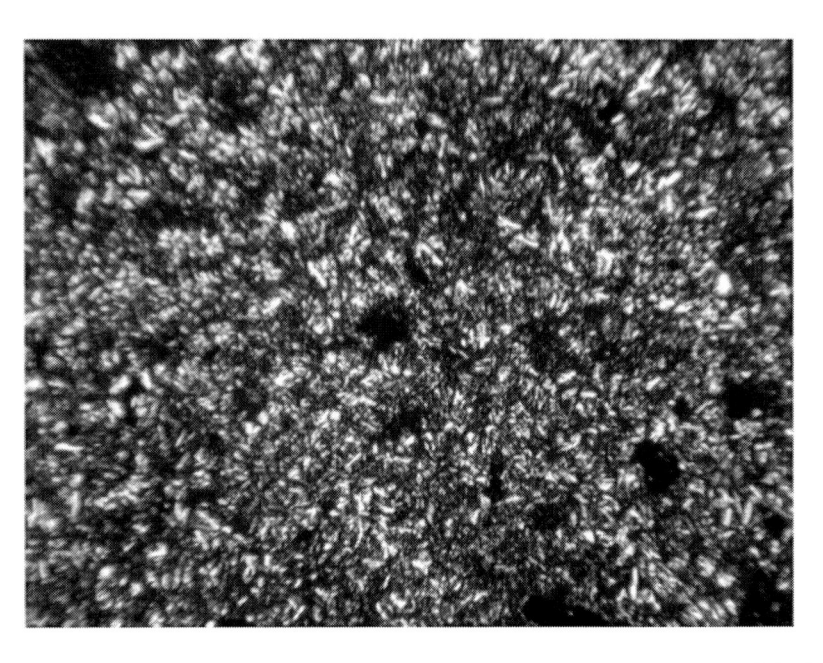

Figure 2 Crosslinked Photomicrograph

The crystals exhibit a narrow particle size distribution and are significantly smaller in size than the large crystals (lower melting phase) in the non-crosslinked product.

Commercial Crosslinked Polymer Products

Typical of the type of materials that can be made using the citrate polyester technology are the following products. They replace materials made using vinyl chemistry in which the products are neither green nor free of vinyl reactive monomers, replace silicone for aesthetics or replace no polymeric esters that may not enjoy REACH acceptance (See **Table 1**).

Waterproofing Study

Lott Research, Inc. undertook a study to determine if Cosmosurf CE-150 could be used as a waterproofing film former for sunscreen products.

Table 1
Materials without REACH acceptance

Product	INCI	Description
CosmoSurf® CE-100	octyldodecyl citrate Crosspolymer	Liquid lower viscosity (ECOCERT Approved)
CosmoSurf® CE-100HV	octyldodecyl citrate Crosspolymer	High molecular weight (ECOCERT pending)
CosmoSurf® CE-140	octyldodecyl stearyl citrate Crosspolymer	Soft wax (ECOCERT pending)
CosmoSurf® CE-150	octyldodecyl stearyl citrate Crosspolymer	Medium hardness wax (ECOCERT pending)
CosmoSurf® CE-250	octyldodecyl behenyl citrate Crosspolymer	Hard Wax (ECOCERT pending)

Method

Formulas for three different products were prepared as shown in **Table 2**.

The manufacturing procedure was basically the same for all three formulations.

1. Parts A and B were heated separately to about 160°F
2. Part B was added to part A while rapidly stirring
3. Parts A and B mixture was cooled with stirring to approximately 105°F
4. Part C was added with stirring

All three formulations were SPF tested using a single port Solar Light Model 15S Xenon Arc, Solar Simulator lamp, which has a continuous light spectrum in the UVA and UVB range (290-400 nanometers). The spectral output of the solar simulator is filtered so that it meets the spectral output requirements for testing sunscreen drug products for over-the-counter human use (Proposed Amendment of Final Monograph, CFR Part 352.70 (b) Light Sources, Federal Register, Vol. 72, No. 165, Aug. 27, 2007 and the International Sun Protection Factor (SPF) Test Method, May 2006).

Table 2
Water Resistance Study using Citrate Ester Polymers

Ingredient	LRI A80 %	LRI A220 %	LRI A175 %
Part A			
Water	74.2	72.2	82.9
Carbomer	.25	.25	.25
Disodium Ethylenediaminetetraacetic Acid	.05	.05	.05
Triethanolamine	1	1	1
Part B			
Octocrylene	3	3	3
Octisalate	3	3	3
Oxybenzone	2	2	2
Avobenzone	1	1	1
Stearic Acid	2	1	1
Sorbitan Isostearate	0	1	1
Polyglyceryl-3 Distearate	0	1	1
Glyceryl Stearate Self Emulsifying	3	0	0
Benzyl Alcohol	1	1	1
Dimethylpolysiloxane	.5	.5	.5
VP/Eicosene Copolymer	0	0	2
Methylparaben	0	.2	.2
Propylparaben	0	.1	.1
Finsolv TN	8	0	0
Cosmosurf CE-150	0	2	0
Part C			
Liquipar PE(Phenoxyethanol, Isopropylparaben, Isobutylparaben, and n-Butylparaben	1	0	0

The SPF test for all three formulations was performed on the same subjects. The only difference was that LRI A80 was performed as a static, non-water-resistant test and LRI A220 and LRI A175 were performed as 80 minute VWR tests.

All three formulations were submitted to an independent analytical lab, Allied Analytical Laboratory Services.

Results

The average values for the SPF tests as reported by Florida Suncare Testing, Inc. (*http://flsuncaretesting.com/*) were as follows:

LRI A80	< 19 (static)	No waterproofing agent
LRI A220	28.85 (VWR)	VP/Eicosene Copolymer
LRI A175	29.05 (VWR)	Cosmosurf CE-150

The analytical results for the formulations are shown below to verify the actual amount of sunscreen in the formulation (given in % by weight).

	Octocrylene	Octisalate	Oxybenzone	Avobenzone
LRI A80	3.03	3.12	2.02	1.04
LRI A220	2.94	3.04	1.95	0.95
LRI A175	3.04	2.96	1.99	1.00

Discussion

All three formulas were targeted as an SPF 25. For an SPF 25 the lowest number obtainable is a SPF 19. Four of the subjects tested for SPF had MED responses at the SPF 19 level. When this happens it means the actual value is at a maximum SPF 19. Based on discussions with the Florida Suncare Testing, Inc. investigator, the values would probably have been considerably lower than 19. The investigator estimated that the actual value would probably have been closer to SPF 12–15 based on the responses at SPF 19. For a five subject tested for SPF in the study, the values obtained for LRI A220 and LRI A175, with standard deviations of 2.53 and 4.12 respectively are not statistically different.

Conclusion

Based on the results of these SPF tests, CE-150 has significant value as a SPF waterproofing agent when compared to a control formula without a waterproofing film former. Based on the results of this study, SurfaTech Cosmosurf CE-150 was equivalent to the well-known waterproofing film former, VP/Eicosene Copolymer.

SPF Improvement

Additional studies were undertaken using a different formula to test improvement in SPF values.

Formula A
SPF 31.55 (a total of five individual subjects)

Ingredient	Code	Percent
Part A	Water	67.2000
	Ultrez 21	0.2500
	EDTA	0.0500
Part B	TEA	1.0000
Part C	Octocrylene	3.0000
	Octisalate	3.0000
	Oxybenzone	2.0000
	Avobenzone	1.0000
	Stearic Acid	2.0000
	GMS SE	3.0000
	Benzyl alcohol	1.0000
	DC 200-200	1.5000
	Finnsolv TN	8.0000
	Spider Ester ®ESO	5.0000
	Cosmosurf ®CE-100	2.0000
Part D	Lipuipar PE	1.0000
Total		100.00

Formula B
SPF 18.87 (five subjects)

Ingredient	Code	Percent
Part A	Water	67.2000
	Ultrez 21	0.2500
	EDTA	0.0500
Part B	TEA	1.0000
Part C	Octocrylene	3.0000
	Octisalate	3.0000
	Oxybenzone	2.0000
	Avobenzone	1.0000
	Stearic Acid	2.0000
	GMS SE	3.0000
	Siltech F-200	1.0000
	DC 200-200	0.5000
	Finnsolv TN	15.0000
Part D	Lipuipar PE	1.0000
Total		100.00

SPF tested using a single port Solar Light Model 15S Xenon Arc, Solar Simulator lamp, which has a continuous light spectrum in the UVA and UVB range (290-400 nanometers). The spectral output of the solar simulator is filtered so that it meets the spectral output requirements for testing Sunscreen Drug Products for over-the-counter human use; Proposed Amendment of Final Monograph, CFR Part 352.70 (b) Light Sources, Federal Register, Vol. 72, No. 165, Aug. 27, 2007 and the International Sun Protection Factor (SPF) Test Method, May 2006.

Hair Care Applications

The citrate polymers also find application in shampoos as oils used in coacervate products replacing silicone fluids (see **Table 3**). CosmoSurf CE-100 together with a silicone complex Silplex J-2S has been found to be an effective agent for the formation of a coacervate in shampoos.

Properties

The shampoo had the following characteristics:

Viscosity (cps)	12,000
pH	5.70
Appearance	Opaque white cream

Shampoo Foam

The shampoos were evaluated with the same procedure. A 1000 mL cylinder with 10 mL increments was used. All samples and distilled water were prepared at 25°C. 1.00 gram of test material was used and 100 ml distill water was added to dissolve the test material in a 250 ml beaker. After the test material was totally dissolved, the solution was transferred into the cylinder. An outlet of air pump was located on the bottom of the cylinder to generate the bubbles. Recorded the foam height within 20 seconds for each test material, each material was evaluated three times and their averages were documented.

The scale for Foam Height of 1000 ml is considered outstanding and 100 mL is very poor. The type of foam was also noted whether it is tight or loose. Bubbles were generated by electronic air pump. The foam generated was then measured in mL (see **Table 4**).

Table 4

Sample (Bubble for 20 sec)	Initial Reading (Average, ml)	Two Minute Reading (Average, ml)	Five Minute Reading (Average, ml)
FH183D	700	690	670

Table 3
Shampoo Formulation
2 in 1 Shampoo (Coacervate) FH183D

Phase	Description	INCI Name	Weight
A	D.I. Water	Aqua	22.000
	Carbopol Aqua SF-1 Polymer (1%)	Acrylates copolymer	2.500
	TEA 99%	Disodium EDTA	0.100
	Na2EDTA	Disodium EDTA	0.100
	Sodium Laureth Sulfate	Sodium Laureth-2 Sulfate	27.500
	Cocamidopropyl Betaine	Cocamidopropyl Betaine	6.000
B	D.I. Water	Aqua	18.000
	Sodium Laureth Sulfate	Sodium Laureth-2 Sulfate	5.500
	Cocamidopropyl Betaine	Cocamidopropyl Betaine	4.000
	Ninol COMF	Cocamide MEA	1.200
	EGDS	Ethylene Glycol Distearate	3.000
C	Silplex J2-S (Siltech LLC)	Silicone Quaternium-20	1.000
	Cosmosurf® CE-100 (SurfaTech)	Octyldodecyl citrate crosspolymer	1.000
	Wheat Protein	Wheat Protein	0.500
	Hemp Seed Oil	Cannabis Sativa (Hemp) Seed Oil	1.000
	Nipaguard DMDMH	DMDM Hydantoin	0.500
D	Decyl Glucoside	Decyl Glucoside	3.000
	Amphosol 2C	Disodium Cocoamphodiacetate	3.000
	Citric Acid (40% aq)	Citric Acid	q.s.
	Sodium Chloride (if needed)	Sodium Chloride	q.s.
	Crothix (Croda) (if needed)	PEG-150 Pentaerythrityl Tetrastearate	q.s.
	Fruity Herbal	Fragrance	q.s.
		Total	100.00

Procedure: The shampoos were made using the following procedure:
1. Into a clean and sanitized stainless steel container equipped with propeller mixer, add water in phase B
2. Add SLES-2 and Betaine, heat up to 70°C to 75°C, slowly add Cocamide MEA and EGDS, mix slowly while minimizing air incorporation. Mix until uniform, then cool down to room temperature.
3. In another clean and sanitized stainless steel tank equipped with propeller mixer, add water and the rest of ingredients of phase A one by one while minimizing air incorporation. Mix until uniform.
4. Add phase B slowly into phase A. Mix until uniform.
5. Premix Silplex J2-S and Cosmosurf CE-100 until uniform, then add into phase A+B and mix well. Add the rest of ingredients in phase C one by one into phase A+B until homogeneous while minimizing air incorporation.
6. Add ingredients in phase D one by one. Adjust pH by using citric acid to pH = 5.5–6.5, and adjust viscosity to 6,000 cps–12, 000 cps by adding q.s. NaCl and Crothix. Add fragrance if necessary.

Shampoo Wet Comb

All products were evaluated on 10-inch virgin brown hair. Two x 2-gram swatches were used for each material tested, all from the same lot. All swatches were wet with 25°C water and one gram of test material was used for each swatch. Swatches were washed and then rinsed for at least one minute per swatch. Wet comb evaluation was then performed. No blow-drying of hair was done. All swatches were air-dried, and then the dry comb evaluation was performed once hair was completely dry. Scale used was 1 to 5, 5 being the best. Used for wet and dry combing (see **Tables 5** and **6**).

Table 6
Shampoo Dry Comb

Evaluation Sample:	Control Water Only	FH183D
Wet Comb	1.0	4.5
Rinse Off	3.0	4.5
Clean Feel (scroop)	2.0	4.5
Shine Feel	2.0	3.0
Residual	2.0	3.0
Average	2.0	3.9

Shampoo Dry Comb

Table 6
Shampoo Dry Comb

Evaluation Sample:	Control Water Only	FH183D
Dry Comb	3.0	4.5
Dry Feel	3.0	4.5
Clean Feel/Look	2.0	4.5
Shine	2.0	3.0
Fullness/Manageability	1.0	3.0
Fly-away	1.0	3.9
Residual	1.0	3.5
Static	2.0	4.0
Average	1.75	4.12

Salt Tolerance, pH, Viscosity, Ease of Formulation, Effect on Formulation Stability

Scale used was 1 to 5, 5 being the best, only for salt tolerance, ease of formulation, and effect on formulation stability. Viscosity was tested by using Brookfiled, LVT, #4 spindle, 12 rpm. See **Table 7**.

Table 7
Salt Tolerance, pH, Viscosity, Ease of Formulation, Effect on Formulation Stability

Evaluation Sample:	FH183D
Salt Tolerance	2.5
pH	5.70
Viscosity, cps	12,000
Ease of Formulation Stability	4.0
Effect of Formulation	4.5
Average	3.67

Antiperspirant with Cosmosurf CE-100 and Silwax CR-1

Addition of the citrate ester together with a silicone to lower surface tension (Silwax CR-1) results in an antiperspirant with outstanding properties, that is D5 free. See **Table 8**.

Conclusion

Citrate ester polymers are a new class of materials that find application in a variety of personal care applications. The ability to alter the structure to change the properties makes this class of compounds very flexible.

References

1. US Patent 4,868,236 to O'Lenick issued September 19, 1989.
2. US Patent 7,723,456 to O'Lenick et al issued May 25, 2010.
3. US Patent 7,569,607 to O'Lenick et al issued August 4, 2009.
4. US Patent 7,473,707 to O'Lenick et al issued January 6, 2009.
5. US Patent 7,462,729 to O'Lenick et al issued December 9, 2008.

Table 8

Phase	Ingredient	INCI Name	% w/w
Part A			
Reach AZP-908 (Summit Research)		Aluminum/Zirconium Tetrachlorohydrex-GLY	24.00
Silsurf DMC-AP (Siltech)		PEG/PPG 18/6 Dimethicone	2.50
Part B			
Silwax CR-1 (Siltech)			25.00
Cosmosurf CE 100			5.00
Part C	Fancol IH-CG (Fanning)	Isohexadecane	9.00
	Probutyl 14 (Croda)	PPG-14 Butyl Ether	9.00
	Castorwax NF	Hydrogenated Castor Oil	2.50
	Protomate 400-DSPEG-8	Distearate	1.00
	Crodacol S-95 NF	Stearyl Alcohol	18.00
Part D	270764 Talc USP 300	Talc	3.00
	Cab-O-Sil M-5 (Cabot)	Silica	0.50
Part E	Fragrance Blue Musk	Fragrance (Parfum)	0.50
			100.00

Procedure:
1. In a side vessel, combine phase A ingredients. Impeller mix to uniformity.
2. In main vessel, heat phase B ingredients to 70°C under agitation. Continue mixing and add phase A. Bring to 75°C.
3. Combine phase C in side vessel, heat to 85°C under impeller agitation and mix to uniformity.
4. Add phase C to AB under homogenization. Maintain batch at 80°C.
5. Pre-combine phase D. Add to batch under homogenization. Begin cooling.
6. Add phase E at 70°C under homogenization. Continue cooling.
7. Pour batch into sticks at 65°C.
8. Heat-treat surfaces.

Credits

The photomicrographs and conclusions provided in this section were provided by:
  Microtrace LLC
  790 Fletcher Drive
  Suite 106
  Elgin, IL 60123-4755

Index

A

absorption 323-4
AC *see* acrylates copolymer
acetone 152, 155-6
acid 10, 26-7, 29, 43, 70, 155, 182, 290, 389
  succinic 63, 66-7, 72
acrylamide 131-2, 145
acrylates 88, 93, 126, 133, 137, 139, 210, 220-2, 254, 256, 341, 343
acrylates copolymer (AC) 91, 93-4, 222, 339, 342-9, 428
acrylates copolymer, acrylates/hydroxyesters 95-6
acrylates/octylacrylamide copolymer 339, 341-5
Acrylates/octylacrylamide copolymer solutions 341-2
acrylic acid 24, 26, 33, 126, 128, 131, 136-8, 407-9, 412
acrylic-based film-forming polymers 339, 347-8
Acrylic copolymer 125, 134
Acrylic Film-forming Polymers to Enhance SPF Water Resistance 343
ACTH 293-4
Aculyn 137-9, 256, 258
AFM (atomic force microscope) 22, 32, 173, 247-8
agents, antidandruff 186, 193
AIBN 6
alcohols 9, 12, 102, 151, 155-6, 312, 341, 343, 418
  stearyl 416, 418
alkyl 130, 137, 256, 309, 328-9, 331, 384

alkyl acrylate copolymer 210
alkyl acrylate crosspolymer 91-4, 99, 256-7, 342, 344, 346
alkyl benzoate 303-4, 311, 335, 349, 358, 361-2
alkyl dimethicone compounds 329, 377, 381, 387
alkyl dimethicone copolyol compounds 384-5
alkyl dimethicones 328-9, 331, 377, 381-2, 386-7
alkyl silicones 328, 330-3, 386
alkylmethylsiloxanes 352, 355, 359, 368
amide 10-12
amines 10-11, 109, 168
amino acids 12, 165, 233, 289-94, 296-8
amodimethicone 111, 367
amphiphilic diblock copolymer 133, 413
amphoteric 135, 138
AMSs 355-6
aniline pentamer (AP) 21
anionic 100-1, 127, 129, 131, 135, 137, 183, 192, 223
anionic polymerization 127, 134
anionic polymers 99-100, 131, 134, 180, 221
anionic rheology modifiers 206, 209
anions 234, 404-5
aroma 17-18
associative polymers 91, 93, 137-8, 147
atomic 22, 31-2, 146, 185, 247-8
atomic force microscope *see* AFM
ATRP (Atom Transfer Radical Polymerization) 4-5
avobenzone 335, 342, 360, 366, 424-6

B

bacteria 16, 26, 76-7, 297
bases, oxidation 147
BASF 125-7, 133-4, 222, 249, 257-8, 358
behenyl dimethicone 329-31, 333, 336
Benzophenone-3 342, 345-6, 349
bimodal polymers 100-1, 103
Biomacromolecules 16, 33-4
biopolymers 15, 17, 19, 21, 23, 25, 27, 29, 31, 33, 49, 162, 173
bleaching 106, 143, 233, 235, 240, 245, 266
blends 33, 156, 208, 290, 307, 320, 331-4, 353, 362, 365
block copolymers 24, 122, 124-8, 134, 147, 375-6, 409
borage oil 316, 320-5
 viscosity of 320, 322
Brassica campestris 317, 325-6
bubbles 37, 317, 427
build-up 198-9
Butyl methoxydibenzoylmethane 344-5, 358, 362, 365
butylaminoethyl methacrylate 222
butylene glycol 108, 263-4, 292

C

CAB 28
CAPB 191, 194, 199, 265
caprylyl dimethicone 322-3, 326
carbomer 42, 93, 96-7, 99, 136, 206-14, 217, 256, 335, 346, 358, 365, 424
carbomer film 212
carbomer gels 128, 207-8, 210, 213

carbon atoms 72, 241, 329, 383, 385
carboxylic groups 9-10, 26, 80
carrageenans 17-19, 35
castor 66-8
castor isostearate succinate 73-4
castor oil 63-8, 72, 74, 336
 hydrogenated 106, 257-8
catalyst 4, 389-93, 395
cationic 99-100, 103, 130-2, 135, 137, 180, 233, 248, 263
cationic conditioning polymer 180, 203
cationic guars 118-19, 190-1, 194-5, 198-200
cationic polymer 114-15, 117, 131, 145, 147, 175, 178, 180-1, 183-4, 186-7, 194, 203, 233-4, 244, 246
cellulose 32, 147, 190
centistokes 388, 390
Cerotyl dimethicone 382-3
Cetearyl alcohol 73-4, 344
cetyl dimethicone 315, 317-20, 322-3, 325-6, 355-7, 359
CFCs (chlorinated fluoro carbons) 102, 150-1
chains 12, 38, 49, 60, 78, 80, 100, 122, 126, 289-90, 296-7, 305, 406
chitosan 23, 32-3
chloride, cetrimonium 217, 264-5, 268-9, 271
chlorinated fluoro carbons (CFCs) 102, 150-1
cholesterol 27-9, 34, 45
cholesterol rings 28
Ciba 88-90, 132, 134, 146, 180, 185
Citrate Polyesters 415, 417, 419, 421, 423, 425, 427, 429, 431
Citric Acid 264, 416, 428
classes 8, 12, 32, 121, 129, 151, 190, 328, 341, 352, 356, 377-8, 381, 385, 387, 407

clear gel systems 90
CLSM (confocal laser scanning microscopy) 262-3
CMC (critical micelle concentration) 114, 140, 177, 183, 380-1, 405, 409-10
coacervate 113-14, 118, 120, 179, 181, 185-6, 427-8
cocamidopropyl betaine 44-5, 191, 202, 264-5
collagen 21, 33, 290-2, 295, 297
collagen gels 22
color 106, 136, 144, 146, 184, 201, 266, 268-71, 334, 336, 369, 372, 374-5
color molecules 271
color retention 87, 111, 135, 144, 367
color values 268
combing 100, 111, 121-2, 128, 133, 161, 164-6, 168, 183, 192, 195, 236-7, 251, 254, 284
conditioners 35, 106-10, 121, 131-2, 165-6, 169, 171-2, 233, 236, 261-2, 264, 266-7, 269-70, 302, 366-7, 378
conditioning 66, 87, 108-9, 111, 121, 125, 175, 183-4, 190, 197-8, 261, 267, 273, 378, 380-1
conditioning benefits 126, 132, 177, 180-3, 209, 367
conditioning polymers 104, 108, 180, 189-92, 200, 202
conditioning shampoos 113-15, 117, 119, 175-7, 179, 182-3, 185, 203
  2-in-1 200, 202
  modern 114, 175, 177-8
copolymer blends 16
copolymerization 276, 370, 407
copolymers 16, 21, 28, 88-9, 94, 97, 107, 125, 131-2, 138, 145-6, 222, 234, 249, 276, 349

new 89, 133
octylacrylamide 341, 343
silicone-free 280
copper 4-5
Cosmosurf 423, 426, 428
Cosmosurf CE-150 422, 424-5
crotonic acid/vinyl 275, 277-8, 280-2, 286
crystal-clear gel systems 88
crystals 133, 256, 334, 420-2
curl retention 93, 104-5, 253-7
curls 96, 102, 104, 208, 211, 253-4
cyclopentasiloxane 110, 315, 317-20, 323, 325-6, 349, 353-5, 357-8, 363-5
cytokines 297-8

D

dehydroxanthan gum (DG) 128, 134, 339, 347-50
DG *see* dehydroxanthan gum
dimethicone 102, 110, 126, 193-8, 200-2, 217, 236-7, 239, 316-17, 325, 329, 331, 336, 352, 354, 357
Dimethicone copolyol 181, 257-8, 328, 378
dimethicone crosspolymer 109-10, 363, 365
dimethicone deposition 193-4
dimethicone emulsion 189, 194-6, 199-200, 202-3
  submicron 189, 193-5, 202
dimethyl ether 102, 155-6, 281-2
Dimethypabamidopropyl laurdimonium tosylate 263-4
Divinyldimethicone/dimethicone copolymer 108, 183, 362
DSC (differential scanning calorimetry) 40, 267, 273, 280, 404

DSC measurements 269, 273
dye precursors 135-7, 139, 146
dyes 136, 145, 179, 192, 199, 266, 268
  demipermanent 269-71
  fluorescent 145, 147

E

Elaeis guineensis 317, 325-6
elasticity 81, 111-12, 213, 226, 228, 275, 283, 287
elastin 290-2, 295, 297
elastomers 125, 128, 352, 369-70
electrical stimulus 21
electrochemical 177, 289
electrolyte 37, 39-40, 42, 47, 114
emulsifier/thickener systemse 56, 58-9, 61
emulsifiers 53, 55-8, 72, 106-7, 153, 342, 378, 384
emulsions 45-6, 49-51, 53, 55-61, 81, 84, 106, 112, 193, 196, 344, 360, 362, 385
  nonionic 108-9, 362
  stable oil-in-water 72
  vitro-tested 344, 346, 349
enzymes 11-12, 291, 294, 297-8
esters 9-10, 64, 104, 316, 360, 384
  citrate 415-16, 420, 430
ethanol 46-7, 97, 123, 151-2, 155, 210, 221, 226, 228, 230, 265, 276-7, 281, 341-2, 345, 371

F

fatty acids 27, 70, 72, 233, 316
FDA (Food and Drug Administration) 335, 343, 345

fermentation 75, 416
fermentation broth 78
FH183D 427-30
fiber 34, 122, 124, 144, 162-4, 168, 170, 173, 176, 196, 262, 266, 268, 279
fibronectin 290, 295, 297-8
film-forming polymers 133, 339-45, 347, 349
films 17-18, 21, 23, 31-2, 96-7, 122, 127, 208-9, 212, 220, 226, 228, 249, 259, 328, 340-1
  hydrocolloid 17
  uniform 91, 336, 340-1
  waterproofing 422, 425
fixative polymer 100, 121-2, 125, 150
flocculate 190, 192-4, 196
flocculation 49, 56-7, 61, 189-91
fluid 40, 110-11, 304, 355-8, 362-3, 365, 389
  silicone carbinol 354, 368
fluid gels 35-6, 40-1, 47
fluorescence 25, 29, 147, 243, 263
foams 394, 407-8, 412, 427
Food and Drug Administration (FDA) 335, 343, 345
Formula 44-7, 72-4, 101-2, 216-17, 257-8, 264-8, 280-5, 304, 312, 325-6, 335-6, 344-5, 347-8, 354-8, 360-3, 384-5
formula stability 301-2, 312
formulas 3, 99, 125, 153, 155-7, 223, 225, 229-30, 255, 263, 284, 289, 335-7, 344-9, 361, 425-6
  hairspray 223
  standard 372-3
formulation stability 197, 207, 430
formulation variables 177, 179
formulations 91-4, 108-10, 113-16, 254-5, 280-2, 326-30, 337, 340-3, 345-8, 353-7, 362-3, 365-6,

371-5, 377-9, 423-5, 430
conditioner   131, 171, 266, 268, 270, 272
hair relaxer   130
hairspray   226
nail polish   369
test hair spray   283
water-based   152-3
fragrance   17-18, 45-6, 73, 107, 111, 153, 245-6, 257-8, 305, 312, 325-6, 357, 371
free-radical polymerization   127
living   24, 121, 187
friction   180, 207, 214-15, 236-9, 247, 251, 259, 276, 279
friction coefficient   207, 214, 235, 237, 239, 251
frizz   109-10

G

gel formulations   89-90, 211, 247
various hair   207
gel layer   233, 236, 242-3
gel permeation chromatography analysis   393-4
gelation   39-40, 60, 409
gelation temperature   39, 42, 408-9
gels   17, 24-7, 39-43, 47-51, 60-2, 80-1, 122, 152-4, 156, 205-7, 209-11, 213-15, 217-18, 252-5, 405-6, 408
adhesive protein-free synthetic polymer   34
alkyl acrylate copolymer   210
crystal-clear   89-90
diluted   253
excess   253
mucoadhesive   15, 25-6
non-sheared   40

reversible   49-50, 60
tested   252-3
thixotrophic   328, 331, 333
gloss   66, 70, 72-3, 101, 181, 301, 305-6, 311-12, 315, 369, 374, 379
glucose   36, 38, 49, 78, 84, 416
Glucovis   44-7
Glycerin   45-7, 344, 346, 349, 355, 357, 361-2
glyceryl stearate   50, 335, 346, 349, 358, 362, 365
graft copolymers   121, 123-4
guar hydroxypropyltrimonium chloride   114, 117, 175-6, 179-80, 182, 190, 203
gums   48-50, 59, 61-2, 64, 145

H

hair   94-101, 106-12, 121-3, 129-37, 144-7, 161-73, 175-7, 179-84, 192-203, 222-5, 228-31, 233-4, 236-43, 245, 275-6, 366-7
coloring   146-7
combability of   238, 251
damaged/oxidized   196-7
dimethicone-treated   239
dyed   261, 269, 273
polyquaternium-64-treated   239
polyquaternium-7-treated   239
silicone-treated   276
hair bleaching   197, 240
hair care   87, 89, 91, 93, 95, 97, 99, 101, 103-5, 107-9, 111, 133, 135, 146, 259, 261
hair care applications   104, 108, 427
hair care compositions   134, 147, 159
hair care formulations   110, 163, 273
hair care polymers   87, 248

hair color   106, 266-7, 273, 367
hair conditioners   72-3, 133, 378
hair conditioning   113, 117, 121, 131, 133, 175, 189-90, 194-5, 197
hair dyes   106, 135, 267
hair gel formulations   248
hair gels   46, 133, 205, 247, 252, 255-6
hair shine   152, 189, 202-3
hair softness   177, 180
hair sprays   72, 94, 103, 121, 149, 152-3, 155-6, 158-9, 229, 275-6, 284, 286
hair straightening   121, 130
hairsprays   221-2, 224, 229, 287
HEUR-thickened systems   142-3
HHCR (high-humidity curl retention)   93, 98, 103-4, 284
high humidity curl retention   205, 207-8, 221, 284
high-humidity curl retention *see* HHCR
homopolymers   28, 122-3, 131, 133
  crosslinked acrylic acid   145
  dimethylaminoethyl methacrylate   145-6
hybrid polymers   276-7, 281-2, 286
  new   275, 282-3, 286
  organic-silicone   279, 282, 285
  silicone-organic   368
hydrocolloids   17, 48-50
hydrogels   15, 22-4, 33
hydrophilic   24, 29, 141, 192, 201, 276, 329, 354
hydrophilic polymers, modified   397, 409
hydrophobic   24, 88, 126, 141, 192, 201, 329
hydrophobic properties   276-7
hydroxyethylcellulose   136-8, 185

I

inert hydrogels   23
inflection points   402
Interpolymer   99-102, 104
irradiation   170, 238, 241, 262, 266-7
isoalkyl esters/VA/bis-vinyldimethicone crosspolymer   277, 281-2, 284
isoalkyl esters/VA/bisvinyldimethicone crosspolymer   275, 278, 280
isododecane   303-5, 309, 311, 353-4

K

keratin   106-7, 161-2, 166, 241, 290-2
keratin biopolymer   162-6, 169-73
keratin IFP   163, 166, 168, 171

L

LCST (lower critical solution temperature)   24, 397, 399-400, 403-6, 411-12
LCST polymers   406-7
lipids, natural   315-16, 326
lotions   81, 98-9, 136, 221, 302, 333, 353-4, 362, 367
  sun   46-7, 356

M

macromolecules   48, 62, 134, 139-40, 147, 277, 279, 411-13
menthol   82-3

methacrylate copolymer   88-90, 139, 210, 256
  beheneth-25   88
methacrylic acid copolymer   137, 187
methicone, caprylyl   315, 317-22, 326
mineral oil   303-4, 308, 311-12, 356, 360, 382, 384
molecules   8-11, 27-8, 37, 65, 78, 80-1, 84, 124, 141-2, 291, 331, 354-5, 382, 384, 406, 417-18
  active   81-2
  glycerin   316
  linking   142-3
  pectin   19-20
  receptor   294
  water-binding   292, 298
monomers   1, 4, 6, 8, 66, 122-3, 127, 134, 276-7, 407, 419
  nonionic   129-31
mucoadhesion   26-7
multi-domain silicones   333-6

N

nail polishes   369, 371-5
nails   371-3
natural ingredients   36, 303, 315, 416
Natural Polymers   35, 37, 39, 41, 43, 45, 47
nonionic   58, 128, 131-2, 135, 138
nonionic surfactants   49, 61-2, 408-9, 413
nuclear magnetic resonance (NMR)   78, 406

O

Octisalate   335, 342, 424-6
Octocrylene   335, 342, 346, 349, 424-6
Octylacrylamide/acrylates   222
octyldodecanol   47, 74, 416, 418, 420
oils   45, 50-1, 58-9, 63-4, 129, 183, 196, 302-5, 307, 309, 312, 317, 319-20, 323, 325-8, 331
  cosmetic   319
  natural   315, 327-8, 337
  safflower   303-4, 308, 311
  seed   312, 315-17, 325-6, 428
  soybean   65, 330
oligopeptides   12, 290, 292, 295, 297
organic polymers   276, 281-2, 286
organic-silicone hybrid polymer crotonic acid/vinyl   284
organic sunscreens   356, 359-60, 363, 365-6, 368
organogels   26-7
Oxybenzone   74, 335, 342, 424-6

P

palmitate, isopropyl   303-4, 308, 311
PCR (percent curl retention)   103-4
pectins   19-20, 23, 35, 146
PEG/PPG dimethicone compounds   377-8, 380, 387
peptide bond   12, 290
peptides   12, 29-30, 163, 289-99
peroxide   168, 271
pH   20, 22, 31-2, 37, 43-4, 79-81, 88-9, 91-2, 264, 281, 344, 349, 358, 365, 427-8, 430
  low   43, 407
pH range   88, 90
PLAAP copolymers   21
poly   16, 21, 24, 26-7, 33, 125, 141, 147, 180, 255, 403, 405, 407-8, 411
polyacrylate-14   91-3
polyacrylic acid, cross-linked   247-8, 257

Polyamide-2 263-4
polyamides 8, 10-11, 405
polyesters 8-10, 63, 66, 70, 72, 108, 180, 419
polyethylene 301-4, 306, 309, 311-12
polyethylene/oil bases 303, 305, 307-8
polyimide-1 205-18
  ratio of 212, 214
polyimide-1 formulations 208, 210
polyion 176-7, 407
polyion chain 177
polymer adhesion volume 238, 241
polymer backbone 2, 94, 190, 199, 206, 405
polymer chains 2-3, 7, 60, 79-80, 95, 101, 139, 279, 405, 408-9
polymer composition 101, 400
polymer concentration 398-401
polymer content 281-3
polymer deposition 192, 198
polymer film properties 222, 226, 228, 257
polymer films 122, 211-12, 214, 226, 228, 236, 248-9, 251-3, 259, 275, 277
polymer hydrophobes 140, 409
polymer matrix 409
polymer molecules 20, 94, 101
polymer performance 209, 214
polymer solids 224, 227
polymer solutions 123, 223, 237, 239, 397, 399, 402-3, 405, 411
polymer structure 117, 403, 412
polymer structure effects 404, 412
polymer-surfactant 175, 177
polymeric N-vinyl acetamide 134
polymerization 2, 4-5, 7-8, 66, 126-7, 416

polymers 4-6, 35-7, 66, 76-81, 87-9, 91-7, 113-15, 120-3, 129-31, 133-5, 221-30, 276-8, 341-3, 401-7, 411-13, 417-21
  active 88-9, 91-2
  amphoteric 130, 206
  bimodial 104
  biomedical 15
  cationic cellulose 179
  cationic guar 183
  charged 37, 119
  citrate 416, 427
  hair-setting 156
  multifunctional 91, 93
  synthetic 35, 150, 190, 245, 316
  total 42-4
polypeptides 11-12, 290
polyquaternium-7 130-1, 190, 236-7, 239
polyquaternium-10 131, 175-6, 180, 190
polyquaternium-59 108, 263-4
polyquaternium-64 233-7, 239-45
polyquaternium-69 97-9
polyquaternium-74 189-91, 193-5, 197, 199, 201, 203
polysaccharides 17, 19, 32, 35, 37-8, 48, 61, 75, 84-5, 157, 190, 405, 407
Polysilicone-15 263-4
polysilicone-19 261-4, 273
Polyurethane-14 AMP-Acrylates Copolymer 220-1, 223, 225, 227, 229, 231
polyurethanes 12, 125, 132, 219-21, 225, 228
propylene glycol 74, 153, 217, 355, 358, 365
propylene glycol stearate 263-4
propylparaben 50, 74, 335, 344, 346, 355, 357, 365, 424

proteins 11-12, 17, 21-4, 104, 106-8, 120, 162-3, 168, 173, 187, 233, 289-91, 293-5, 297-9, 404
 hydrolyzed vegetable 107-8

R

radical polymerizations 1-4, 133
 controlled-living 4
 conventional 1-3
 free 2, 66, 127
Radical Polymers 1, 3, 5, 7, 9, 11, 13
radicals 4-5
RAFT (Reversible Addition-Fragmentation Transfer) 4-6, 127
relative humidity *see* RH
resins
 conventional hair spray 123, 128
 organic 363, 365-6
RG *see* rhizobium gum
RG gel 82-3
RG molecules 78
RH (relative humidity) 93, 98, 103, 105, 110, 208-9, 211, 214-15, 236, 238-9, 250-1, 253-4, 256-7, 266, 283-4, 341
rheological measurements 49, 51
rheological properties 26, 46, 78-9, 94, 136
rheology modifiers 30, 88, 90-1, 93, 97, 210, 339, 347, 350
 carbomer-type 90
rhizobium gum (RG) 75, 77-85

S

sensory assessment 248, 252-3, 261, 266, 268, 271

sensory attributes 91, 323, 367
shampoo applications 100, 263, 267, 269-71
shampoo formulations 189, 197, 199, 428
shampoos 35, 44-5, 90, 95, 109, 113-14, 117, 175, 177-85, 189-90, 193-7, 202-3, 261-4, 267, 270, 427-8
silicone acrylate copolymers 351, 353
silicone backbone 262, 332, 355-6, 383
silicone block copolymers 132
silicone blocks 277, 279
silicone compositions 147
silicone compounds 327-8, 377, 381, 384, 387
silicone elastomer blend 363-6
silicone elastomers 351, 363, 365-8, 371, 375
silicone emulsions 108-10
silicone fluids 110, 129, 337, 363, 377-8, 382, 384, 387-9, 391-3, 395
 centistoke 394
 finished 390
silicone glycols 378, 380
silicone microemulsion 182-3
silicone oil 193, 196, 200, 354
silicone polymers 327, 329, 337, 377, 390-2
silicone resins 110-11, 181, 328
silicone-soluble 328-9
silicone surfactants 337, 378, 380
silicone technology 220, 222, 287, 352
silicone/vinyl acetate copolymer 275, 277, 279
silicones 107-11, 144, 180, 182, 186-7, 276, 315-23, 325-9, 341, 350-3, 355-6, 359-60, 366-8, 375, 378-9, 383-4

skin   12, 61, 66, 72, 81-5, 233-4, 237, 245, 319, 323-4, 327, 339-41, 351-3, 355-6, 361-2, 418
  lighter   323
  porcine   237
sodium chloride   39-40, 42-5, 81-2, 355, 361, 428
solar simulator   335, 423, 426
solids   152-3, 223-4
solubility   8, 70, 123, 156, 231, 290, 296, 330, 382, 384-5, 398
SPF (Sun Protection Factor)   335-7, 339-40, 343-52, 354-6, 360, 363, 368, 423, 425-6
SPF retention   345, 348
SPF tests   335, 424-5
SPF values   340-2, 344, 348, 359, 366, 426
spinodal, chemical   402-3
spinodal decomposition   402-4, 406
stability   49, 89-90, 254, 298, 301, 307
stabilization   49-50, 91
stabilizers   48, 53, 57-8, 107
stearyl   331, 417, 420
stearyl dimethicone   356-9, 365, 382-3
styling   87, 97, 100, 102, 111, 121, 183, 195, 199, 219, 225
styling polymers   97, 158, 215, 220, 222, 224, 230, 247, 257
sulfate   117, 179, 181-3, 191
sun care   350-1, 353, 355, 357, 359, 361-3, 365, 367-8
sun care formulations   352, 360, 363, 367
Sun Protection Factor *see* SPF
sunscreen formulations   343-4, 363
sunscreens   46, 336, 342, 346, 350-2, 355-6, 360, 363, 425
  physical   356, 360
  very water-resistant   343, 345

surfactant concentration   114, 139, 177, 409
surfactants   49, 59, 61, 91, 94, 114-15, 119-20, 139-40, 143, 146, 153, 187, 189, 234, 245-6, 408-10

T

tack   129, 219, 225, 247, 249, 251, 259
tackiness   225, 252-3, 256, 259, 317, 323, 353, 361, 363
tacky   100, 129, 156, 253, 275, 277, 282, 286
terpolymers   126, 137
  water-soluble anionic   96
thickeners   17, 35, 57, 61, 99, 129, 135-9, 141, 211, 247-8, 254-5, 397
  associative   129, 135, 137, 146, 410
  non-associative   135, 145
thickening   88, 91, 94, 128, 130
thickening polymers   129, 147, 197
Triethanolamine   131, 217, 257-8, 335, 342, 346, 357, 424
triglycerides   315-16, 353
tripeptides   292-3
tryptophan   165, 167-71
tryptophan content   165, 167, 170, 172

U

UV filters   340-1, 343, 348
UV protection   161-2, 173, 261, 273, 339
UV radiation   150, 165, 172-3, 339, 352, 366-7

V

vegetable oil blend   317-18, 322-5
vegetable oils   315-17, 319-23, 325-6, 360
vinyl acetate-crotonate-neodecanoate copolymer   282
viscosity   37, 51-2, 59, 78-80, 88-9, 91-2, 94, 219-20, 280-1, 320-2, 360-1, 388, 394, 396, 409-10, 430
  intrinsic   19-20
  low   223, 227, 231, 282
  low shear   56-7, 59
  reproducible   45-7
  residual   52, 55
  zero shear   51, 55, 59, 61
VOCs (volatile organic compounds)   95, 99, 123, 149, 151-3, 155, 159, 223, 229-30, 258, 276
volatile organic compounds *see* VOCs

W

water   8, 24-5, 39-40, 43-7, 49-51, 72-4, 95-7, 106-7, 122-3, 128-9, 155-6, 206-8, 257-8, 280-1, 340-6, 357-9
water resistance   208, 339-42, 345, 347-8, 350, 362
water solubility   377, 387, 412
water-soluble   23, 128, 157, 177, 206, 245, 385, 407
waxes   64, 132, 158, 304, 311, 329, 340, 356, 360, 382-4
  synthetic   301-2, 312, 360

X

xanthan gum (XG)   35-6, 39-40, 44-7, 49-50, 52-3, 59-61, 145, 181, 342, 347, 349, 362
xanthan gum, traditional   347-8
Xanthan gums   60-1
xanthan molecules   36-7, 43, 60
XG *see* xanthan gum

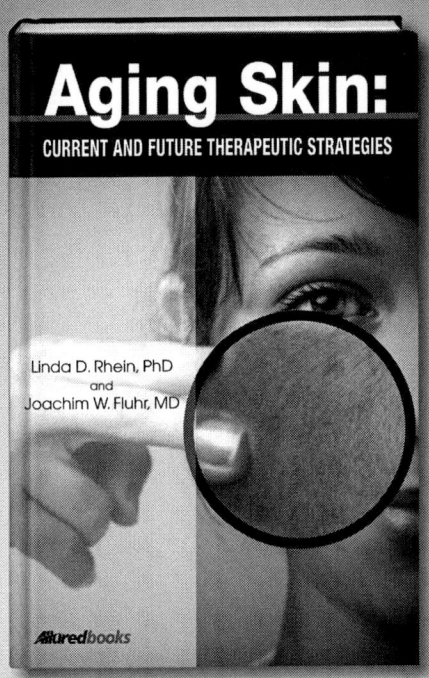

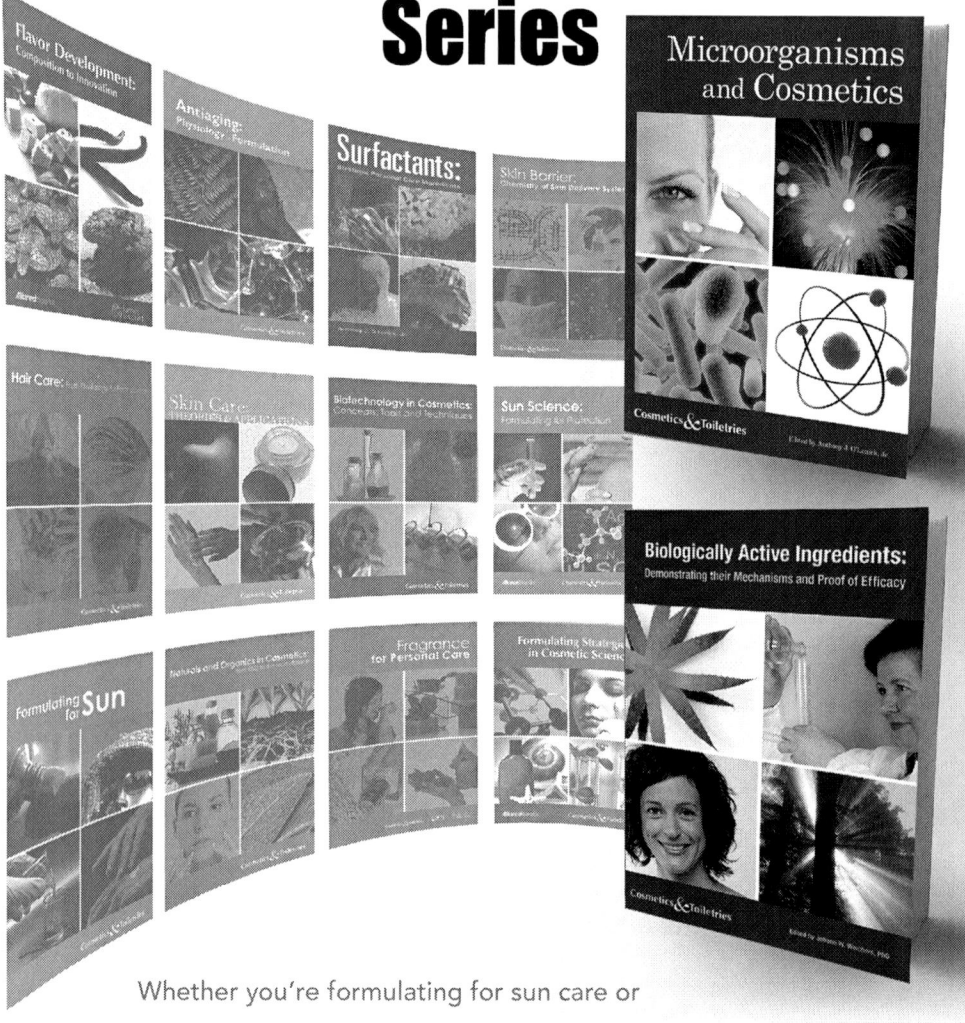

Formulators' Resource Series

Whether you're formulating for sun care or hair care products, antiaging products or personal care, Allured's formulary resources can help you meet your needs.

Order Today!
www.AlluredBooks.com

*Allured*books

New from Alluredbooks

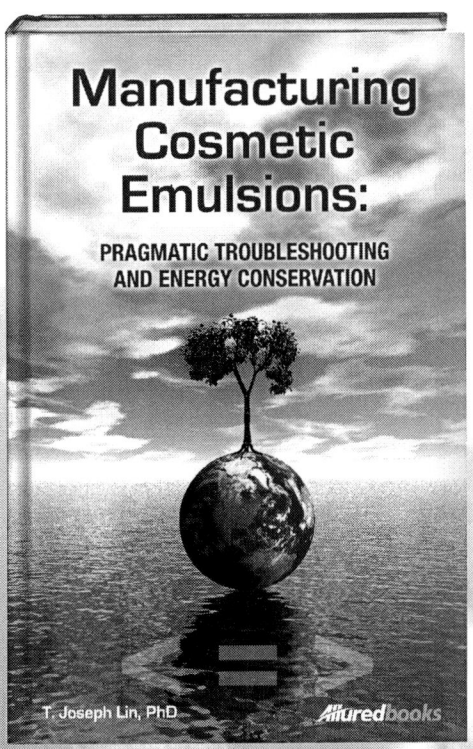

Manufacturing Cosmetic Emulsions: Pragmatic Troubleshooting and Energy Conservation by T. Joseph Lin, PhD

" I urge all people who are involved in the development or production of emulsions to read this book and learn from [Lin's] wealth of knowledge. "

— Ken Klein, President
Cosmetech Laboratories, Inc.

Order Today!
www.AlluredBooks.com

SPECIALTY SCIENCE RESOURCES

Allured books
www.AlluredBooks.com